Register Now for Online Access to Your Book!

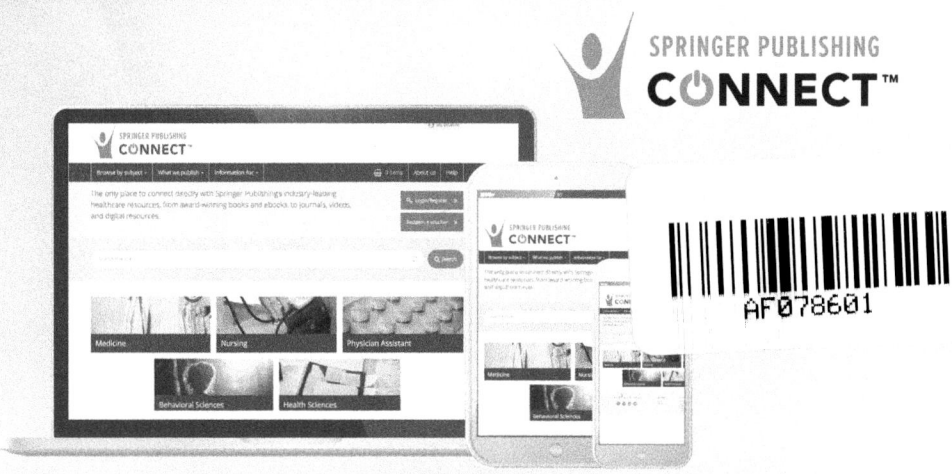

Your print purchase of *EMDR Therapy and Sexual Health* **includes online access to the contents of your book**—increasing accessibility, portability, and searchability!

Access today at:
http://connect.springerpub.com/content/book/978-0-8261-8676-8
or scan the QR code at the right with your smartphone. Log in or register, then click "Redeem a voucher" and use the code below.

K2V8NTA5

Scan here for quick access.

Having trouble redeeming a voucher code?
Go to https://connect.springerpub.com/redeeming-voucher-code

If you are experiencing problems accessing the digital component of this product, please contact our customer service department at cs@springerpub.com

The online access with your print purchase is available at the publisher's discretion and may be removed at any time without notice.

Publisher's Note: New and used products purchased from third-party sellers are not guaranteed for quality, authenticity, or access to any included digital components.

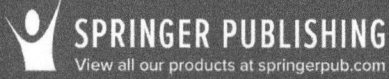

EMDR THERAPY AND SEXUAL HEALTH

Stephanie Baird, LMHC, has provided therapy, assessment, and educational talks and programs on trauma, self-care, and stress reduction in various mental health settings such as prisons, hospitals, clinics, and private practice since 1999. Her private practice specialties include EMDR therapy, trauma/PTSD, sexual health, and treating mental health professionals. She became an EMDRIA Approved Consultant in 2016 and runs monthly EMDR therapy consultation groups. She joined the Western Massachusetts EMDRIA Regional Network Board of Directors in 2012, serving as Treasurer and Regional Co-Coordinator until late 2018.

Regarding sexual health, Ms. Baird attended a Sex Therapy Consultation Group at the Northampton Sex Therapy Associates (NSTA) from 2016 through 2019. Most recently she became an OWL (Our Whole Lives) certified sex educator in April 2018, for grades 7 through 12. In March 2019 she became certified to teach the Adult OWL (young adult, adult, and older adult) curriculum. In 2020 she attained her Advancing Clinical Sexuality Excellence certification.

Ms. Baird loves bringing sex-positive information and sexual health into her EMDR therapy practice and especially loves bringing clients through healthy sexuality EMDR Future Templates and resources. Furthering her goals of empowered sex-positive and pleasure-positive sexual health education she writes a monthly column called "Sex Matters" for the local *Montague Reporter* newspaper.

Lastly, she has a lifelong love of writing from both sides of her brain. This first professional book, *EMDR Therapy and Sexual Health: A Clinician's Guide*, very much engaged her right brain. Writing prose and poetry (since her teens) engrosses her left brain. She recently published her first poetry chapbook *Duets: Love Poems and Prayers* (2020) available through Orchard Street Press (https://orchpress.com/index.php/en/). When not writing or working, she loves road bicycling and planning trips, and traveling with her family or friends.

EMDR THERAPY AND SEXUAL HEALTH

A Clinician's Guide

Stephanie Baird, LMHC

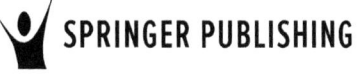

Copyright © 2023 Springer Publishing Company, LLC
All rights reserved.

No part of this publication may be reproduced, stored in a retrieval system, or transmitted in any form or by any means, electronic, mechanical, photocopying, recording, or otherwise, without the prior permission of Springer Publishing Company, LLC, or authorization through payment of the appropriate fees to the Copyright Clearance Center, Inc., 222 Rosewood Drive, Danvers, MA 01923, 978-750-8400, fax 978-646-8600, info@copyright.com or at www.copyright.com.

Springer Publishing Company, LLC
11 West 42nd Street, New York, NY 10036
www.springerpub.com
connect.springerpub.com/

Acquisitions Editor: Kate Dimock
Compositor: Amnet

Cover photo: © Ben Sears. Used with permission.

ISBN: 978-0-8261-8675-1
ebook ISBN: 978-0-8261-8676-8
DOI: 10.1891/9780826186768

SUPPLEMENTS:
Supplemental Materials ISBN: 978-0-8261-8689-8

21 22 23 24 / 5 4 3 2 1

The author and the publisher of this Work have made every effort to use sources believed to be reliable to provide information that is accurate and compatible with the standards generally accepted at the time of publication. The author and publisher shall not be liable for any special, consequential, or exemplary damages resulting, in whole or in part, from the readers' use of, or reliance on, the information contained in this book. The publisher has no responsibility for the persistence or accuracy of URLs for external or third-party Internet websites referred to in this publication and does not guarantee that any content on such websites is, or will remain, accurate or appropriate.

Library of Congress Cataloging-in-Publication Data

Names: Baird, Stephanie, author.
Title: EMDR therapy and sexual health : a clinician's guide / Stephanie
  Baird.
Description: New York, NY : Springer Publishing Company,
  LLC, 2022. | Includes bibliographical references and index.
Identifiers: LCCN 2021045631 (print) | LCCN 2021045632 (ebook) | ISBN 9780826186751
  (paperback) | ISBN 9780826186768 (ebook)
Subjects: MESH: Eye Movement Desensitization Reprocessing—methods | Sexual Health
  | Sexual Trauma—therapy | Sexual Dysfunctions, Psychological—therapy
Classification: LCC RC556 (print) | LCC RC556 (ebook) | NLM WM 425.5.D4
  | DDC 616.85/830651—dc23
LC record available at https://lccn.loc.gov/2021045631
LC ebook record available at https://lccn.loc.gov/2021045632

Contact sales@springerpub.com to receive discount rates on bulk purchases.

Publisher's Note: New and used products purchased from third-party sellers are not guaranteed for quality, authenticity, or access to any included digital components.

Printed in the United States of America.

This book is dedicated to my best friend and life partner, Ben Sears. Without his support I never could have found and prioritized the time to write this book. This book is also dedicated to my daughter, Lyra. It is my hope that books such as these, as well as the entire canon of sex-positive information, will help pave the way for the healthiest, brightest, and most empowered sexual future for her and all children everywhere.

Contents

Contributors	*ix*
Foreword Jamie Marich, PhD, LPCC-S, LICDC-CS, REAT, RYT-500	*xi*
Preface	*xiii*
Acknowledgments	*xix*

1. Sexual Health Frameworks *Stephanie Baird* 1
2. Sexual Health Information, Arousal and Desire Research, and Sexual Styles *Stephanie Baird* 27
3. Sex Therapy Frameworks and Sexual Problems, Dysfunctions, and Disorders *Wendy Stock* 61
4. Applying EMDR Therapy to Sexual Health Targets *Stephanie Baird* 101
5. Sexual Health EMDR Future Templates and Resources, Body Image, and Pornography *Stephanie Baird* 131
6. Considering Gender With All EMDR Clients *Michelle M. Marchese* 165
7. EMDR Therapy and Sexual/Affectional Orientation: Relationship and Pregnancy Status *Stephanie Baird* 191
8. Other Marginalized Populations, Sexual Health, and EMDR Therapy *Stephanie Baird* 217
9. Aging Sexual Health and EMDR Therapy *Ashley L. Mader* 243

10.	Spirituality, Sexual Health, and EMDR Therapy *Jeanne C. Folks*	267
11.	Sexual Health Resources for EMDR Therapists and Their Clients *Stephanie Baird*	295

Index — *319*

Contributors

Jeanne C. Folks, DMin, LPC, Clinical Director, Connecticut Psychotherapeutic Resources, Avon, Connecticut

Sabrina Herman, LICSW, Psychotherapist, Independent Practice, South Hadley, Massachusetts

Ashley L. Mader, PhD, LICSW, Sex Therapist, Consultant and Educator, Founder/Blogger of Ourshine.org, Northampton, Massachusetts

Michelle M. Marchese, LICSW, PhD candidate, Smith School for Social Work, Director of Counseling Services, Smith College, Adjunct Professor, Smith College, Northampton, Massachusetts

Jamie Marich, PhD, LPCC-S, LICDC-CS, REAT, RYT-500, Founder & Director, The Institute for Creative Mindfulness, Warren, Ohio

Robert Miller, PhD, President, Image Transformation Psychological Institute, Del Mar, California

Wendy Stock, PhD, Clinical Psychologist, Independent Practice, Berkeley, California

Foreword

When I made the transition from agency work to a group practice in 2008, I immediately became known as "the EMDR specialist," and I was promptly referred an abundance of cases directly related to trauma. I soon began getting any person who presented with an overt concern around sex, sexuality, or spirituality as well. While I had some training in pastoral counseling and considered spiritual abuse one of my specialties, I became concerned that, without much specific training in sex therapy, I was becoming the "go-to" person for whatever felt like too much for my fellow clinicians. Because I was willing to *go there*, and because in my other specialty of addiction I made very public challenges about the need to address sexual health in addiction care, my colleagues saw me as the one to take these cases. Yet I soon called out the problem both in my group practice and later in EMDR communities—we all have to be willing to *go there*.

I am delighted that Stephanie Baird has taken the charge, together with other skilled collaborators, to write this important book for the EMDR community. As she aptly observes, the vast majority of EMDR therapists work with sexual abuse and sexual trauma in some way (certainly every therapist I've met encounters sexual abuse). So why aren't we, as a community, having larger conversations about sexuality and assisting our clients in moving toward sexual health? Why aren't more of us willing to *go there*? Stephanie gently yet directly points out that many of us, even as EMDR therapists, have perhaps never examined our own attitudes about and issues with sex and sexuality. She and her collaborators provide an inviting framework that allows us to start doing some of this introspective work while also learning some of the basic education about sex and sexuality that most of us did not get in graduate school.

I am also excited to see so much content in this book about working with the broad spectrum of people who identify as LGBTQ+. As a bisexually identified individual, I have experienced microaggressions within the EMDR community among my peers, and I can still viscerally react when I hear the manner in which some of my colleagues talk about LGBTQ+ folks. Indeed, many of these comments come from a place of ignorance and not outright bigotry. As Eastern mystics have long observed, *ignorance ends when knowledge begins*. To the open-minded and open-hearted EMDR therapists picking up this book, you are invited to receive a great deal of knowledge that will enhance your clinical effectiveness with those who are traditionally marginalized.

The content in this book on spirituality is also essential. For many of our clients, sexual trauma, gender or sexual identity discrimination, and religious trauma are so intermingled. Using the wisdom of the Adaptive Information Processing model combined with insight that addresses these major components of wounding, Stephanie and her colleagues will help you to conceptualize your cases with enhanced critical thinking. Similar to how helping clients move toward a healthier or more adaptive framework for sexual health is critical, so it also goes with spirituality. The spiritual self, which is so much greater than anything religious or dogmatic, can receive a great deal of healing through properly and sensitively delivered EMDR therapy.

Stephanie helps you pull all of these pieces of the puzzle together in *EMDR Therapy and Sexual Health: A Clinician's Guide*. To Stephanie and to her colleagues, the EMDR therapy community owes you a debt of gratitude. Thank you for *going there*.

Jamie Marich, PhD, LPCC-S, LICDC-CS, REAT, RYT-500
Founder & CEO, The Institute for Creative Mindfulness
Warren, Ohio

Preface

At this point in my career, I remain first and foremost an eye movement desensitization and reprocessing (EMDR) clinician and consultant focusing on helping clients heal from sexual violence and trauma. The Centers for Disease Control and Prevention (n.d.) defines sexual violence as "sexual activity when consent is not obtained or not given freely. Anyone can experience SV [sexual violence], but most victims are (cis)female. The person responsible for the violence is (often) (cis)male and usually someone known to the victim."

Most therapists are too familiar with the general statistics that one in three females, one in six males, and that 50% of transgender individuals experience sexual violence at some point in their life (often before the age of 18). Most of our caseloads are overwhelmingly comprised of sexual trauma survivors, yet sexuality is barely mentioned in the many volumes of books now published in the EMDR therapy field (despite most of our clients presenting for these obviously sexual health–related reasons). Unfortunately, this general silence should not be surprising given the sorry state of sex education in this country. Only about 20 states mandate some amount of public school sex education, usually equaling just a few hours.

An interest in sexual health and empowerment has been a strong undercurrent throughout my entire conscious life since early college, thanks to my first teacher of sex education, Dr. Wendy Stock (who authored Chapter 3, "Sex Therapy Frameworks and Sexual Problems, Dysfunctions, and Disorders"). I recall having my mind blown nearly every class meeting in "Human Sexuality," circa 1993, at the mostly conservative Texas A&M University. I will never forget seeing my classmates' stereotypes and myths smashed to smithereens, day by day, very calmly, by the plethora of equalizing, enlightening, and normalizing research and accurate information Dr. Stock shared. That may have been the first time I heard the word "clitoris."

I continued to seek information on sexuality, as well as women's studies, in my upper level classes and took all graduate level sexuality-related classes available to me in the University of North Texas Counseling Psychology master's program (a whopping three classes, I believe). I followed beloved sexuality writers like Betty Dodson. I also volunteered at rape crisis programs during this time and wrote a thesis on vicarious traumatization of sexual and domestic violence volunteers. This focus turned my attention from pure sexual health to sexual trauma. Everywhere I looked I met someone who was a survivor of trauma, fueling an urgency to help this population.

During postgraduate school I worked in prisons with sex offenders, looking at the other side of trauma, then returned to working with sexual trauma survivors from 2001 on. I got trained in EMDR therapy (2009), falling in love with this highly effective and efficient way of treating sexual trauma survivors.

I never forgot my interest in sexual health and earnestly began seeking, obtaining, and integrating fresh sexual health information a few years ago. During that process I became astounded at the lack of sexual health discussion and education at psychotherapy conferences and events, with very few books available for clinicians. This lack of sexual health discussion within the EMDR therapy model and community is also astonishing when you think about it.

It is my hope that this first professional book of its kind will fill this 30-year gap, integrating sexual health concepts in one's EMDR therapy practice, helping EMDR therapists become literate in modern sexual health. Most EMDR therapists handily complete the Eight Phase EMDR protocol with sexual trauma survivors, but often discharge clients once that final negative target is completed. This is due to many reasons including a lack of sexual health classes in graduate school, our general erotophobic culture, and worries about therapist/client boundaries.

Many EMDR clients want permission to explore and discuss their sexual health and how their prior history of disturbing events may have negatively impacted their sexual health. My hope is that this book will help EMDR therapists gain updated knowledge and confidence to address current sexual health within the EMDR therapy framework. This book also assumes that readers have received the full EMDR basic training and therefore does not go into detail about the Adaptive Information Processing (AIP) model or the EMDR Eight Phase protocol, unless specifically linking these concepts to sexual health. There are many books available that specifically dive into the inner workings of EMDR therapy.

Chapter 1, "Sexual Health Frameworks," provides a basic literacy in current sexual health, addresses therapists' potential discomfort in addressing sexual health with clients, and introduces the idea of the therapists' own Sexological Worldview. The PLISSIT (Permission, Limited Information, Specific Suggestions, Intensive Therapy) model of sexual health communication is detailed, as well as important foundational elements of sexual health from the longstanding, reputable *Our Whole Lives* and Planned Parenthood curricula. Gina Ogden's 4-D Wheel of Sexual Health is explored as a helpful clinical sexual health framework. These frameworks are then integrated into the AIP model.

Chapter 2, "Sexual Health Information, Arousal and Desire Research, and Sexual Styles," provides basic sexual anatomy, development, and essential sexual health information (sexually transmitted infections [STIs], HIV, pregnancy prevention, safer sex) that every EMDR therapist needs to know for sexual health literacy. This chapter also explores the history of sex research and current 21st century understanding of the Dual Control Model of arousal, as well as spontaneous and responsive desire. Sexual styles are explained. The sexual styles questionnaire is provided for therapists to administer to their clients, helping clients learn about their own sexual style. Erotic templates (often formed in childhood and adolescence) and how they relate to EMDR targets are also discussed.

Dr. Stock's Chapter 3, "Sex Therapy Frameworks and Sexual Problems, Dysfunctions, and Disorders," describes modern sex therapy frameworks, acquaints the EMDR therapist with basic sex therapy information (correcting misconceptions and providing accurate information), and provides information about what occurs when clients are referred for sex therapy. Commonly reported sexual health dysfunctions are defined with suggestions of how EMDR therapists can work adjunctly with sex therapists.

Chapter 4, "Applying EMDR Therapy to Sexual Health Targets," provides a brief refresher on EMDR therapy and the AIP model, integrating sexual health into this framework. Resources particularly helpful for sexual health (including two new resources, Bubble Boundary and Self-Compassion Container) are shared. Positive and negative EMDR cognitions related to sexual health are provided, as well as lists and case examples of EMDR sexuality-related targets. Highlights from the EMDR Protocol for Sexual Dysfunctions are included. The Feeling State Addiction protocol and *out of control* sexual behaviors (e.g., "excessive" porn viewing, unwanted sexual behaviors) are discussed, with a contribution from Dr. Robert Miller. Resources are provided for how therapists can handle potential complex dissociation that may come up as sexuality is addressed.

Chapter 5, "Sexual Health EMDR Future Templates and Resources, Body Image, and Pornography," provides a refresher on EMDR Future Templates and several case studies using Future Templates to address sexual health. Improving sexuality-related concerns related to self-esteem and body image, via EMDR therapy, will be addressed, as well as the impact of social media and pornography on self-image. Also included is a new EMDR resource on "Strengthening a Confident and Joyful Sexual Self" designed to help clients spend more time mindfully and positively developing and experiencing their sexuality.

Michelle Marchese's Chapter 6, "Considering Gender With All EMDR Clients" examines how gender is a social construct that exerts pressure on every individual within their culture. This pressure can take the form of narratives, roles, and expectations. Someone's gender can impact their experience of trauma, their access to care, how they have learned to express or process emotions, and how they react to a variety of situations. This chapter examines some of the ways that gender can impact cisgender and transgender women, cisgender and transgender men, and gender-diverse individuals in the context of trauma treatment. It also offers specific ways to address some common gender-related challenges within Phases 1 to 6 of EMDR therapy. Current concepts and language for a variety of genders is shared, with cultural humility and intersectional understanding continuously encouraged for every unique therapeutic context. Information on how to respect transgender and gender non-conforming (TGNC) clients' lead in discussing more specific sexual health concerns is provided.

Chapter 7, "EMDR Therapy and Sexual/Affectional Orientation: Relationship and Pregnancy Status," shares current information about sexual/affectional/romantic orientation (including *bisexual*, *asexual*, and *demisexual*), relationship status (e.g., monogamy, affairs, and consensual non-monogamy), and pregnancy. Sabrina Herman, LICSW, explores pregnancy loss, sexual health, and EMDR therapy in depth. Case studies are provided to illustrate the intersection of EMDR therapy and sexual health for demisexuality, infidelity, and pregnancy loss.

Chapter 8, "Other Marginalized Populations, Sexual Health, and EMDR Therapy," provides fundamental information about additional culturally and/or erotically marginalized populations and communities. Specifically this chapter addresses information and EMDR therapy considerations regarding the sexual health of people with physical and/or intellectual disabilities. This chapter shares information about erotically marginalized clients that may engage in kink/bondage and discipline, dominance and submission, sadism and masochism (BDSM), fetishes, and/or paraphilias. Brief considerations about sex work are shared. Lastly, a brief section on encountering clients that report sex offending is also included. EMDR therapy case studies are provided to illustrate the intersection of sexual health regarding physical disability, kink/BDSM, sex work, and an adjudicated sex offender. With regrets this initial first edition is not able to cover the breadth and depth of all marginalized populations.

Ashley Mader's Chapter 9, "Aging Sexual Health and EMDR Therapy," discusses the needs of older adults. Aging and sexuality is not often considered in the field of mental health, even though it is something that we are all doing everyday. Older adults face menopause, sexual dysfunction/changes, and changes in body functioning and image. Internalized ageist myths and stereotypes can prevent these adults from having a positive outlook on the aging process. It is extremely important that these views do not prohibit older adults from getting help from healthcare providers. All healthcare providers need to be open and comfortable with talking about sex and aging. EMDR therapy and sexual health suggestions are integrated throughout, ending with a case study featuring an older adult, sexual health, and EMDR therapy.

Dr. Jeanne Folks contributed Chapter 10, "Spirituality, Sexual Health, and EMDR Therapy." Spiritual themes of ecstasy, guilt, fear, shame, freewill, surrender, control, sacrifice, safety, and belonging are integral parts of a client's experience of self and others. These equally qualify as sexual themes. Integration of a client's spiritual understanding broadens and empowers therapeutic response to their sexual issues. Skillful access to and utilization of the client's spiritual lexicon equips the EMDR therapist to address the convergence of spiritual and sexual injury and recovery, especially when viewed through the lens of relationship and attachment. Five case studies illustrate the benefits of working concurrently with this intersection, enhancing EMDR processing.

Chapter 11, "Sexual Health Resources for EMDR Therapists and Their Clients," provides a comprehensive, but not exhaustive, list of sexual health resources. As the field of human sexuality continues to expand and interface more positively with mental health, physical health, and our culture at large, increasing numbers of helpful resources are becoming available for sex educators, lay folks, and anyone seeking updated and positive information. This final chapter provides lists (with synopses of the most useful and relevant) essential sexual health-related websites, TED Talks, podcasts, books, and educational resources for EMDR therapists and clients. National and regional sexual health training organizations are listed for further learning. Additionally, although directly addressing children and their sexual health was out of the scope of this book, educational resources for children and teens regarding sexual health are included in this chapter.

Please keep in mind that as the field and agents of sexual health continue to expand, these resources may quickly become outdated or replaced by more current versions. Always locate the most current websites and/or editions of the listed resources to learn about updates or revisions.

May every reader of this book emerge feeling much more informed, confident, and sex-positive with the integration of sexual health in their own EMDR therapy practice.

Terms: In this book the term *man* generally refers to individuals with a penis, testes, prostate, and so on, and/or socialized into a masculine gender (generally speaking, *cismen*). The term *woman* refers to individuals with a vulva, labia, clitoris, vagina, ovaries, and uterus, and/or socialized into a feminine gender (generally speaking, *ciswomen*). This particularly pertains to how researchers have categorized individuals in the studies mentioned throughout, as well as some of the self-identified gender of individuals featured in case studies. However, a transman who may not yet have all of the biological anatomy generally associated with a cisman (penis, testes, etc.) also receives masculinized gender socialization. Similarly for transwomen. Throughout this book transgendered individuals are generally referred to as transfemale, transwoman, transmale, and/or transman. Case study individuals that identify as gender nonconforming and/or gender nonbinary are labeled as such. As gender terminology is rapidly (and happily) changing, some of this terminology may be outdated once this book comes out in print.

Case Studies: For case studies, names, ages, and many identifying details have been changed and/or recombined for total anonymity. Many of the case studies feature individuals from non-White identities, and/or LGBTQIA+ individuals.

Working Definition of Sex and Sexual Activity: For the purposes of this book, *sex* and *sexual activity* may refer to any behavior that involves any amount of sexual interest/desire, and/or arousal, among any configuration of consenting individuals and genders. This non-exhaustive list of behaviors includes kissing, deep kissing, making out, outercourse (any non-penetrative activity), touching sensitive and/or erogenous areas like breasts and genitals, erotic/sensual massage, masturbation, solo or mutual masturbation, giving and/or receiving oral sex, penis–vagina intercourse, anal sex, manual stimulation, consenting adult kink/BDSM activities, and/or sex toy use with adults of any consenting gender and/or genitalia configuration.

Stephanie Baird

REFERENCE

Centers for Disease Control and Prevention. (n.d.). *Sexual violence.* https://www.cdc.gov/injury/features/sexual-violence/index.html

Acknowledgments

I wish to first thank George Abbott, Denise Gelinas, Mark Nickerson, Farnsworth Lobenstine, and Caryn Markson for all their EMDR therapy wisdom and guidance on my journey toward becoming EMDR certified and an EMDRIA-approved consultant. Once that step was attained, I felt I could finally shift back to my first love, sexual health.

I wish to acknowledge the general support of our very vibrant Western Massachusetts EMDR community. Involvement in the Western Massachusetts EMDR Regional Network's Board of Directors for many years provided lovely connections, including meeting Michele Marchese, LICSW (previous Board President), who authored Chapter 6, "Considering Gender With All EMDR Therapy Clients." I met Jeanne Folks, DMin, LPC, when she gave a presentation at our annual Western Massachusetts EMDR Conference on EMDR and Spirituality. She enthusiastically jumped on board to write Chapter 10, "Spirituality, Sexual Health, and EMDR Therapy."

Other EMDR therapy community members Sabrina Herman, LICSW, and Sandy Murphy, LICSW, contributed important sections and case studies. Nancy Simons, LICSW, contributed her wonderful Self-Compassion Resource. Dr. Robert Miller agreed to contribute a helpful and informative section on his Feeling State Addiction Protocol. Melanie Peele, LPC, wrote up the recent research on EMDR Therapy and Intellectual Disabilities.

Delightedly, Dr. Jamie Marich graced this book with her foreword—thank you, Jamie! Much appreciation to Sheryl Knopf (Greater Boston EMDRIA Regional Network) and Marilyn Luber (writer and editor extraordinaire) for giving positive endorsement in the beginning stages of this book proposal.

After taking Vera Basford's training on *A Beginners Guide to Sex Therapy* at Smith College School for Social Work (2016), I joined Basford's sex therapy consultation group via the Northampton Sex Therapy Associates from September 2016 through August 2019. I owe sincere thanks to Vera and this group for facilitating my transition back into the world of sexual health. During this consultation group I learned about the Sexual History Questionnaire and The Sexual Styles Survey, incredibly helpful questionnaires, incorporating their use into my practice. I thank Jassy Casella Timberlake, LMFT, at NSTA for giving permission to include the Sexual History Questionnaire. I thank Dr. Kathy McMahon for giving permission to include the Sexual Styles Survey.

It was at the Sex Therapy Consult group's suggestion that I present on *Integrating EMDR and Sexual Concerns*, thus laying the groundwork for presenting *Let's Talk About Sex: Bringing Sexual Health Into Your EMDR Practice* at both the Western Massachusetts EMDR Conference (2019) and the National EMDRIA Conference (2019). I also made several lovely connections within that group, including Dr. Ashley Mader, LICSW, expert on sex and aging, who contributed her expertise with Chapter 9, "Aging Sexual Health and EMDR Therapy."

During this time of increased focus on sexual health I was also fortunate to attend many presentations facilitated by the Northeast American Association of Sexuality Educators, Counselors, and Therapists–Northeast. Dr. Jane Fleishman was the regional president during this time and brought many excellent guest speakers including Emily Nagoski (author of *Come as You Are*), Gina Ogden (author of *Expanding the Practice of Sex Therapy*), and Roz Dischiavo (author of *The Deep Yes: The Lost Art of True Receiving*). I owe gratitude to Dr. Fleishman for helping to round out my education with these fascinating and cutting-edge presenters.

I wish to acknowledge and thank Dr. Rosalyn Dischiavo, founder of the Institute for Sexuality, Education, and Enlightenment (ISEE). ISEE offered many classes in my region, including the essential SAR (sexual attitude reassessment) class. It was always an intellectually exciting highlight to take classes from Dr. Dischiavo and her colleagues at ISEE. I was grateful to receive my Advancing Clinical Education in Sexuality (ACES) via ISEE in 2020.

I owe a debt of gratitude to my home UU society, the Unitarian Society of Northampton and Florence and Jessica Harwood, Director of Religious Education and Faith Development. At her suggestion I received the *Our Whole Lives* (OWL) sex educator training in April 2018 (for grades 7 through 12), as well as the Adult OWL training (Young Adult, Adult, and Older Adult) in March 2019. I enjoyed finally being on the side of prevention: co-teaching many sex education classes until the 2020 COVID-19 pandemic brought in-person instruction to a screeching halt.

Teaching and taking so many classes in sexual health gave me the gumption to approach Nina Rossi, Features Editor at the local *Montague Reporter* newspaper, about writing a sex-positive column on sexual health. I jumped for joy when both Nina and Mike Jackson (Editor) loved the idea, one of my lifelong dreams. I have been enthusiastically writing this monthly column since September 2019. Thank you for this fun and meaningful opportunity, Nina and Mike!

Somehow this curious feminist human from conservative Texas landed at a geographic nexus of EMDR and sexual health—it was only a matter of time before integration of the two frameworks occurred.

I wholeheartedly thank friend and EMDR colleague Veronica Hartman and my cousin Liz Sears. Both of these gracious humans allowed me to stay at their rural properties for days at a time (on a dime!), affording me precious alone time and mental space to accomplish the bulk of this writing. If I had not had these opportunities to think and write, I would never have been able to finish this manuscript during a pandemic, with myself, my spouse, and my young child stuck in a small house 24/7. Thank you for keeping me sane, Veronica and Liz. Thank you also to Jamie Sullivan who provided a flurry of last minute formatting edits before I turned in the manuscript to Springer Publishing.

I also wish to thank my editors at Springer Publishing, Mehak Massand and Kate Dimock. Thank you, Kate, for sending that wonderful email out of the blue, asking if I was interested in turning my initial EMDRIA 2019 presentation into a book. That was the most exciting email I have ever received! And thank you, Mehak, for always promptly answering my many questions and providing ongoing support and encouragement.

Finally, I wish to thank all my brave clients over the years that have inspired me on a daily basis with their courage, resilience, insight, and tenacity in fighting through the aftereffects of sexual trauma, especially those clients who were my first initial EMDR clients! Each and every client is truly on a hero's journey. I am in awe to be in witness with them and to learn anew how hope is always within reach, no matter how bleak things may seem. And I hold special appreciation for the clients who brought their sexual health questions to our sessions. This drove the point home that we EMDR clinicians need to be much more informed and comfortable in *going there* when our clients ask that of us.

This book has been a collaborative labor of love, birthed by many midwives/midspouses.

Although I belong to certain marginalized or historically oppressed groups (bisexual/omnisexual, ciswoman appearing), I must acknowledge that my White, educational, and professional privilege has allowed me to pursue this project with relative ease, even during a difficult pandemic. Lastly, I respectfully acknowledge my places of home and work, where much of this manuscript was created, are within the ancestral, unceded homelands of the Pocumtuck and Nonotuck peoples.

1

Sexual Health Frameworks

Stephanie Baird, LMHC

LEARNING OBJECTIVES

- EMDR clinicians gain an introductory understanding of modern sexual health.
- EMDR clinicians learn about factors interfering with discussing sexuality and increase their own comfort with addressing sexual health.
- EMDR clinicians explore their own *Sexological Worldview.*
- EMDR clinicians fully define *consent* and the PLISSIT (Permission, Limited Information, Specific Suggestions, Intensive Therapy) model of sexual health communication.
- EMDR clinicians learn about several positive sexual health models (OWL, Planned Parenthood, 4-D Wheel, Global Declaration of Sexual Rights and pleasure).
- EMDR clinicians will begin integrating sexual heath information into the EMDR Adaptive Information Processing (AIP) model.

INTRODUCTION TO SEXUAL HEALTH

Congratulations on taking this next step to empower yourself and your clients toward full healthy sexual functioning. If you are like me, and most Western psychotherapists, your education and background included very little information about sexual health. Perhaps you were able to take one class on human sexuality in graduate school; maybe you were lucky enough to enjoy two classes. Most of us received zero to just 6 hours of basic sex education in our grade school, and depending on the decade and geographic region of our middle school, our education likely only mentioned menstruation and abstinence.

Even pursuing advanced specialization and/or certification in eye movement desensitization and reprocessing (EMDR) therapy, a therapy that every day helps thousands of folks overcome sexual (and other) trauma, does not bring automatic access to sex-positive information. Additionally, the statistics regarding sexual assault remain sobering. One in three ciswomen, one in four cismen, and two out of three transgender individuals will experience sexual assault in their lifetimes, much of it by the age of 18 (National Center for Injury Prevention and Control, Division of Violence Prevention, 2021).

Over the years I have learned that the majority of clients seeking psychotherapy have a history of sexual trauma and find this to be true in my own private practice. These high statistics informed my drive to become a trauma-focused EMDR therapist and now inform my drive to integrate and share positive sexual health information, resources, and healing in our work with survivors. This chapter provides a foundation of sexual health, introducing you to the several uplifting paradigms.

What Is "Sexual Health"?

The World Health Organization (WHO, n.d.) defines sexual health as "a state of physical, emotional, mental, and social well-being related to sexuality: it is not merely the absence of disease, dysfunction, or infirmity. Sexual health requires a positive and respectful approach to sexuality and sexual relationships, as well as the possibility of heaving pleasurable and safe sexual experiences, free of coercion, discrimination, and violence. For sexual health to be attained, the sexual rights of all persons must be respected, protected, and fulfilled."

The Office of the Surgeon General and Office of Population Affairs (2001) defines sexual health as "inextricably bound to both physical and mental health. Just as physical and mental health problems can contribute to sexual dysfunction and disease, those dysfunctions and diseases can contribute to physical and mental health problems. Sexual health is not limited to the absence of disease or dysfunction, nor is its importance (sic) confined to just the reproductive years … It includes freedom from sexual abuse and discrimination and the ability to integrate their sexuality into their lives, derive pleasure from it, and to reproduce (if one wishes)."

Working Definition of Sex and Sexual Activity

For the purposes of this book, *sex* and *sexual activity* may refer to any behavior that involves any amount of sexual interest/desire, and/or arousal among any configuration of consenting individuals and genders. This non-exhaustive list of behaviors includes kissing, deep kissing, making out, outercourse (any non-penetrative activity), touching sensitive and/or erogenous areas like breasts and genitals, erotic/sensual massage, masturbation, solo or mutual masturbation, giving and/or receiving oral sex, penis-vagina intercourse, anal sex, manual stimulation, consenting adult kink/bondage and discipline, dominance and submission, sadism, masochism (BDSM) activities, and/or use of sex toys with any consenting gender and/or genitalia configuration. And while individuals and organizations have been studying sex, sexuality, and sexual health for decades, in my work with clients I often come back to Peggy Kleinplatz's direct and arresting research question "What kind of sex is worth wanting?" (2009).

DECLARATION OF SEXUAL RIGHTS AND PLEASURE

Since 1978 the World Association for Sexual Health (WAS) has worked towards sexual health and rights. Thousands of members attend global biennial congresses and in recent years have made declarations for sexual rights.

Declaration of Sexual Rights

This is adapted from the the World Association for Sexual Health (WAS). (2014, March). *Declaration of Sexual Rights*. Retrieved from https://worldsexualhealth.net/wp-content/uploads/2013/08/declaration_of_sexual_rights_sep03_2014.pdf.

1. The right to equality and freedom of sexual expression.
2. The right to make decisions about one's body in regard to sexuality.
3. The right to be safe from all forms of sexual violence and coercion, and be free from inhumane treatment or punishment because of one's sexual or gender expression.
4. The right to accurate scientific information and education about sexuality and sexual health.
5. The right to freely create and dissolve marital and other similar relationships.
6. The right to family planning resources.
7. The right to organize freely to promote sexual rights and health.
8. The right to privacy regarding sexual matters.
9. The right to judicious laws and remedies regarding sexual rights.
10. The right to the highest attainable standard of sexual health, including sexual safe and pleasurable sexual experiences.

Declaration on Sexual Pleasure

At WAS's congress in Mexico City (October 2019) they improved their previous declaration by adding a separate *declaration on sexual pleasure* adapted from a definition from the Global Advisory Board for Sexual Health and Wellbeing (GAB, 2016)

> *Sexual pleasure is the physical and/or psychological satisfaction and enjoyment derived from shared or solitary erotic experiences, including thoughts…dreams, [and autoeroticism]. Self-determination, consent, safety, privacy, confidence and the ability to communicate and negotiate sexual relations are key… factors for pleasure to contribute to sexual health and well-being. Sexual pleasure should be exercised within the context of sexual rights…[including] equality and non-discrimination, autonomy and bodily integrity, and the right to the highest …standard of health and freedom of expression. The experiences of human sexual pleasure are diverse and sexual rights ensure that pleasure is a positive experience for all concerned and not obtained by violating…. human rights and well-being. (GAB, 2016)*

Some of WAS's declaration includes:

- Sexual pleasure is a fundamental part of sexual and human rights and includes the possibility of diverse sexual experiences.
- Access to appropriate sources of sexual pleasure is part of human well-being.
- Sexual health and well-being include pleasurable and safe sexual experiences free of discrimination, coercion, and violence.
- Sexual pleasure shall be globally integrated into education, health services, research, and advocacy and contributes to global health.

I list these various sexual guidelines and declarations to emphasize the importance of including sexual health as a vital and essential piece of our clients' healing and lives. Van der Hart and others (2006) often describe healing from trauma as a three-phase comprehensive approach. Phase One involves stabilization (resourcing, grounding, etc.). Phase Two includes the nitty-gritty of treatment (including EMDR therapy Phases 3–8). Phase Three of overall trauma treatment includes improving intimacy, sexual health, and self-actualization.

If we all had been lucky enough to receive sex education reflecting WAS values (as well as the OWL and Planned Parenthood values mentioned later in this chapter), from early childhood, I believe the sexual trauma statistics would be greatly reduced and all of us would happily exist in "Phase Three" of overall treatment: empowered and fulfilling sexual health and intimacy.

CULTURAL AND INDIVIDUAL FACTORS INTERFERING WITH BRINGING SEXUAL HEALTH INTO THE EMDR THERAPY OFFICE

Despite most of us walking by magazine covers at the grocery store touting advice like "fifty ways to spice up your sex life" or "achieve your most powerful orgasm yet," our culture as a whole remains erotophobic, shaming, and "puritanical" when it comes to embracing sexual pleasure and health. "Erotophobia" is a term used by sex educators Rosalyn Dischavio (2016) and Marty Klein (2010), among others, to refer to our society's fear of anything sexual.

We have now had several decades of sex-positive activism, ramping up in the 1960s with the sexual revolution and burgeoning forms of birth control, continuing through the second wave liberation-oriented feminism of the seventies, surfacing again in the nineties with third wave feminism (partially in response to right-wing Christian/Reaganomic backlash in the eighties and the rise and stigmatization of HIV/AIDS). The nineties' third wave feminism increased public awareness of sexual assault and emphasized intersectionality of race, culture, class, gender, sexual orientation, and so forth. The nineties also brought an army of sex-positive feminists activists like Susie Bright (sex-positive essayist and author of Sexual State of the Union [1997]), Carol Queen (popular sex educator, adult toy store co-owner, and author of *Real Live Nude Girl* [2002]), and Tristan Taormino (writer, activist, filmmaker), along with the mainstreaming of feminist sex toy stores like Good Vibrations in California. Safer sex discussions also increased in response to the HIV/AIDS crisis. Much of the mainstream can thank Dr. Ruth Westheimer (2012) for all of her trailblazing work candidly and openly tackling any sexual matter thrown her way, from the 1980s to the present.

Increasingly available internet pornography burst onto the scene in the late 1990s and early 2000s, single-handedly misinforming millions of individuals about average sizes of body parts and once again locking folks into stereotypes of masculine individuals actively seeking and receiving sex, and feminine individuals "happy to oblige" others' desires, passively neglecting their own. The widespread availability of e-readers plus steamy erotic fanfiction (e.g., the problematic *Fifty Shades of Grey* published in 2011) allowed feminine individuals to catch up with masculine individuals in viewing and engaging with erotic material.

The #metoo movement is one of our most recent cultural sexual history developments. Initially beginning in 2006 when Black, Indigenous, and People of Color (BIPOC) sexual assault survivor and activist Tarana Burke developed the phrase, it erupted in 2017 when actress Ashley Judd accused Harvey Weinstein of sexual assaulting her. This accusation soon unleashed a torrent of disclosures from other famous and non-famous ciswomen (and some cismen) against (mostly) cismen in power. The #metoo movement has also brought with it much needed discussion of consent, which will be discussed in more detail shortly.

However, despite this ever-widening spiral of positive sexual health awareness, our puritanical and shaming culture is not going out without a fight. This means that despite the availability of more sex-positive television shows such as *Mrs. Fletcher* (HBO), *Sex Education,* and *Bridgerton* (Netflix), several factors continue to interfere with psychotherapists (even EMDR therapists who regularly discuss sexual trauma) addressing positive sexual health with clients. Some of these factors include therapists' own discomfort in discussing sexuality, therapists' own unexplored/unresolved issues regarding sexuality, and/or therapists' own traumatic histories or propensity for vicarious traumatization (Saakvitne & Pearlman, 1996).

Even if we feel comfortable and confident discussing sexual health, we may harbor uncertainty about our clients' own comfort levels and interest, worrying that introducing sexual health material might make our clients uncomfortable. Other concerns for us may include perceived boundary issues, potential lawsuits, potential attraction/arousal, our own appropriate versus inappropriate curiosity, misspeaking a term, or introducing a topic on which we have less expertise. However, according to Kevin Gallagher (2014), overall research shows that many clients want to bring up and discuss sexual concerns, yet most prefer their providers inquire first. Gallagher noted that, in fact, most clients rarely ever bring up their concern at all, likely due to concerns about whether they are "normal." In 2020 Klein noted that a typical view of "normal" sexuality includes: "sex when tired, too high or too low expectations, and awkwardness and self-consciousness," versus a joyful, fulfilling, and positive part of life.

Bringing sexual health into our intakes and conversations with our EMDR clients not only gives them likely much-needed permission to mention sexual concerns, it also combats erotophobia in our society at large. In turn our clients will be able to embrace a personal vision of their sexuality that goes beyond "normal," "typical," or "average" into the joyful and pleasurable extraordinary.

Finally, while perusing the *Psychology Today* therapist directory listings in 2020, *sex therapy* was not available as a psychotherapy focus/topic (thankfully EMDR is an option). As of May 2021, I am happy to report *sex therapy* is now an option.

CONSENT

The concept of consent is relevant in all ways as we continue on our journey toward integrating sexual health. Hopefully you are enthusiastically consenting to read and integrate the information in this book. As we work with clients, particularly utilizing EMDR therapy, we ideally constantly ask for and obtain consent as we move through the EMDR eight stages. The #metoo movement has helped generate increased and essential discussion about sexual consent.

As someone who came of age in the eighties and nineties, not much was discussed or even known about active negotiation of sex-related activities. During my work in the late nineties, primarily working with sexual assault survivors, *consent* concepts emerged in clinical work as well in rape crisis educational campaigns. However, most of these campaigns centered around the "no means no" concept. This, of course, is paramount. Humans being able to say no to unwanted activities is the foundation from which we can later say yes to wanted activities.

Much of the twentieth century stereotypical cismale and cisfemale gender expression involved the idea that a cisgender man should always want and try for sex, and that a "good" cisgender woman should be a "gatekeeper," saying no often, but eventually "giving in" (like Scarlet O'Hara and Rhett Butler in "Gone With the Wind"– he forcibly dragged her, kicking and fighting, upstairs for sex, and then the next scene shows her post-sex, looking content). It wasn't okay for a woman to outright want and ask for sexual activity - that desire somehow put the woman in a "slut" category. Luckily our wonderful twenty-first century has brought increased activism with folks naming "slut-shaming" as a bad thing, along with the creation of the problematic term "man-slut" (which I dislike), in an attempt to equalize notions of sexual desire.

Now that we are one-fifth into the twenty-first century, with #metoo solidly in place, humans thankfully continue to expand the conversation around consent. At a minimum, for a person to legally consent to any sexual activity (physical, verbal, or otherwise), the person needs to be of age (16 is the youngest age for any type of intercourse in Massachusetts; this varies state by state).

Consent has further evolved into the acronym *FRIES*. According to the Planned Parenthood website (https://www.plannedparenthood.org/learn/relationships/sexual-consent), modern full consent is:

1. **Freely** given. "Consenting is a choice you make without pressure, manipulation, or under influence of drugs or alcohol."
2. **Reversible**. "Anyone can change their mind about what they feel like doing, anytime. Even if you've done it before" and you are preparing to do it again.
3. **Informed**. "You can only consent if you have the full story. For example, if someone says they'll use a condom, but don't, then there isn't full consent."
4. **Enthusiastic**. "When it comes to sex, you should only do things you WANT to do, not things you are expected to do."
5. **Specific**. "Saying yes to one thing (like going to the bedroom to make out) doesn't mean you've said yes to other" things (like intercourse).

I personally love the addition of *enthusiasm*, as this concept finally equalizes desire within all the genders. No longer does sex have to reflect the Western stereotype of a cisman being socialized all his life to seize any opportunity of sex (a concept resented by many cismen and others). Now women and other genders can seize the permission, and the imperative, to enthusiastically ask for what they want.

INCREASING EMDR THERAPIST COMFORT WITH ADDRESSING SEXUAL HEALTH

Two of the best ways to increase one's comfort level with addressing sexuality involve self-reflection (examining one's own biases and stereotypes) and continuously seeking information and education. Reading this book, if this is your first foray into accurate and empowering sexual health, is a great step toward education. This book mentions many more resources that will hopefully find its way onto your office bookshelf or bookmarked on your web browser. Stephanie Buehler's indispensable primer *What Every Mental Health Professional Needs to Know About Sex, Third Edition* (2021) recommends topics for the professional to journal at the end of each chapter, another wonderful step toward self-reflection and sexual health acclimation.

There are many organizations and individuals that offer specific training and workshops on sexual health. The national organization that addresses sex education and counseling is the American Association of Sexuality Educators, Counselors and Therapists (AASECT). For anyone wishing to pursue further sexuality certification, taking a three-day SAR (sexual attitude reassessment) class is required. SARs are designed to "inundate participants with sexual material in order to bring awareness to areas of discomfort or bias, and through exploration and discussion, ease participants into greater comfort and confidence in approaching this work" (South Shore Sexual Health Center, n.d.). I highly recommend signing up for a SAR class if you wish to expand your comfort with sexuality-related concerns. Not only will you learn about every imaginable sexual topic, often through videos, guest speakers/panels, interactive learning, and relevant readings, you will meet a group of open-minded folks also willing to explore the outer limits of current societal norms. Completing a SAR will tackle both the self-reflection and educational piece, as well.

Another very effective strategy, one that I greatly benefited from in the years leading up to writing this book, includes receiving regular consultation or supervision regarding your sexuality-related cases. I was fortunate to gather monthly with a small group of clinicians meeting at a sex therapy practice. These meetings provided education, validation, and space for reflection on bias and discomfort, as well as internalizing and integrating many of the concepts you will be reading further about in this book.

THERAPIST'S SEXOLOGICAL WORLD VIEW

A Sexological Worldview (Sitron & Dyson, 2012) is the "result of the socialization process that is comprised of values, beliefs, opinions, attitudes, and concepts specific to sexuality, including any and all sexual behavior and identities." This socialization comes from television, films, books, schools, the news, media, social media, pornography, religion, peers, and family, and so on. As therapists it is crucial that we continuously examine our own worldviews, remain aware that clients may not inhabit our worldview, and set aside our own biases in order to best help our clients. Our goals for ourselves, and ultimately our clients, include moving away from a rigid right or wrong dualistic way of thinking, toward a more relativistic evolution of a changing, progressing world, with room for greater sexual diversity and acceptance of others' realties. This larger worldview helps provide the foundation for a culturally competent sexual health practice. Additionally, embracing the concept of *polysemicity* can help us attain this greater worldview. Poylsemicity essentially means that someone else's experiences may not be what ours would be, even if we do the exact same thing (Klein, 2010). For example, two cismen can report very different experiences regarding the exact same sexual activity.

PLISSIT MODEL OF ADDRESSING SEXUAL HEALTH

One of the first concepts I learned in my foray into sexual health involves the PLISSIT model developed by Annon in 1976. The PLISSIT initials stand for Permission, Limited Information, Specific Suggestions, and Intensive Therapy.

Permission is considered a first level intervention in which the therapist provides *permission* for the client to discuss/talk/ask questions and/or disclose client feelings and concerns related to specific sexual health issues. "By encouraging clients to share their thoughts, questions, etc., you validate the issue as a legitimate health matter" (Annon, 1976). This may be the most important step and help we can provide certain clients that have been searching for answers or validation for years. You can explicitly provide permission by asking clients verbally or in your intake paperwork if they have any sexuality-related concerns. You can also make mention of your experience and comfort with sexual health on your website or listings. By having sex-positive posters, books, or pamphlets displayed in your waiting room and office, you can provide an environment that says "we can talk about sex here."

Limited Information is a second level intervention, goes beyond the *permission* obtained in first step, and provides basic *information* about the topic. During this step you might provide handouts, dispel myths and preconceptions, and refer clients to books and websites. This book references many educational tools and resources you can add to your library of knowledge.

Specific Suggestions comprises the third level and involves advanced level of knowledge or *specific* expertise. If you are not comfortable or able to provide these, and the client continues to report sexual difficulty, even after accomplishing all the relevant EMDR therapy targets (sexuality-related included), you may need to refer your client to a certified sex therapist, pelvic floor physical therapist, midwife or sex-positive ob/gyn, or other sexual health specialist.

The fourth level intervention of *Intensive Therapy* (if needed) is typically provided by an outside specialist (e.g., sex therapist or pelvic floor physical therapist) for a particular issue, such as continued pelvic pain or erectile dysfunction.

POSITIVE MODELS OF SEXUAL HEALTH

Since being on this journey of integrating sexual health into my own EMDR practice, I have discovered many wonderfully positive models of sexual health. My favorites are mentioned in this section.

Our Whole Lives Sexuality Education Curriculum

I fell in love with Our Whole Lives (OWL) after my local Unitarian Universalist (UU) congregation asked me if I wanted to attend a weekend training for seventh through twelfth grade curriculum in 2018, with the intent of volunteering to teach the 9-month long curriculum to our congregational youth. I jumped at this lifelong chance to proactively prevent sexual trauma by inoculating youth (and later, adults) with as much factual, educational, and sex-positive information as the curriculum could provide.

The concepts and guidelines that inform this curriculum grew from the research of the Sexuality Education Task Force in the early nineties and from the work of many educators and UU and UCC (United Church of Christ) congregations who saw a lack of evidence and factual-based sexuality education for youth, developing curriculum for the life-span. You don't have to be a UU or UCC member to receive training to teach the various OWL curricula (broken into these age ranges: Kindergarten through First Grade, Fourth through Sixth Grade, Seventh through Ninth Grade, Tenth through Twelfth Grade, Young Adult, Adult, and now Older Adult). Like taking a SAR, becoming OWL trained is a good way to open up one's mind and sexological worldview.

Keeping in mind these OWL program values, assumptions, and circles of sexuality makes excellent guidelines for a sex-positive therapy practice.

OWL Program Values

Self-Worth: "Every person is entitled to dignity and self-worth, and to their own attitudes and beliefs about sexuality" (Wilson, 2014).

Sexual Health: "Knowledge about human sexuality is helpful, not harmful. Every person has the right to accurate information" (Wilson, 2014). Healthy sexual relationships are consensual, non-exploitative, mutually pleasurable, safe (low or no risk of sexually transmitted infections (STIs), emotional pain, unintended pregnancy), developmentally appropriate, based on mutual expectations and caring, respectful. Any type of sexual intercourse is only one of the many valid ways of expressing sexual feelings with a partner.

Responsibility: We enrich our lives by expressing sexuality in ways that enhance human wholeness and fulfillment and can express love and pleasure. "All persons have the right and obligation to make responsible sexual choices" (Wilson, 2014).

Justice and Inclusivity: "People of all ages, sexual identities, races, ethnicities, genders, income levels, abilities, and sexual orientations must have equal value and rights. All of the following are natural in the range of human sexual experience: being romantically and sexually attracted to more than one gender (bisexual), the same gender (homosexual), another gender (heterosexual), and/or to those with a more fluid understanding of their own and others' gender (pansexual), and experiencing no sexual attraction (asexual)" (Wilson, 2014). There should be no coercion or exploitation in sexual relationships, nor should humans be subjected to double standards or stereotypes.

OWL Assumptions

It can be helpful to hold these OWL assumptions in mind:

"All humans are potentially sexual beings from before birth until death. It is natural to express sexual feelings in a variety of ways. Sexuality is a good part of the human experience and includes much more than sexual behavior. People engage in healthy sexual behavior for a variety of reasons including to express caring and love, experience intimacy and connection with another, share pleasure, bring new life into the world, and have fun and relax. Sexuality in our society is damaged by violence, exploitation, alienation, dishonesty, abuse of power, and the treatment of persons as objects. It is healthier for young teens to postpone forms of intercourse" (Wilson, 2014).

OWL Circles of Sexuality

This diagram adapted by OWL depicts the overlapping and intersecting circles of sexuality, which permeate human experience, according to OWL (see Figure 1.1). Dennis Dailey originally developed this for a youth education curriculum in 1995. It remains a solid framework from which to explore sexuality.

Planned Parenthood Model of Sexual Health

Planned Parenthood sex educators base their curriculum on material developed by ETR (Education, Training and Research) whose goal is to advance to health equity. ETR's textbook *Sexuality Education: Theory and Practice* (Bruess & Schroeder, 2018) provides a wealth of history and information regarding sexuality education and lists several major guidelines for comprehensive sexuality education such as the United Nations Educational, Scientific and Cultural Organizations' (UNESCO) and the Sexuality Information and Education Council of the United

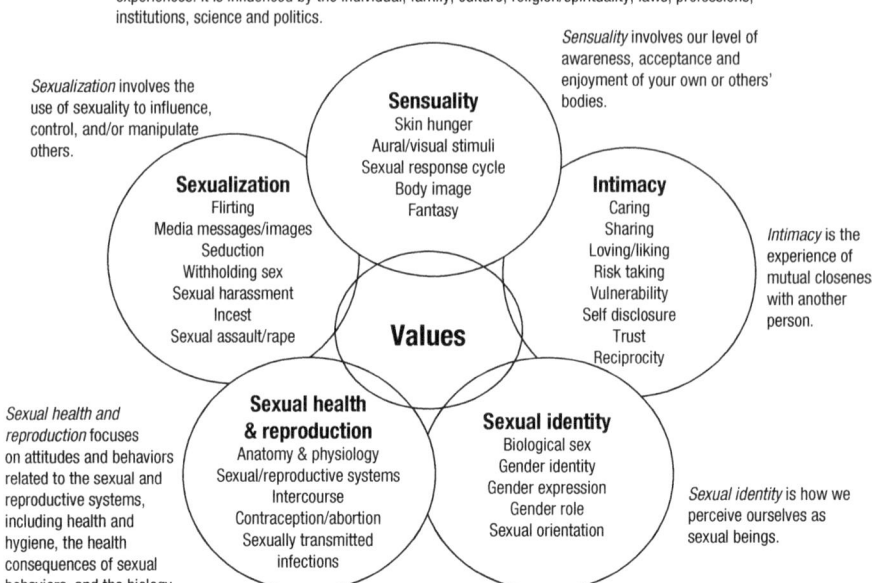

FIGURE 1.1 Circles of Sexuality.

Source: Adapted from *Life Planning Education*, 1995, Advocates for Youth, Washington, DC, Advocatesforyouth.org, based on the original work of Dennis Dailey, Professor Emeritus, University of Kansas.

States' (SIECUS) guidelines as helpful psychoeducation. We can share these with our clients, pointing out that most of us never received any sex education at all, let alone comprehensive sex education adhering to these fairly extensive guidelines. Acknowledging the global and pervasive lack of helpful sex education can reduce our clients' sense of shame or inadequacy around any sexual health gaps they may posses.

UNESCO's (2018) sexuality education goals are "to equip children and young people with knowledge, skills, attitudes and values that will empower them to realize their health, well-being, and dignity; develop respectful social and sexual relationships; consider how their choices affect their own sexual well-being and that of others; and understand and ensure the protection of their rights throughout their lives." UNESCO advocates for both formal and non-formal settings, both in-school and out-of-school settings and includes scientifically accurate information, incremental (building through development), age and developmentally appropriate, based on a curriculum, inclusive of human rights, and culturally appropriate and relevant.

SIECUS (2004) lists four main goals of sexuality education: (a) provide accurate information about human sexuality, (b) provide an opportunity for people to develop and understand their values, attitudes, and insights about sexuality, (c) help people develop relationships and interpersonal skills, and (d) help people exercise responsibility with regard to sexual relationships (including abstinence, contraception use, and coping with sexual pressure).

SIECUS (2004) also includes thirty characteristics of sexually healthy adults. Here are just a few: appreciate one's own body, interact with all genders in respectful ways, express love and intimacy in appropriate ways, avoid exploitative or manipulative relationships, take responsibility for one's own behavior, enjoy and express one's sexuality throughout one's life, reject sexual stereotypes and promote acceptance of diverse sexualities.

GINA OGDEN'S 4-DIMENSIONAL WHEEL OF SEXUAL HEALTH

Gina Ogden has developed a wonderfully comprehensive and holistic approach to sexual health, worth learning about briefly here and more on your own as this approach links well with EMDR therapy concepts. Ogden's 4-Dimensional Wheel of sexual health consists of four quadrants: Physical, Mental, Emotional, and Spiritual, similar to EMDR's three-prong approach of body, mind, and emotions. See Figure 1.2.

The *Physical* quadrant involves the person's range of sensory experience (smell, touch, taste, sight, hearing), movement and stillness, comfort and safety, arousal, orgasm, and other physical pleasures/sensations. This quadrant can be characterized by heightened senses. The "shadow side" can contain pain, disgust, numbness, and dysfunction (Ogden, 2016).

The *Emotional* quadrant contains the person's range of feelings (love, passion, yearning, anger, hatred, and fear), empathy, self-compassion (described by Dalai Lama as the ability to "love yourself and others no matter how conflicted your feelings may be"), trust (the ability to let go of control), open-heartedness, and heightened feelings. The shadow side can include disappointment, anxiety, depression, restriction, anger, boredom, shame, and guardedness (Ogden, 2016).

The *Mental* quadrant includes beliefs and messages about sexuality and spirituality, including religious messages. Ogden also includes imagination, intuition, memory, dreams, waking dreams and fantasies, along with wishes, intentions, anticipations, and expectations. This quadrant can involve a curious open-mind, problem-solving, increased understanding, and expanded beliefs. The shadow side may contain negative messages and rigid attitudes about what sex should be like (Ogden, 2016)

The *Spiritual* quadrant involves a deep sense of connection with one's self, partner(s), and/or "higher power." It can include inner visions, communication

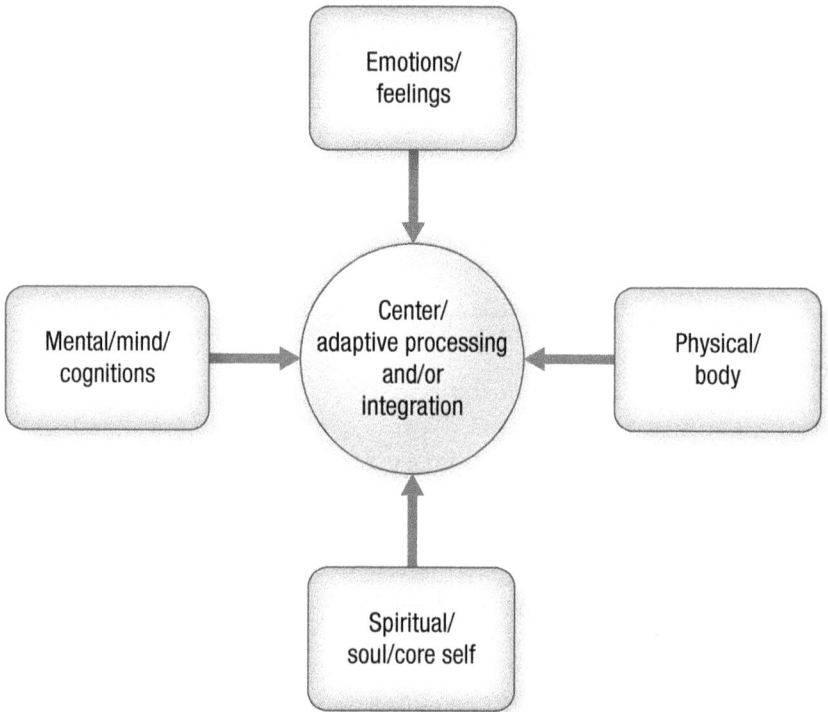

FIGURE 1.2 The Dimensions of Sexual Experience.
Source: Adapted from Ogden, G. (2016, May). *Exploring the 4-D wheel of sexual health*. Workshop presented at the AASECT Northeast Region Meet and Greet. Florence, MA.

with divine forces, experiencing oneself as part of all that is sacred. It can be characterized by ecstasy, increased energy, lasting satisfaction, connection, and transcendence. The shadow side can include a profound sense of isolation, depression, and paralysis (Ogden, 2016).

The *Center* of these four quadrants converging positively varies by individual. Some folks may report that visiting this center feels like a "high-definition Oz." The center "may feel like place of mystery and paradox where opposites emerge in an uncanny way." The person "may experience one-ness, integration, shape-shifting, timelessness, light, and/or lightness of being." They may report communing "profoundly" with self and/or partner. The center may feel like a "place of clarity, vision, vastness, and unconditional love." As with the four quadrants, the center has a shadow side: hopelessness and despair (Ogden, 2016).

You can have your client explore and address an issue or potential EMDR target using the four dimensions of the wheel. As with EMDR, you will want to create a sense of safety in the office, perhaps in one specific area (or one specific area in their home, if you are doing teletherapy). Invite your client to try a movement to address the issue. Help your client develop a ritual. If possible, you may want to apply slow bilateral stimulation (BLS). Concretize abstract concepts with tangible objects (feathers, rocks, shields, pillows, etc.) and have the client hold them while receiving the BLS and holding positive cognitions related to the concept.

Please refer to Ogden's 2018 book *Expanding the Practice of Sex Therapy* for full instruction on incorporating her 4-D Wheel into your client work. Consider completing the 4-D training and joining the 4-D network.

INTEGRATING SEXUAL HEALTH INTO THE EMDR ADAPTIVE INFORMATION PROCESSING MODEL

When Francine Shapiro began developing EMDR therapy in the late 1980s, she initially posited a theoretical model called "Accelerated Information Processing" to explain the framework and efficacy of EMDR therapy. Over time the name evolved to *Adaptive Information Processing (AIP)* while retaining many of the original hypotheses and principles (Shapiro, 2018). The main tenets of the AIP model focus on healing using the client's resources and innate ability to process maladaptive information to complete integration. Ideally a human brain can usually process information satisfactorily, filing that data away appropriately and neatly, like in a file cabinet. However, if this "information system is impaired, the memory will be stored in a raw, unprocessed, and maladaptive form" (Hase et al., 2017).

This means that this disturbing event will have difficulty connecting to other memory networks that hold adaptive information. Therefore, "when a memory is encoded in such excitatory, state-specific form, the original perceptions can be triggered by a variety of internal and external stimuli" (Hase et al., 2017). These dysfunctionally stored memories then form the basis for future maladaptive responses and possible psychopathology. Activating these memories, even years later, can lead to a variety of symptoms from post-traumatic stress disorder (PTSD) to anxiety to "barely noticeable intrusions" (Hase et al., 2017).

I summarized the AIP model to help us understand how a client's sexual health can be negatively impacted at any point in time, leading to sexual unease, discomfort, or dysfunction. From a yet-to-be-born child experiencing domestic violence vicariously through their parent's stress hormones to a child witnessing a parent's sexual coercion to a pre-teen noticing the lack of physical affection from or between parents—these are all events and atmospheres that can negatively impact a client's sexual health. Add in a shaming and sexually punitive society, and it's a miracle that any child can make their way to adulthood with an empowered pleasurable sex life.

EMDR therapy has been an amazing force of good in righting so many wrongs via alleviating suffering and unlocking adaptive cognitions and futures for clients, particularly related to sexual traumas. However, we all can do better to look for the thousand tiny cuts our clients have likely sustained from negative messaging around sexuality, and find EMDR targets related to early misinformation, lack of information, shaming of emerging sexuality, and the million other ways our puritanical culture shames individuals for being sexual beings.

Here is a just a small list of potential EMDR targets related to negative sexual socialization or lack of appropriate sexuality education:

1. An adult cismale client reveals he was caught masturbating as a youth and remains mortified.
2. An adult cisfemale client recalls an abusive first boyfriend that criticized her "slutty" outfits in public.
3. An adult discloses first learning about sex through pornographic magazines discovered in the woods, resulting in continued confusion.
4. An adult who went to Catholic primary school mentions how there was no sex education at all. When they began menarche, they were treated with scorn.
5. A gender non-binary adult described how her parents simultaneously shamed her growing interest in dating AND emphasized and enforced feminized notions of beauty (make-up, dresses, body shape, etc.), creating confusion and shame.

> **Case Study 1.1: Lily: Sexual Trauma, EMDR Therapy, Sexual Health, Sexual Rights and Values, PLISSIT, Consent, 4-D Wheel**

The following case composite example draws from many clients for the purpose of illustrating the aforementioned sexual health frameworks, demonstrating how these additional lenses can help an EMDR clinician search for EMDR and sexual health–related targets. Mostly sexual frameworks are touched upon in this example. The following chapters explore the intersection of EMDR therapy and sexual health in greater detail.

Lily sought EMDR therapy to process and treat pre-teen sexual trauma by slightly older neighbors, early college sexual assault, and current sexual dissatisfaction. Lily has a full-time job in Human Resources, is a lesbian-identified ciswoman in her late thirties, is bicultural (Puerto Rican and Irish heritage), a practicing Catholic, and is in a committed long-term monogamous relationship with another ciswoman. She also reported an abortion related to the college sexual assault.

Placing her life experience within the Circles of Sexuality, she experienced Sexualization (unwanted sexual activity), Reproductive Concerns (she continues to harbor shame and guilt about the abortion), Intimacy Concerns (difficulty trusting her partner), and Sensuality Concerns (current lack of pleasure with touch, infrequent orgasms, poor body image, and lack of sexual fantasy). She reports comfort with her sexual identity as an out lesbian and ciswoman.

After working on all the obvious EMDR targets of the pre-teen sexual abuse and the college sexual assault, we determined that there were many small trauma ("small t") targets around the negative messaging of sexuality she experienced within her family culture as well as from the religious Catholic culture in which she was raised. We found numerous EMDR targets that rated three or higher on the Subjective Units of Distress scale (SUDs) such as nuns at her Catholic school shaming make-up, her mother's disapproval of her clothing choice, calling her "a slutty dresser," and the neighborhood boys catcalling her (she had developed slightly earlier than her cisfemale peers). She had never received any accurate sex education other than "don't have sex." No one in her family instructed her about menarche; menstrual pads simply showed up in her bathroom drawer one day.

Broadly speaking, she had not been provided with any healthy or accurate sexual education or framework. She had no idea, even through her late twenties, that she was entitled to a "positive and respectful approach to sexuality" (WHO, n.d.), a life free from sexual abuse, nor was she aware of the basic tenets of consent.

Throughout the therapy, Permission (from the PLISSIT) was often given for Lily to discuss her trauma and all of her sexuality concerns and questions. Often Limited Information was provided in the form of sexuality-related self-help resources such as books on women's sexuality. As she had reported some numbing in her genital region, she was referred to a respected sex-positive ob/gyn to rule out any medical condition.

A great many sessions were spent on normalizing sexual health and sexuality, including the right to engage in sexual behavior simply for pleasure and connection. Keeping in mind SIECUS's thirty characteristics of sexually healthy adults, the positive cognitions of "I am normal and can enjoy my body," "I have the right to enjoy and express my sexuality," and "I can identify and ask for what I want" were identified and frequently used. Her negative cognitions included: "Something is wrong with me," "I can't be vulnerable," and "I don't have choice or voice."

Once all these "small t" EMDR targets were addressed, we then used Ogden's 4-D Wheel to identify any lingering difficulties or challenges. Physically Lily continued to report some difficulty identifying arousal and other pleasurable signs. Emotionally she noticed continued fear and shame. Mentally she continued to harbor lingering messages of guilt around sexual enjoyment from her Catholic background, particularly in light of the homophobia she went through in her coming out process. These generated even more "small t" appearing targets, which ended up rating higher on the SUDs upon further activation, pushing them into more "big T" territory. Spiritually she reported a lack of deep connection to her body and her partner.

We were able to find more recent and current EMDR targets based on the 4-D Wheel categories. For example, Lily noted that when her partner approached her from behind to hug her, she froze and went numb, essentially shutting down. Once we processed these more current/present targets, we developed and processed several EMDR Future Templates to navigate through any lingering negative experiences of her sexuality.

Additionally, Lily and her partner had joined an Episcopalian "welcoming" congregation a couple of years ago (specifically welcoming to LGBTQ folks). She was now able to parse out her own spiritual identity, retaining the pieces similar to her Catholic upbringing that continued to feel meaningful and positive (her relationship to Jesus and Mary), as well as enjoy a new comfort during church services knowing that she was "normal," loved, and enthusiastically accepted as herself.

At discharge Lily noted consistent sensation perception throughout her body, including her genitals, more orgasms, and a greater interest and ability to receive and enjoy sexual connection with her partner. She was now able to more easily access the "center" of her 4-D Wheel, experiencing timelessness, unconditional love, and integration of Mental, Physical, Emotional, and Spiritual quadrants.

Lily also chose to "install" more resources via BLS including a cherished Celtic cross given to her by a nurturing and open Irish grandmother (representing unconditional love and spiritual connection), shells found in Puerto Rico (representing openness and sensual connection), and her engagement ring from her supportive partner (representing trust, healthy risk-taking, mutual sharing, and pleasure). Lily reported consistently being able to identify and ask for what she wanted, not only sexually, but in her profession, family of origin, and friendships. At the mutual decision of client and therapist, Lily discharged from EMDR therapy with many sex-positive resources and messages, plus full encouragement and support.

SUMMARY

WHO and the Office of the Surgeon General and Office of Population Affairs both have helpful definitions of sexual health. A working definition of sexual activity is provided, and the uplifting and affirming WAS's Declaration of Sexual Rights and Pleasure is shared.

Many individual and cultural factors (e.g., erotophobia) impact therapists' potential comfort and discomfort in addressing sexual health with their clients. Therapists also bring their own *Sexological Worldview* into the session; therefore, gaining knowledge and familiarity with sexual health is critical. There are many ways therapists can increase their comfort with sexual material, including training such as a SAR workshop.

The concept of *consent* (particularly FRIES) is extremely important, not only regarding clients' experiences with sexual activity, but for ourselves as therapists as we inquire about our clients' sexual health. The PLISSIT model is an excellent model for sexual health communication and intervention.

The *Our Whole Lives* and the Planned Parenthood curricula embrace many sex positive values (e.g., dignity and self-worth, knowledge, choice, equal rights and value), which we can keep in mind in our work with clients. Gina Ogden's 4-D Wheel of Sexuality (Mental, Physical, Emotional, Spiritual, and Center dimensions) also offers a helpful clinical framework and is easily integrated into the AIP Model.

REFERENCES

Advocates for Youth. (1995). *Life planning education: A youth development program.* Author.

Annon, J. S. (1976). The PLISSIT model: A proposed conceptual scheme for the behavioral treatment of sexual problems. *Journal of Sex Education and Therapy, 2*(1), 1–15. https://doi.org/10.1080/01614576.1976.11074483

Bright, S. (1997). *Sexual state of the union.* Touchstone.

Bruess, C., & Schroeder, E. (2018). *Sexuality education: Theory and practice, seventh edition.* ETR.

Buehler, S. (2017). *What every mental health professional needs to know about sex, second edition.* Springer Publishing Company.

Dailey, D. (1995). Circles of Sexuality as depicted in *life planning education: A youth development program* (Dr. Dennis Dailey, DSW, Professor Emeritus, University of Kansas, 1111 East 19th Street, Lawrence, KS 66046-3205).

Dischavio, R. (2016). *The deep yes: The lost art of true receiving.* Spanda Press.

Gallagher, K. (2014, October). *Pandora's Box: Sex from A to Z in clinical work* [Presentation]. Brattleboro Retreat, Holyoke, MA.

Global Advisory Board for Sexual Health and Wellbeing. (2016). *Working definition of sexual pleasure.* https://www.gab-shw.org/our-work/working-definition-of-sexual-pleasure/

Gruskin, S., Yadav, V., Castellanos-Usigli, A., Khizanishvili, G., & Kismödi, E. (2019). Sexual health, sexual rights and sexual pleasure: Meaningfully engaging the perfect triangle. *Sexual and Reproductive Health Matters, 27*(1), 29–40. https://doi.org/10.1080/26410397.2019.1593787

Hase, M., Balmaceda, U., Ostacoli, L., Liebermann, P., & Hofmann, A. (2017). The AIP model of EMDR therapy and pathogenic memories. *Frontiers in Psychology, 21.* https://doi.org/10.3389/fpsyg.2017.01578

Klein, M. (2010, April). *When sex gets complicated: Pornography, kink, cybersex, and other clinical challenges* [Workshop]. AASECT, Florence, MA.

Kleinplatz, P. J., Menard, A. D., Paquet, M.-P., Paradis, N., Campbell, M., Zuccarino, D., Mehak, L. (2009). The components of optimal sexuality: A portrait of "great" sex. *The Canadian Journal of Human Sexuality*, *18*(1-2).

Mexico City World Congress of Sexual Health. (October 15, 2019). Declaration on Sexual Pleasure. https://worldsexualhealth.net/declaration-on-sexual-pleasure/

National Center for Injury Prevention and Control, Division of Violence Prevention. (2021, February 5). *Preventing sexual violence*. Centers for Disease Control and Prevention. https://www.cdc.gov/violenceprevention/sexualviolence/fastfact.html

Office of the Surgeon General & Office of Population Affairs. (2001). *The Surgeon General's call to action to promote sexual health and responsible sexual behavior*. Office of the Surgeon General. http://www.ncbi.nlm.nih.gov/NBK44216

Ogden, G. (2016, May). *Exploring the 4-D wheel of sexual health*. Workshop presented at the AASECT Northeast Region Meet and Greet, Florence, MA.

Ogden, G. (2018). *Expanding the practice of sex therapy: The Neuro-update edition – An integrative approach for exploring desire and intimacy* (2nd ed.). Routledge.

Queen, C. (2002). *Real-live nude girl: Chronicles of sex-positive culture*. Cleis Press.

Saakvitne, K. W., Pearlman, L. A., & Staff. (1996). *Transforming the pain: A workbook on vicarious traumatization*. W.W. Norton & Company, Inc.

Sexuality Information and Education Council of the United States (2004). *Guidelines for comprehensive sexuality education, 3rd edition: Kindergarten through 12th grade*. National Guidelines Task Force.

Shapiro, F. (2018). *Eye movement desensitization and reprocessing therapy: Basic principles, protocols, and procedures, third edition*. Guilford.

Sitron, J. A., & Dyson, D. A. (2012, March 13). Validation of sexological worldview: A construct for the use in the training of sexologists in sexual diversity. *SAGE Open*. https://doi.org/10.1177/2158244012439072

South Shore Sexual Health Center. (n.d.). Retrieved September 23, 2021, from https://www.sssexualhealthcenter.com/getcertified#sar

United Nations Educational, Scientific and Cultural Organizations. (2018). *International technical guidance on sexuality education*. UNESCO Joint United Nations Programme on HIV/AIDS, United Nations Populations Fund, United Nations Children's Fund, United Nations Entity for Gender Equality and the Empowerment of Women, World Health Organization.

Van der Hart, O., Nijenhuis, E. R. S., & Steele, K. (2006). *The haunted self: Structural dissociation and the treatment of chronic traumatization*. W.W. Norton and Company.

Westheimer, R., Grunebaum, A., & Lehu, P. (2012). *Sexually speaking: What every woman needs to know about sexual health*. John Wiley and Sons.

Wilson, P. (2014). *Our whole lives: Sexual education for grades 7–9, 2nd edition*. UUAC.

World Health Organization. (n.d.). *Sexual and reproductive health*. Retrieved September 23, 2021, from http://www.who.int/reproductivehealth/topics/sexual_health/sh_definitions/en

SUPPLEMENTAL MATERIALS FOR CLIENTS

I have included here a helpful article I wrote for my monthly column, *Sex Matters*, that can be handed out to clients to further explain consent and pleasure.
Consent and Pleasure
By Stephanie Baird, LMHC
(Originally published December 2019 in the *Montague Reporter* newspaper monthly *Sex Matters* column.)

Let's talk about consent and pleasure. As someone who came of age in the eighties and nineties, not much was discussed or even known about active negotiation of sex-related activities. During my work in the late nineties, primarily working with sexual assault survivors, "consent" concepts emerged in clinical work as well in rape crisis educational campaigns. However, most of these campaigns centered around the "no means no" concept. This, of course, is paramount. Humans being able to say no to unwanted activities is the foundation from which we can later say yes to wanted activities.

Much of the twentieth century stereotypical male and female gender expression involved the idea that a cisgender man should want and try for sex, and that a "good" cisgender woman should be a "gatekeeper," saying no often, but eventually "giving in" (like Scarlet O-Hara and Rhett Butler in "Gone With the Wind," he forcibly dragged her, kicking and fighting, upstairs for sex, and then the next scene shows her post-sex, looking content). It wasn't ok for a woman to outright want and ask for sexual activity—that desire somehow put the woman in a "slut" category. Happily our wonderful twenty-first century has brought increased activism with folks naming "slut-shaming" as a bad thing, along with the creation of the problematic term "man-slut" (which I dislike), in an attempt to equalize notions of sexual desire.

Now that we are one-fifth into the twenty-first century, with #metoo solidly in place, humans continue to expand the conversation around consent. At a minimum, for a person to legally consent to any sexual activity (physical, verbal, or otherwise), the person needs to be of age (16 is the youngest age for any type of intercourse in Massachusetts, this varies state by state).

Consent has further evolved into the acronym **FRIES**. According to Planned Parenthood, modern full consent includes

1. **Freely** given. "Consenting is a choice you make without pressure, manipulation, or under influence of drugs or alcohol."
2. **Reversible**. "Anyone can change their mind about what they feel like doing, anytime. Even if you've done it before," and you are preparing to do it again.

3. **Informed**. "You can only consent if you have the full story. For example, if someone says they'll use a condom, but don't, then there isn't full consent."
4. **Enthusiastic**. "When it comes to sex, you should only do things you WANT to do, not things you are expected to do."
5. **Specific**. "Saying yes to one thing (like going to the bedroom to make out) doesn't mean you've said yes to other" things (like intercourse).

I personally love the addition of enthusiasm, as this concept finally equalizes desire within all the genders. No longer does sex just have to be a dude being trained all his life to seize a moment of sex whenever opportunity is there. Now women and other genders have been given permission, and the imperative, to enthusiastically ask for what they want.

In November 2019 I heard acclaimed journalist Peggy Orenstein speak on "Girls and Sex: From Risk and Danger to Responsibility and Joy" (Boston), and learned some helpful terms and alarming statistics.

She noted that research psychologist Sarah MacLelland coined the term *"intimate justice'*: the idea that sex has political as well as personal components, reflecting issues of gender inequality, economic disparity, violence, and mental health. Intimate justice asks: Who is entitled to engage in a sexual experience? Who is entitled to enjoy it? How does each partner define good enough?"

Orenstein shared research that looked at cisfemale self-objectification (girls trying to attain an "effortless perfection" of "hotness and sexiness" for the "male gaze") and found that higher self-objectification correlated with reduced sexual satisfaction among cisfemales. It is also linked with depression, anxiety, eating disorders, negative and reduced cognition, and political participation. She noted that many heterosexual teens and young women seemed to undergo a *psychological cliterodectomy*, preferring to give rather than receive any kind of pleasure, mostly for status, security, and notions of power. However, the "orgasm gap" disappears among lesbians.

One antidote for this lopsided quandary of who gets to receive pleasure can be found in an encouraging book by local author Dr. Rosalyn Dischiavo called *The Deep Yes: The Lost Art of True Receiving* (2016). At a talk she gave, one of the first things Dischiavo asked was if we remembered our last shower. She pointed out that folks often mindlessly rush through their showers, sometimes even forgetting if they have shampooed, when showering is a great opportunity to say yes to mindful sensuality with oneself.

Her book explores the original *yin* energy of receptivity as one of "drawing in ... allowing," and incredibly active in its "power to receive." In India, "the Goddess Shakti, the embodiment of all power, is the *yin* principle." Within the white yang of the yin-yang symbol is *Spanda* (the yang-feminine): spontaneous movement, birthing, and power. Dischiavo applies these ideas to saying yes to sleep, mindful eating, our beautiful bodies, and pleasurable sex with oneself and others.

After hearing Orenstein's alarming review of the pleasure disparity, and her mention that even modern sex educators fail to mention clitoris to their children at early ages, I found a diagram of female genitalia that included the clitoris and gave my nearly 9-year-old daughter a quick clitoris lesson, telling her that it's the only organ whose sole purpose seems to be fun and pleasure. Her eyes widened with interest as she said, "you mean it's something that's supposed to feel good and it's a good thing to touch it?" I answered with a resounding "yes" (and advised her that alone time in her bedroom is a great way to explore).

DECLARATION OF SEXUAL RIGHTS, PLEASURE, AND CONSENT HANDOUT

Since 1978 the World Association for Sexual Health (WAS) has worked toward sexual health and rights. Thousands of members attend global biennial congresses and in recent years have made declarations for sexual rights.

Declaration of Sexual Rights (Adapted from WAS, 2014)

1. The right to equality and freedom of sexual expression.
2. The right to make decisions about one's body in regard to sexuality.
3. The right to be safe from all forms of sexual violence and coercion, and be free from inhumane treatment or punishment because of one's sexual or gender expression.
4. The right to accurate scientific information and education about sexuality and sexual health.
5. The right to freely create and dissolve marital and other similar relationships.
6. The right to family planning resources.
7. The right to organize freely to promote sexual rights and health.
8. The right to privacy regarding sexual matters.
9. The right to judicious laws and remedies regarding sexual rights.
10. The right to the highest attainable standard of sexual health, including sexual safe and pleasurable sexual experiences.

[*Source*: Adapted from the World Association for Sexual Health. (2014, March). *Declaration of Sexual Rights*. https://worldsexualhealth.net/wp-content/uploads/2013/08/declaration_of_sexual_rights_sep03_2014.pdf.]

Declaration on Sexual Pleasure

Sexual pleasure is the physical and/or psychological satisfaction and enjoyment derived from shared or solitary erotic experiences, including thoughts, dreams, and autoeroticism. Self-determination, consent, safety, privacy, confidence…communicating and negotiating sexual relations are key…factors for pleasure to contribute to sexual health and well-being. Sexual pleasure should be exercised within the context of sexual rights… (including) equality, non-discrimination, autonomy, bodily integrity, and the right to the highest…standard of health and freedom of expression. The experiences of human sexual pleasure are diverse and sexual rights ensure that pleasure is a positive experience for all concerned and not obtained by violating…human rights and well-being. (Gruskin et al., 2019)

Some of WAS's Declaration of Sexual Rights include:

- Sexual pleasure is a fundamental part of sexual and human rights and includes the possibility of diverse sexual experiences.
- Access to appropriate sources of sexual pleasure is part of human well-being.
- Sexual health and well-being include pleasurable and safe sexual experiences free of discrimination, coercion, and violence.
- Sexual pleasure shall be globally integrated into education, health services, research, and advocacy and contributes to global health.

Consent

According to the Planned Parenthood website, modern full *FRIES* consent is:

1. **Freely** given. "Consenting is a choice you make without pressure, manipulation, or under influence of drugs or alcohol."
2. **Reversible**. "Anyone can change their mind about what they feel like doing, anytime. Even if you've done it before," and you are preparing to do it again.
3. **Informed**. "You can only consent if you have the full story. For example, if someone says they'll use a condom, but don't, then there isn't full consent."
4. **Enthusiastic**. "When it comes to sex, you should only do things you WANT to do, not things you are expected to do."
5. **Specific**. "Saying yes to one thing (like going to the bedroom to make out) doesn't mean you've said yes to other" things (like intercourse).

2

Sexual Health Information, Arousal and Desire Research, and Sexual Styles

Stephanie Baird, LMHC

LEARNING OBJECTIVES

- EMDR clinicians will familiarize themselves with basic sexual anatomy and development (in utero to geriatric), as well as basic sexual health information (STIs, HIV, pregnancy prevention, safer sex).
- EMDR clinicians will learn about twentieth century sexual research (Kinsey, Masters and Johnson, Basson's non-linear model).
- EMDR clinicians will learn about the current 21st century "Dual Control Model" of Arousal and Responsive Desire (Bancroft, J., Graham, C. A., Janssen, E., & Sanders, S. A., 2009).
- EMDR clinicians will learn about spontaneous and responsive desire, arousal concordance and nonconcordance.
- EMDR clinicians will learn about sexual personality styles and how to administer the accompanying questionnaire.
- EMDR clinicians will learn about "Erotic Templates" and how they can relate to EMDR targets.

SEXUAL AND REPRODUCTIVE ANATOMY AND DEVELOPMENT—IN UTERO TO GERIATRIC

Introduction

Hopefully you have one or two sexuality-related books in your possession, but if this is your first book addressing sexual health, this chapter provides some basic medical and scientific reference information, including reproductive/sexual systems. Again, other books go into much greater detail including *Our Bodies, Ourselves* (2011), *What Every Mental Health Professional Needs to Know About Sex, Third Edition* (Buehler, 2021), and *The Guide to Getting It On* (Joannides, 2017).

In Utero

In a college level Women's Studies class, in conservative Texas in the early 1990s, I learned that all human embryos start out with undifferentiated bipotential reproductive organ morphology. If there were no Y chromosome and/or low testosterone, the initially ambiguous gonadal material usually defaulted into commonly "female" grouped organs such as ovaries, vulva, and clitoris. My mind was blown. The professor explained that as the embryo grows, around week 7 or 8, the specific chromosomes indicate which sex hormones will begin releasing. I had always suspected that we humans had a lot more in common with each other, versus differences. And here was proof that we all start out with similar formats!

Biology has continued to evolve with a much more complex picture of embryonic development (Toulson & Landon, 2021a). More specifically, initial "primordial structures include egg-shaped organs" and tissues. These structures later differentiate into "generative and erectile organs" including gametes where androgens (hormones) such as testosterone, estrogen, and progesterone will be produced (Toulson & Landon, 2021b). Additionally, "two pairs of ducts will differentiate into the tubes that gametes travel through when they leave the gonads, along with other urinary and reproductive structures" (Toulson & Landon, 2021b). Sex chromosomes alone do not dictate which structures develop. Hormones, cellular receptors, *and* the environment (particularly industrial and pharmaceutical chemicals, which can act as androgen or anti-androgen mimics) *also greatly* influence reproductive and tissue differentiation (Toulson & Landon, 2021b).

Therefore, generally speaking, for an XY chromosomal presence, the ambiguous gonadal genitalia will morph into testosterone-producing testes, as long as specific levels of androgens and cellular receptors enable the cells to respond to these hormonal signals (Toulson & Landon, 2021b). If the chromosomes are XX, with appropriate androgen levels and cellular receptors, the gonadal material develops into the labia and vulva (versus scrotum) and the clitoris (versus penis).

Folks born with intersex or ambiguous genitalia may have chromosomal variations (XXY, XO, XXX, XYY, etc.) or have experienced different hormonal influences while in the womb, which can result in less commonly seen combinations of external and/or internal sex organs.

Gross External Sexual Anatomy: Clitoris, Vulva, Labia, Perineum

Someone who experiences an estrogen-dominant body and puberty develops external genitalia that generally include "the *mons pubis* (fatty pad below the abdomen), the *vulva* (consisting of the *labia majora* [large "lips"] and *labia minora* [smaller lips]; the *clitoris*; and the *introitus* (entrance to the vagina). The *perineum* is the strip of skin between the vagina and anus and can be sensitive to touch. The *external urethral orifice* (exit for urine) is located between the clitoris and vagina (Buehler, 2017). See Figure 2.1.

An article in *The Guardian* reported recent research by El-Hamamsy and colleagues (2021) that half of nearly 200 British patients in hospital waiting rooms surveyed could not identify the urethra, while 37% mislabeled the clitoris—regardless of their gender (Geddes, 2021). Only 46% of this sample correctly identified that people with vaginas have three "holes" (vagina, urethra, and anus). Additionally, the respondents were given diagrams of external and internal sexual and reproductive anatomy to label. Only half even attempted to label the diagram, and of those who did, just 9% labeled the requested structures correctly. Many respondents confused the urethra with the clitoris, and vice versa. Based on my own clinical practice with clients over the years, I have little reason to think that folks on this side of the pond would do much better with these diagrams. Such a poor understanding of sexual anatomy does not bode well for self-advocacy, informed consent, or even basic health seeking (El-Hamamsy et al., 2021).

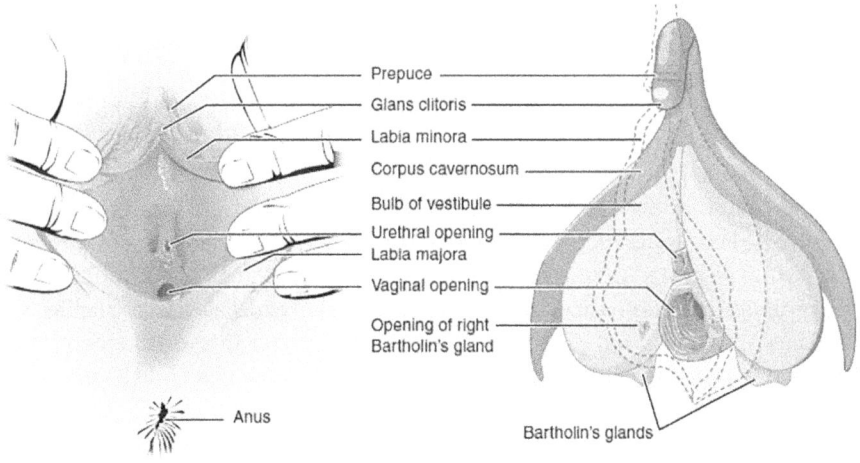

FIGURE 2.1 Vulva, external anterior view and internal anteriolateral view.

Source: Courtesy of OpenStax, Rice University, https://openstax.org/books/anatomy-and-physiology/pages/27-2-anatomy-and-physiology-of-the-female-reproductive-system

Clitoris (Erectile Organ)

The clitoris, an incredibly sensitive organ with thousands of nerve endings, is the only organ in any body that appears to have an exclusive pleasure function and not play double duty. Due to this high concentration of nerve endings (the highest in any organ), the clitoris (an external glans) is covered by a "hood" of skin that can retract when aroused. The clitoris was only recently discovered to be much larger than believed, having two leg-like extensions that are contained internally within the pelvis (Pauls, 2015) and connected to the vulva. Therefore, it is more of dual organ, configured both externally and internally. Internally this system possesses a "root, crura, and bulbs." The overall size resides within a 4-inch range. The dorsal nerve of the clitoris, part of the pudendal nerve, is responsible for "clitoral somatic innervation" (Pauls, 2015).

Some clients may report a lack of sensitivity in their clitoral area. If possible, refer your client for a full genital evaluation by a respected and preferably feminist-oriented skilled sex-positive midwife or ob/gyn in your area. [Be careful with your referrals as many clients disclose uncomfortable experiences at gynecologist offices.] If medical causes are ruled out, this numbness may be related to overall body numbness from dissociative symptoms. Often, once the eye movement desensitization and reprocessing (EMDR) targets are worked through, a sense of comfort or safety can be established within the client's own physical home and mind, allowing them to get more in touch with bodily sensation. Additionally, with the PLISSIT (permission, limited information, specific suggestions, and intensive therapy) model in place (giving clients permission to feel and explore their anatomy, plus psychoeducation about the clitoris and orgasm), sensitivity may return to the clitoris.

Many of us have heard of female genital mutilation (FGM) practices, most commonly occurring in Africa, the Middle East, and Asia, and even in very religiously conservative sects in the United States and other "developed" countries. The World Health Organization (WHO) estimates that around 300 million women alive today have been subjected to some form of FGM. Thankfully, much activism has brought attention to and reduced these torturous and debilitating cliterectomy practices.

The notable journalist Peggy Orenstein, in interviewing 70 teen girls for her book on *Girls and Sex* (2016) coined the term "psychological cliterectomy." This refers to the lack of instruction to females about the existence and role of the clitoris in sexual pleasure, leaving essentially a blank space in their sexual functioning. This omission de-emphasizes and decenters female sexual pleasure, placing the emphasis on male sexual pleasure. Of note, it was either in the aforementioned Women's Studies college class, or in another Human Sexuality college-level class (circa 1993), when I first heard the word "clitoris" uttered out loud. Although I was 20 years old at the time, I knew very little about my own anatomy. [Much of modern medical research has mostly been conducted on cismale-gendered bodies. Only in the recent decade have scientists even begun to research pregnancy!] Paul Joannides (2017) corroborates that even recently, in the late 2010s, when he asks large college audiences how many of them learned about the clitoris from a parent, very few students raise their hands.

Case Study 2.1: Richita, Genital Numbness

This brief EMDR and sexual health case example illustrates the return of genital sensation.

Richita, a ciswoman restaurant chef, sought EMDR therapy for adolescence sexual abuse targets. She reported being raised by "overprotective, rigid," and non-communicative Southeast Asian professional immigrant parents in a suburb of Boston. She also reported abuse by an older male cousin, which was never disclosed until now. As a result of this perceived parentally oppressive environment, plus the sexual abuse, she reported "acting out" sexually in her late teens and early twenties, yet deriving no sexual sensation, pleasure, nor satisfaction. She also began engaging in substance use during this time, to help "numb" out.

Now in her early thirties, Richita reported success with obtaining and maintaining sobriety from substances. At this point in her recovery she wanted to heal from the sexual trauma and get in touch with her sexual body. As we worked through the EMDR targets relating to the sexual abuse, her parents' oppressive parenting behaviors, and many of her negative experiences with addiction and sexuality, she reported beginning to notice sensation in her genitals. Sensation had largely been absent for many years. She was referred to Betty Dodson's book on learning how to have orgasms, called *Sex for One: The Joy of Self-Loving* (1996). Between EMDR therapy and sexual health psychoeducation, she noted a gradual increase of sensation, eventually reporting pleasurable masturbation accompanied by orgasms. Additionally, she became more comfortable with explaining her sexual needs to current partners, thereby increasing her presence, sensual enjoyment, and positive genital experience with said partners.

Labia (Appears to Swell Due to Erectile Clitoral Bulbs)

Labia have sensitive nerve endings and can appear to engorge and deepen in color with stimulation. Due to the rise of easily available pornography, some people have become self-conscious about their labia color or size and have fallen prey to surgical procedures such as "labiaplasty" (to change the shape and/or size of the labia) or even "vaginoplasty" (to supposedly tighten a loosened vagina). These costly procedures are neither medically necessary nor recommended, as genitals come in all shapes and sizes, and surgery may cause lasting scarring and interfere with sexual function and pleasure (American College of Obstetricians and Gynecologists [ACOG], 2007). If your clients report any dissatisfaction with the appearance of their genitalia, these dissatisfactions may be good EMDR targets.

Nipples (Erectile)

For many bodies (of any gender), breasts/chests and nipples may show sensitivity and harden when stimulated. Some folks may feel self-conscious of their nipple color or the size of the areolas (the dark area around the nipples), as well as breast/chest size (clients may consider this area too big, too small, too "unusually" shaped, or too saggy). These concerns might generate good EMDR therapy targets to work on.

Other Clitoral Orgasm and Knowledge Concerns

Unfortunately, despite all the consciousness-raising groups in the 1970s where ciswomen examined their genitalia with hand mirrors, very few ciswomen have ever visually inspected their genitals to this degree. People with penises have frequent opportunities (typically during urination or masturbation) to observe their genitals. I, and many other authors of sexual health books, recommend that folks with clitorises, vulvas, and labias consider bringing a mirror to this region regularly for general health inspection and awareness of appearance and condition, similar to monthly breast self-examination. For bonus self-appreciation folks can articulate positive affirmations and intentions to this area (e.g., "My clitoris is an important source of pleasure, which I treasure" or "I take care of my vulva, labia, clitoris, and vagina by bringing it love and pleasure"). Clients could add slow Butterfly Hug tapping bilateral stimulation (BLS) or listen to audio BLS to intensify positive feelings.

Additionally, despite the prevalence of those *Cosmopolitan* magazine covers claiming "top 10 tricks for stronger orgasms," many ciswomen continue to report lack of orgasm during sexual activity, even with the progress in de-emphasizing so-called "vaginal orgasms." I have found that a small but persistent number of my own cis-female-identified clients have never or rarely masturbated to orgasm. Those who have masturbated often have yet to share their preferred technique or strategies with a partner, out of embarrassment, fear of hurting their partner's feelings, or placing a greater value on their partner's needs. I highly recommend Dodson's book *Sex for One: The Joy of Self-Loving* (1996), a classic for assisting those with a clitoris, vulva, and vagina to learn how to have orgasms and share that information more easily with others.

Gross Internal Sexual and Reproductive Anatomy: Vagina, G-Spot, Pelvic Floor, and So Forth

Internal parts that often develop together in an estrogen-dominant body and environment include the *introitus* (vagina's entrance), *vagina, Grafenberg* or *G-spot, cervix, uterus, Fallopian tubes*, and *ovaries* (see Figure 2.2). Ovaries are the gonads that produce and release eggs during the menstrual cycle and also produce sex hormones. A released egg travels the Fallopian tube to the uterus, where, if fertilized by sperm, it can implant and become an embryo. The cervix is tissue that connects the vagina to the uterus. The *urethra* (tube from which the body releases urine) in this anatomical configuration is usually located between the clitoris and the vagina.

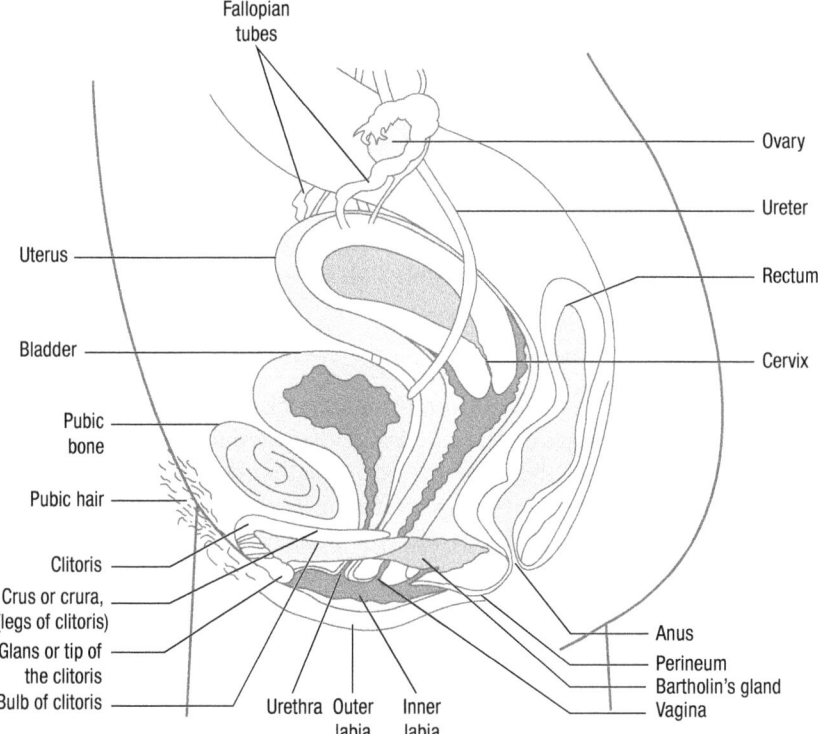

FIGURE 2.2 Vulva, anterolateral view.

The *hymen* is a very thin piece of tissue that in many bodies nearly covers the vagina until it is worn away from exercise, injury, or, infrequently, intercourse (Buehler, 2021). At different eras throughout history intact hymens have been associated with "virginity" and used to accuse individuals of being impure if a hymen appeared to be absent before marriage. On the other hand, some individuals may possess a very thick hymen that may require surgery to allow comfortable penetration.

Vagina (Generative Organ)

The vagina (the canal through which menstruation, birth, and/or semen can travel) automatically strives to maintain a certain pH-level for daily health and functioning, as well as for comfortable intercourse. Sexual stimulation (whether mental or physical) can result in lubrication of the vagina lining via pores (and can occur in 30 seconds or less). However, some vaginas may not discharge lubrication (possibly due to hormonal interference such as birth control, or even something like cold and flu medicine), despite mental or physical sexual stimulation. This presence or lack of lubrication can create difficulties for bodies with vaginas, particularly if the lubrication (or lack of) is in opposition to a desired activity.

Becoming familiar with water-based lubrication can resolve some of these situations. The vagina is not known to be very sensitive to touch or pressure and contains much fewer nerve endings than the clitoris or labia.

Aging clients may report dissatisfaction with the tightness (or looseness) of the vaginal wall. Non-surgical "vaginal rejuvenation" uses radiofrequency to increase tightness, which may help with urinary incontinence as well. Clients should obtain second opinions from sex-positive medical practitioners before proceeding with any of the aforementioned procedures, and could benefit from in depth exploration in therapy to look for possible EMDR targets.

G-Spot Area (Erectile Area)

The G-spot area, once viewed with complete skepticism, is reported to be about two inches inside the vagina on the anterior side (toward the upward front of the body), and may be part of the clitoral system. Anatomists remain divided about the shape, purpose, and area. Biology professor Toulson (2021, personal communication) believes it is analogous with the prostate. Stimulation of this area, whether via penis, fingers, or sex toy, can result in female ejaculation and/or orgasmic sensation for some bodies. This "vaginal" orgasm may actually be related to the clitoral structure. Other bodies may find this stimulation painful or related to feeling the need to urinate (Buehler, 2021). Every body is different and normal, and should not be pathologized.

Pelvic Floor

"The *pelvic floor muscles*" hold up the uterus and other organs in the abdomen, and are responsible for "*continence* (the ability to retain or evacuate urine and feces)" (Buehler, 2021).

The pelvic floor is an area that has recently begun to receive more attention in the medical establishment within the last couple of decades. The pelvic floor muscles act like a basket holding in and up the internal organs. They form a diagonal path supporting the clitoris, urethra, vagina, and anus. "For optimal sexual health, the pelvic floor muscles must be in a good tone. Muscles that are too tight, or *hypertonic*, can contribute to a variety of medical problems, including painful intercourse. Muscles that are loose, or *hypertonic*, can make it difficult for a woman to experience appropriate stimulation," potentially leading to weak or no orgasms (Buehler, 2021).

Thankfully, some physical therapists have specialized in pelvic floor physical therapy for decades and have been busy helping folks regain sexual health and functioning, as well as improve continence. Bodies that have given birth often suffer for years, involuntarily urinating while sneezing and coughing, believing that nothing can resolve their incontinence. Directing such a client to a well-informed pelvic physical therapist can not only reduce or eliminate the incontinence, but the exercises learned and practiced may also result in regaining orgasmic strength. Also, many of our sexually traumatized clients hold tremendous physical and emotional pain in their pelvis, particularly in the form of constant (usually unconsciously) tensing of these muscles. Pelvic physical therapy will help these clients retrain their muscles to a more balanced tension, ultimately allowing for fuller and enhanced sexual health. For some clients, this referral may be the best thing that can come out of psychotherapy.

Many folks have heard of learning and practicing Kegel exercises to improve continence and decrease post-childbirth vaginal wall slackness. Clients should make sure they have accurate information and instructions. I myself suffered from reduced continence, 7 years after giving birth vaginally. My own physical therapist, Stacy Troy, MS, PT, noted that most people learn and perform Kegels inaccurately, and emphasized the importance of learning and practicing Kegel exercises correctly. The proper exercise involves pulling up and squeezing the pelvic floor muscles for both short and longer periods. It does *not* involve practicing stopping urine mid-stream (although that can be helpful to *initially* identify these muscles) nor does it involve squeezing your abdomen or butt cheeks together. The Mayo Clinic website (Mayo Clinic Staff, 2021) has a very helpful and accurate guide to performing Kegel exercises (https://www.mayoclinic.org/healthy-lifestyle/womens-health/in-depth/kegel-exercises/art-20045283).

Menstruation, Menopause, and Beyond

The average age of menarche and puberty for estrogen-dominant people with ovaries in the United States is around 12.75 years of age (with children as young as age 8 having their first period). In menstruation, about once a month the body releases an egg from the ovary into the Fallopian tubes where it eventually lands in the uterus that is prepared with extra lining. Should fertilization occur by a sperm, a pregnancy may develop. If there is no fertilization, then the lining will be released as menstrual blood. Breasts are also developing during puberty, along with other secondary sex characteristics such as body hair, body odor, and widening of the hips.

Inquiring as to your clients' experiences with development, menstruation and pregnancy may also reveal potential EMDR targets as some clients may have had very little information about menstruation prior to menarche, may report embarrassing memories about their development (having their first period while wearing white shorts, being teased for having small or large breasts, etc.) or may have had difficult pregnancies or deliveries that still elicit disturbance of mind and body in their recollections.

Menopause on average occurs around the age of 51 to 53 in the United States. However, clients may enter peri-menopause as early as 35. Either way, clients undergoing menopause may experience decreased estrogen, hot flashes, night sweats, vaginal dryness or changes, and sometimes a lower sex interest. Testosterone also declines, possibly contributing to lower sexual interest and less sensation in erogenous zones such as nipples and clitoris. Forty to 60 percent of post-menopausal clients experience atrophic vaginal symptoms (Resh, 2018). Resh (2018) has also observed symptoms such as labial fusion, or even the "labia minora completely vanish."

Many clients do not report these changes and may not schedule a gynecology appointment as often as they did earlier in life, missing opportunities to bring up such changes to health professionals. Not all peri-menopausal, menopausal, or post-menopausal clients report lower sex interest. Some older clients, especially ciswomen, may finally feel free enough to explore their sexuality at this stage in life. It can be good practice to inquire with permission and curiosity about your clients' experiences with hormones, aging, and so forth, versus making assumptions or stereotypes based on generalities. Chapter 8 on aging has more information regarding aging vaginal and vulvar health.

Gross External Sexual Anatomy: Penis, Scrotum, Perineum

Testosterone-dominantly developed external genitals usually include the penis, scrotum, and perineum (see Figure 2.3).

Penis (Erectile and Generative Organ)

The penis is comprised of three main parts: the *root* (contained internally) the *shaft* (the main part that extends from the body), and the *glans penis* (the top or "head" of the penis; Buehler, 2021). Penises naturally come with a *prepuce* (foreskin) at birth, yet, as circumcision is the most common surgery worldwide, many penises no longer have foreskins.

The *urethra* (internal tube that carries urine and/or semen) opening appears at the glans penis' tip. "On the underside of the nonerect or flaccid penis, the corona (meaning "crown" in Spanish) appears as a ridge. The frenulum is a cordlike structure also on the underside of the penis that connects the corona to the shaft.

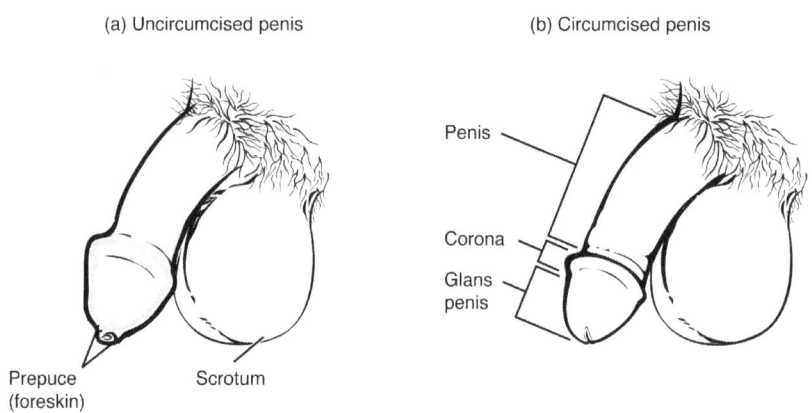

FIGURE 2.3 External sexual anatomy: penis and scrotum.

Source: Courtesy of OpenStax, Rice University, https://openstax.org/books/anatomy-and-physiology/pages/27-1-anatomy-and-physiology-of-the-male-reproductive-system.

The entire glans penis is the most sensitive part of the penis, filled with nerve endings that help with arousal and orgasm" (Buehler, 2021).

Some clients may struggle with questions about their penis size and specific memories of feeling belittled or shamed. It is important to validate that penises come in a range of sizes and circumferences, and offer EMDR help with any size-related concerns, doubt, or shame. It may also be important to provide psycho-education for heterosexual cismen about clitoral sexual anatomy, expanding their sexual repertoire to understand the importance of the clitoris in sexual pleasure. This can help reduce the pressure they may have placed on themselves about penis size and performance.

Scrotum and Perineum (Sensitive)

The "sack-like" external *scrotum* contains the *testes*, the organs that produce sperm and sex hormones. When cold, "the scrotum pulls close to the body to keep the testicles warm, and when warm, the scrotum hangs away from the body. The *perineum* is the strip of skin that is visible from behind the scrotum to the anus" (Buehler, 2021). Most scrotums and perineums enjoy stimulation. Scrotums also typically pull up close to the body just prior to ejaculation, enhancing the orgasm experience.

Medical Trauma or Injuries

Some clients report medical trauma regarding penises or scrotums, perhaps relating to injury, early surgeries, badly performed circumcisions (especially if the child receives a circumcision after the age of one year), or adult medical problems (e.g., Peyronie's disease can result in scarring of penis tissue). If the client reports these events as currently disturbing, then EMDR therapy may help to reduce the emotional/mental disturbance associated with the difficulty.

Gross Internal Sexual Anatomy: Chambers, Testicles, Seminal Vesicles, Prostate

Penis Chambers (Erectile and Generative)

The penis includes three interior chambers: two *corpus cavernosum* (very erectile) and one *corpus spongiosum* (slightly erectile). The two "*corpus cavernosum* are parallel tubes in the penis that fill with blood during an erection, causing the penis to become rigid" (Buehler, 2021). The *corpus spongiosum* (mostly generative, but also erectile) is a "structure of spongy tissue that runs the length of the front of the penis" and expands with blood during an erection. When someone becomes aroused, "nerves cause blood vessels in a healthy penis to expand. Other chemical changes occur that cause more blood to flow into the penis, than out" (Buehler, 2021). Blood is "retained in the penis until either stimulation ceases" or ejaculation occurs (Buehler, 2021).

Testes (Generative)

The scrotum contains the testicles (or testes), suspended by a spermatic cord. "The testes contain (long) seminiferous tubules. The epididymis and the vas deferens carry sperm from the testicles to the urethra, the tube that carries sperm or urine from within the body to its exit at the tip of the penis." (Buehler, 2021) See Figure 2.4.

Seminal Vesicles and Prostate (Generative and Sensitive Glands)

The seminal vesicles are located at the back of the bladder and create about 60% to 80% of the ejaculated semen (Buehler, 2021; Joannides, 2017). The prostate (meaning "guard of the bladder") produces the remaining 20% to 40% of fluid (Buehler, 2021; Joannides, 2017). Stimulating the prostate with either anal play or anal penetration can be very pleasurable for gay, straight, and/or bisexual individuals with prostates. Unfortunately the prostate can acquire diseases like cancer or prostatitis (Buehler, 2021). Some individuals may report shame related to desires of receiving anal penetration or prostate stimulation. This shame could be a potential EMDR target.

Intersex

The original Intersex Society of North America website explains the category and definition of "intersex" succinctly. "Intersex" is a general term used for a variety of conditions in which a person is born with reproductive and/or sexual anatomy that doesn't seem to fit the "typical" definitions of "female" or "male." They note

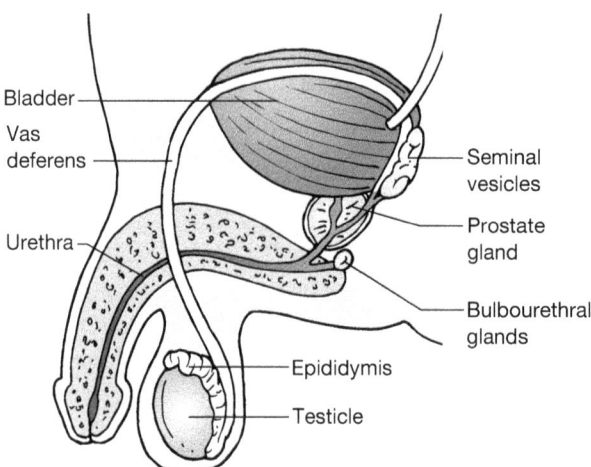

FIGURE 2.4 Gross internal sexual anatomy of penis, scrotum, prostate, and so forth.
Source: Reprinted from Tkacs, N., Herrmann, L., & Johnson, R. (2020). *Advanced physiology and pathophysiology* (1st ed.). Springer Publishing Company.

that it is humans who define what these binary norms are, and that in reality, perhaps penises, clitorises, and vulvas come in a variety of shapes and sizes.

Additionally, humans can have chromosomal combinations other than XX or XY, or can possess internal structures (e.g., ovaries) that don't seem to match external structures (e.g., penis), and are often not discovered until someone tries to conceive or receives an autopsy. Statistically, it seems that about 1.7 infants in every 100 births may be intersex in some way.

InterAct is an activist organization fighting to outlaw any surgeries that could potentially be performed on ambiguous or atypical genitals while the child is still a minor. Many states and organization now recognize that it is best to perform as little surgery as possible (only allowing for life-saving surgeries such as creating a way for urine to exit the body). However, such surgeries have not been outlawed entirely and the medical establishment may still pressure parents to give permission for unnecessary hypospadias repair (the urethra not exiting the gland penis in the expected place), vaginoplasty (removing penis, testicles, and scrotum to create vagina), clitoroplasty (creation of or reduction in size of clitoris), or gonadectomy (removing tests or ovaries). All of these procedures meant to conform organs to the gender binary can have life-long deleterious impact on physical and mental health. Recent standards of care include assigning a gender at birth that makes sense, but being open and honest with the child about what is known about their sexual and reproductive organs, supporting the child in their gender journey, and leaving any surgical options up to them for when they are of consenting age.

I mention intersex concerns as there may be the occasional client that has an experience with this possibility, whether due to childhood surgery, or due to a recent discovery via an infertility clinic of different internal organs than had been assumed. These may be invaluable EMDR targets as you help affirm and validate their experiences.

Sex Hormones: Estrogen, Progesterone, and Testosterone

All healthy bodies produce various levels of estrogen, progesterone, and testosterone at different ages and based on chromosomal and gonadal makeup. Relatively large amounts of testosterone are produced in adult testicles. "Normal" levels of testicle-produced testosterone contribute to good muscle mass, overall energy, and healthy erections. Once a testosterone-dominant individual with a penis and testes turns 35, levels slowly decline over the years and estrogen increases. Some individuals may experience "abnormally low levels of testosterone, which can result in low drive, loss of muscle mass, weight gain, fatigue, and difficulty attaining and maintaining an erection" (Buehler, 2021). As these symptoms can overlap with depression, it is recommended to refer these clients for a physical with testosterone and hormone testing.

Estrogen-dominant clients with vaginas and ovaries may seek therapy complaining of lower energy and interest in sex. They may benefit from a physical as well, although many other factors can also be responsible. Some clients with estrogen-producing ovaries experience a decline in estrogen and testosterone as they age, resulting in vaginal dryness and thinning of the vaginal and vulvar tissue, potentially leading to painful intercourse (Buehler, 2021). Thankfully, there are many potential solutions such as topical estrogen, vitamin E cream, dehydroepiandrosterone (DHEA) cream, barium rings, and water-based lubricants (Resh, 2018). Chapter 8, "Aging Sexual Health and EMDR," has more information.

ESSENTIAL SAFER SEX INFORMATION: SEXUALLY TRANSMITTED INFECTIONS AND PREGNANCY PREVENTION

Sexually Transmitted Infections

For the most updated information, refer to websites such as Planned Parenthood or your local sexually transmitted infection (STI) clinics. However, since some of our clients may mention concerns about STIs or unwanted pregnancy, it is helpful to have a basic understanding of common STIs and protection.

Possible STIs include chlamydia, genital warts, herpes, gonorrhea, human papillomavirus (HPV), pubic lice, scabies, syphilis, trichomoniasis, hepatitis B, and HIV/AIDS. Most of these are very treatable if caught early, so it is recommended that sexually active individuals get tested regularly, regardless if they always use barriers and feel symptom free. Even some skin-to-skin contact that does not include any penetration can spread an STI such as HPV, herpes, pubic lice, or scabies. Using condoms or dental dams can reduce the likelihood of spreading an STI as well as prevent pregnancy, if penile–vaginal penetration is involved. For anal sex, it is important to use water-based lubrication with a condom, increasing the protection a condom provides. To prevent the spread of HIV, using condoms or dental dams is a must. However, if your client is HIV positive, there are now treatments (antiretroviral or ART) that effectively allow an individual to live a long, healthy life, as well as greatly reduce the risk of giving HIV to anyone else. Individuals at risk of HIV exposure can also take PrEP (pre-eprophylaxis), which effectively prevents acquiring HIV.

Unfortunately, despite that fact that millions of people contract an STI sometime in their lives, a great deal of shame continues to accompany these diagnoses. Anywhere you find shame, you find potential EMDR targets, whether it is the moment of diagnosis, when your client told their partner(s) about the STI, or their impending fear about mentioning the STI to a new partner.

Pregnancy Prevention and Abortion Access

Again, consult Planned Parenthood or local family planning clinics for the most updated information. Currently there are many methods available to prevent sperm and eggs from meeting. These methods range from barriers such as condoms and internal condoms to hormonal disruption of the sperm or egg's journey (e.g., emergency contraception such as Plan B, monthly or quarterly birth control pills or injections, some IUDs, implants, birth control patches, vaginal rings) or other methods like diaphragms, birth control sponges, cervical caps, and spermicide. They all have varying degrees of success. Only abstinence from penis–vagina intercourse has a 100% success rate of preventing pregnancy. If a client is most focused on preventing pregnancy, then helping them broaden their view of sex to include outercourse (kissing, massage, dry humping/grinding), oral sex, manual sex, and mutual masturbation (and other kinds of sex play that does not involve sperm potentially meeting eggs) may reduce pregnancy anxiety and enhance overall sexual pleasure.

Abortion involves the termination of the fetus and can happen via a medical abortion (taking the abortion pill within 11 weeks of the pregnancy) or a surgical outpatient abortion, which uses suction and/or medical tools to remove the pregnancy from the uterus, up to 16 weeks after the pregnancy.

Some clients may have experiences related to pregnancy scares, abortions, or partners not using condoms when they were asked to use them. It may be important to inquire about these potential experiences as you look for EMDR targets. Client reports of shame or embarrassment may help to identify these and related EMDR targets.

BRIEF HISTORY OF SEXUAL RESEARCH

In 1940s and 1950s brave early sex researcher Alfred Kinsey demonstrated that most sexual problems were related to ignorance about functioning and variations or deviations from what is considered "the norm" (1948, 1953). Later, Masters and Johnson (1966) specifically set out to understand sexual pleasure, concluding that healthy sexual functioning involves this sequence: *excitement* (i.e., flushing of skin, erections of clitoris and penis, faster breathing), *plateau*, *orgasm*, followed by *resolution* (post-sexual restful state).

Helen Singer Kaplan expanded Masters and Johnson's research, recognizing the cismale focus of their model, into a triphasic model of *desire*, *arousal* (excitement and plateau), and *orgasm*. Desire finally became a critical component, with the understanding that our brains account for a great deal of our sexual response abilities (Kaplan, 1977).

In 2000 Rosemary Basson developed a nonlinear model of emotional intimacy, sexual stimuli, and relationship satisfaction (Basson, 2000). This model includes elements like *spontaneous* desire (e.g., laying in a hammock on a warm sunny day that happens to light up erogenous zones), *sexual motivation* linked to emotional and physical satisfaction, and *responsive* desire. Responsive desire is when partner A may not necessarily be thinking about sexual interaction, but partner B applies all of partner A's favorite courtship rituals and touches, resulting in partner A now developing interest and/or arousal to engage in sexual activity with partner B in that situation. To be clear, responsive desire is NOT about "giving in" (especially in this essential, long overdue #metoo zeitgeist of "enthusiastic and freely given consent"), but rather about being receptive to sexual activity in the context of what one considers to be erotic. "Responsive desire emerges in *response* to pleasure. Spontaneous desire emerges in *anticipation* of pleasure. Both *are* normal" (Nagoski, n.d.).

THE WILLINGNESS MODEL (CONTRIBUTED BY DR. WENDY STOCK)

The Willingness Model, created by Joanne Loulan, a lesbian sex therapist, provides a useful way to help couples with decreased frequency of sex or low desire. Loulan (1984), based on her observations of lesbian couples' sexuality, developed a new model of sexual response that contained a new component—willingness. This model reflects the fact that for many ciswomen, desire does not always occur spontaneously. However, if individuals decide that they are willing and interested in engaging in sexual activity—despite lacking desire—they may find that desire occurs as they become physically aroused and experience pleasure.

True willingness requires consent; it is not an excuse for sexual coercion. The guidance to couples utilizing this technique is for the low desire partner to be willing to engage in physical affection and sexual touching to explore whether their desire can be "kindled." If the flames of arousal catch on, then the couple can proceed to have a sexual encounter, however this is defined. If no "kindling" occurs, the partners do not need to proceed. The higher desire partner must be willing to accept frustration if this happens.

The Willingness Model is helpful for people who know they enjoy having sex with a partner, but are too tired, depressed or stressed to want to initiate sex—they "want to want" sex.

It gives permission to say to one's partner, "I'm not really in the mood, but I might be if we start to fool around," and then see what happens.

PRESENT-DAY "DUAL CONTROL MODEL" OF DESIRE AND AROUSAL

In the late 1990s Erick Janssen and John Bancroft of the Kinsey Institute (Bancroft & Janssen, 2000; Bancroft et al., 2009) developed the Dual Control Model of sexual response. This model consists of two parts: sexual excitation system (SES) and sexual inhibition system (SIS). Emily Nagoski, a sexpert Smith College professor and researcher, has an entire chapter devoted to this in her sexual bible for people with clitorises and vaginas (and the people who love them): *Come as You Are* (2015).

Essentially, Nagoski states that "your central nervous system (brain and spinal cord) is made up of a partnership of accelerator and brakes—like the pairing of your sympathetic nervous system ('accelerator') and your parasympathetic nervous system ('brake')." Therefore, the "brain system that coordinates sex (has) a sexual accelerator and sexual brake," called the sexual excitation system (SES) and sexual inhibition system (SIS).

The SIS has two brakes: an emergency brake that notices all the immediate dangers and turn-offs in the environment such as a child screaming in the next room or a grouchy text from one's supervisor. There is also a second brake that emits more of a "chronic, low-level 'no thank you' signal' possibly associated with a 'fear of performance failure' like worrying about having an orgasm." Humans don't necessarily need to know the specifics of a brake, just that we all have these two brakes, and we all have sexual accelerators. Some humans may have a sensitive SES and/or a sensitive SIS, independent of their environment. Because of how much this model makes sense, I talk almost exclusively with my clients about their sexual accelerator and brakes.

Talking to your clients about the Dual Control Model, as well as the inclusion of elements such as emotional intimacy and sexual responsiveness, can help them figure out how to turn off their sexual brakes and turn on their sexual accelerator. We currently live in a very hectic world that can include juggling parenting and chauffeuring busy children along with work demands, household chores, hobbies, exercise routines, errands, managing finances, and so on.

Sometimes the best therapeutic intervention is giving a client permission to define better boundaries, stake out some private time, or ask for something to change in the environment or their partner's behavior that is impacting their brakes. EMDR therapy relating to the Dual Control Model might include EMDR targets and/or Future Templates of saying no to that 100th task/favor, increasing comfort with resigning from a draining committee or job, asking for household help from a partner or child, and/or setting and important boundary with a relative.

Many clients seeking therapy often mention both a concurrence of a sexual trauma history and a current lack of sexual desire for any sexual activity (whether alone or partnered). In this case we can hypothesize that their sexual brakes are fully engaged and need to be released by using EMDR therapy to treat their sexual trauma. Once their trauma history has been fully processed, their interest in sex may return on its own (the brakes are no longer engaged).

Sometimes clients may still report lower interest in sex, yet no longer feel negatively triggered. In this case they will need to work on identifying and releasing any other limiting brakes (e.g., lack of privacy, overwork), and then identify and engage with their sexual accelerators. This may be a long process for some trauma survivors who rarely have had the chance to freely engage with sexual context solely for themselves. Emily Nagoski now has a companion workbook called *The Come as You Are Workbook: A Practical Guide to the Science of Sex* (2019) that can help folks investigate and expand their sexual accelerator contexts.

Arousal Nonconcordance

All genders during sexual stimulation or fantasy may report or notice increased skin sweat, flushing of the skin, faster breathing, erect nipples, and pupil dilation, along with the genital-specific arousal of clitoral or penile erection, vaginal lubrication, and so on. Unfortunately, many of these responses can occur during unwanted sexual contact, causing a great deal of confusion and distress for sexual trauma survivors who lack this information. Some survivors (regardless of gender identity or anatomical configuration) have reported orgasm during a sexual assault, creating intense confusion and shame.

A very important concept to explain to your clients (especially to clients who have reported erect penises, lubricated vaginas, and/or orgasms against their will) is *arousal concordance* and *nonconcordance*. Arousal concordance is when a person feels aroused physically and reports a strong penile or clitoral erection or noticeable vaginal lubrication *and* also mentally desires to engage in the sexual activity. Arousal nonconcordance is when these two elements do not correspond (i.e., there is "sexually relevant" stimulation, but no sexual response or interest). Cismen have about a 50% overlap of sexually relevant material and confirmed sexual interest, whereas ciswomen have only about a 10% overlap. In other words, in studies showing pornography to adults, cismen's erections correlated 50% of the time with their subjective reports of sexual arousal (Nagoski, 2015).

Sexually relevant stimuli such as an erotic image, nipple stimulation, or kissing does not automatically equal sexually appealing stimuli, and vice versa. What is confusing is that if someone's body seems to be responding to sexual stimulation (because the body interprets the information as sexually relevant), they sometimes believe (or are told) that they want that stimulation. Assailants often tell targets things like, "your nipples are hard" or "you are wet, therefore you want this." Conversely, established consensual partners can notice a lack of lubrication or other arousal signs and therefore question whether the partner really is "turned on." You may have clients who report either of these as traumatic events, deservedly placing them on their EMDR timeline for processing.

A Note on Lubrication

Vaginas differ greatly, and every moment for every vagina is different, depending on the time of day, month, age of person, hormones present or not, where they are in the menstrual cycle, whether peri- or menopausal, daily stress toll, use of alcohol or cigarettes, and generally how hydrated they are that day (the more hydrated the better). Remember, there is no patented direct correlation between lubrication, arousal, and interest in sexual activity at any given moment. Some people may report copious lubrication at all sorts of times, yet not be interested in sexual activity in those particular moments (or any moments). Others may be as aroused as they have ever experienced themselves, yet not secrete any lubrication at all. There may be abundant lubrication that occurs during unwanted sexual activity—possibly the vagina's way of ensuring minimal injury and tears.

There has also been a slight perceived prejudice of "naturally" well-lubricated vaginas over vaginas that benefit from added lubrication. Even a person who every day of their adult life notes regular secretions and fluids may have an off day for any of the preceding reasons.

The simplest solution to any lubrication concern is to keep quality water-based lubrication on hand. Additionally, it is useful to know a little bit about lubrication as clients may report difficulty finding one that does not irritate, therefore experiencing uncomfortable intercourse. It can be helpful to provide some basic consumer education.

There are many different lubrications available, from organic to paraben-free to plant oil-based to water-based to items one can find around the kitchen. Sex educators generally favor water-based lubrications over oil-based as these are least likely to cause allergic reactions, infections, or to dehydrate. Also, they are safe to use with latex condoms and sex toys, keeping the latex and toy material intact.

The badvibes.org website has a wonderfully educational and informative section on lubrication. Osmolality refers to how concentrated are the dissolved particles per unit of water in a solution or serum. Osmolality is important because the "body's natural mucus is constantly trying to maintain homeostasis" (badvibes.org). Osmolality is measured in milliosmoles per kilogram of solvent (mOsm/kg). Ideally vaginas prefer an iso-osmotic lubricant around 285 to 295 mOsm/kg - equal osmotic pressure as the body's hydration level. Badvibes.org notes that Good Clean Love and Sliquid Organics both fall within that "genital-friendly" ideal range.

pH levels are also helpful to consider when selecting lubrication, especially for the vagina. Vaginal pH ranges from 3.8 to 4.6 (and higher if post-menopausal). Individuals should look for lubrications in their general range so as not to disturb the environment more than necessary. Good Clean Love and Astroglide fall right in that sweet spot (although Astroglide has very high osmolality, somewhat canceling out the pH benefit). Slippery Stuff Liquid and Sliquid Organics at 6.8 might be more ideal for the post-menopausal vagina.

Humectants are another ingredient often added to lubricants as preservatives and to increase viscosity. Natural and or organic humectant alternatives that many may find non-irritating can include honey, shea butter, and jojoba oil. Many manufactured lubricants may contain petrochemicals such as "propylene glycol, benzene, benzoic acid" (badvibes.org). These can "dehydrate mucus and cause skin irritation, leaving mucous membrane more vulnerable to bacterial vaginosis or STIs" (badvibes.org). Most medical practitioners recommend avoiding lubrications that contain parabens, petroleum, glycerin, and sugars.

Some manufactured lubricants may contain microbicides to kill or reduce the infectivity of viruses or bacteria added as spermicides. While obviously helpful to kill unwanted sperm, frequent use may also irritate that incredibly self-regulating vaginal environment. (Remember, sperm themselves are chemically not welcome by the vagina, which is why seminal fluid contains a solution of immunosuppressants to neutralize the vagina's environment and help sneak the sperm through.)

Some clients may prefer using naturally occurring products from their cupboards. Sweet almond oil (also helpful for oral and anal sex), virgin coconut oil (con: it can stain sheets), olive oil (con: it can clog pores, so wash off when done), and avocado oil (not as long-lasting as the aforementioned) can be used. Remember that any oil-based lubes should NOT be used if one is using a condom to prevent STIs and/or pregnancy.

Aloe vera is a water-based substance that can be used with condoms and may feel very soothing as well. Less known household lubes include Ghee butter (great for moisturizing, but bad for condoms and must be washed off right away to avoid going rancid) and Nagaimo (a type of slippery yam that is very popular in China, Japan, and Vietnam). Lastly, room-temperature egg whites can be applied with a liquid dropper.

Clients should avoid these household items at all costs: baby oil, petroleum jelly, and any kind of vegetable, canola, or other similarly refined oil. These may have unpleasant chemicals, may increase risk of infections, stain sheets, and degrade condoms or sex toys.

As for anal penetration, lubrication must be used. The anus does not produce any natural lubrication, so to avoid tears, pain, infections, and so on, one must employ a lubrication. Smittenkittenonline.com has a great collection of lubricants recommended for anal play, most made by Sliquid (including an organic option). They also sell "Backdoor balm -anal aftercare" southern butter that contains healing nutrients such as calendula, plantain, chickweed, yarrow, and vitamin E.

SEXUAL PERSONALITY STYLES*

The concept of *sexual styles* was originally observed and posited by Donald Mosher, PhD (1980). Mosher proposed that orgasm quality is mediated by "effective sexual stimulation" that is experienced as "pleasurable sexual sensations" and feeling excited and joyful. Therefore, Mosher suggests that effective sexual engagement results from both pleasurable physical stimulation as well as "involvement" and interest in the activity. Mosher describes three categories of psychological involvement: *sexual trancer, partner engager,* and/or *role enactor* and suggests that most of us gravitate toward one dominant style for ourselves.

Sexual trancers are a bit like the introverts of the Myers-Briggs personality test. They tend to like privacy and freedom from distractions. They enjoy a calm, relaxed, and serene mood. They like slow pacing and repetitive movements, and can be passive, sensual, and inwardly oriented. They prefer less frequent talking during sex so that they might be absorbed more easily into sensations. Their own fantasies may revolve around visual or sensory images.

---

*See the questionnaire at the end of the chapter.

Partner engagers enjoy being psychologically engaged with their partner, preferably involved in what they consider a "good" relationship. They relish a romantic and loving mood, lots of kissing, eye contact, and full body contact. Affectionate sharing, mutual pleasuring, romantic endearments, and love songs can be important parts of their repertoire. They expect their partners to act lovingly toward them, enjoying a flowing, harmonious union with their partner. Their fantasies may include the face of their partner, memories of union with their partner, and other romantic images.

Role enactors are more like the extroverts of the Myers-Briggs and enjoy more interactive sex play. They may show a tendency toward dramatic, possibly even slightly exhibitionist elements, bringing a very playful mood, pride in variety and skill of sexual techniques, and lots of active movement, sound, and facial expressions. Lusty sex talk, dramatic orgasms, novel situations, role-plays, and interest in ecstasy also show up in this style.

Dr. Kathy McMahon later developed a wonderful short Sexual Style Survey (2010) that you can provide to your clients to answer if they are interested in better understanding how they and their partners prefer and experience sexual activity. This survey is at the end of this chapter.

Many folks, just like in the Myers-Briggs personality classifications, can demonstrate flexibility in their sexual personality style. Your client might mostly be a sexual trancer, but if they have a role enactor partner, that person brings out more playfulness and variety. Or perhaps a client's main style is partner engager, with a side of sexual trancer. This client needs to feel connected and mutual with their partner, allowing for the trance state for orgasm.

There is no right or wrong sexual style, just like being a Myers-Briggs' introvert is as valid as being an extrovert. Where trouble can brew is when a sexual trancer client is matched up to a role enactor partner. Those are pretty different styles, which means they might have to work fairly hard to make sure everyone's needs are met. This could look like the role enactor creating an elaborate role-play scenario, bringing in sex toys, props, blindfolds, and so on. The sexual trancer may be requested to engage in this active style for some time to fulfill the emotional and sexual needs of the role enactor. Once fulfilled, the role enactor can more readily and easily provide a distraction-free, sensual focused zone for the sexual trancer's sensation absorption.

Also, just like in life, sexual opposites often attract. So instead of clients thinking, "there is such a big river to cross," we can help them think about how fun it can be to build that sexual bridge with their sexual teammate. This is a great exercise in creative thinking and coming up with ways for differently sexually styled folks to feel satiated, together.

Lastly, long-term partners can notice a waning sex life over time and might jump to a few dozen conclusions about this, whereas it could be as simple as different sexual styles. In romantic beginnings, people easily cross all the bridges of differences, showing high flexibility in moving back and forth between sexual styles. However, as time goes on, and life gets in the way, folks tend to stratify back to their main style. A couple complaining of reduced sex life, or very different interests in sex frequency, might actually be grappling with very different styles. The role enactor is not getting their curiosity piqued, and so has given up on sex. The partner engager has not felt emotionally connected to their partner in some time, so turns to Netflix instead. Helping your clients learn about their own preferred sexual style and asking for their needs to be met can help correct the ship's course.

Some of these incongruous style issues may be addressed through EMDR targeting or specific EMDR Future Templates. For example, an EMDR Future Template can help a client practice speaking up about asking for specific sexual needs, according to their dominant sexual style. If your role enactor client is paired up with a sexual trancer, then a possible EMDR Future Template might go like this:

Clinician: "Imagine yourself effectively asking for your partner to engage in role play or use of props (or talking, etc.) during sex." (Client notes body sensation and BLS is applied until negative sensation becomes neutral, or positive sensation is enhanced.)

Clinician: "Let's pair a positive thought with this event. How about, 'I am worthy and capable of asking for what I need.'" Continue the EMDR Future Template from there.

EROTIC TEMPLATE FORMATION IN RELATION TO EMDR TARGETS

Jack Morin's innovative book *The Erotic Mind* (1995) introduced the concept of *core erotic themes* (CETs). He posits that these CETs develop during infancy and childhood from sexual or sensual triggers or events and lay the groundwork for our future sexual experiences. Specifically, these CETs form the bases of the specific types of feelings (not necessarily scenarios) we require for sexual engagement. Examples of feelings that one's CET might contain include a desire to be ravished, dominating, submissive, taboo, spiritually merged, and so on.

Patrick Carnes (2001) discusses the "sexual arousal template" which can include "thoughts, images, behaviors, sounds, smells, sights, fantasies, and objects" that sexually arouse an individual. While his take on "sex addiction" has been taken to task in recent years by more affirming and sex-positive therapists, there is some reality to the overexposure to internet pornography and how this easy access to what were once fringe and/or illegal images might be shaping clients' erotic templates into something they are ashamed or dismayed by, resulting in behaviors that feel "compulsive" or "out of control" to them. Additionally, it is worth noting that many individuals first stumble upon internet porn around the age of 9 or 10, endangering them toward developing unrealistic or negative associations with sexuality.

One such case example is "Travis," a senior cismale college student who sought EMDR therapy due to lingering feelings of disgust around seeing sexual images. As we developed our EMDR target list, several targets of early exposure (around age 8) and viewing of internet pornography were discovered. Working through these targets allowed him to have mental and emotional room to sort out for himself his own sexual likes and dislikes, without the accompanying disgust. He went on to have enjoyable sexual experiences with a new partner.

Another case example involved a young cisfemale child "Mackenzie" around the age of 12. She had been exposed to pornographic images unwillingly at an earlier age (around age 6). Her presenting complaint was seeing unwanted flashes of the imagery in her mind and feeling anxious in general. After completing EMDR on the identified targets and difficulty life circumstances relating to the early exposure (i.e., parents divorcing), she reported no longer experiencing the interfering thoughts and felt more "peaceful" and at ease.

Compassionately helping your adult clients explore their erotic templates (images, feelings, and themes) by using an open-minded, nonjudgmental, and curious stance can help them gain insight into the origins. If these CETs are truly distressing to the client or are illegal (such as looking at under-age or violent pornography), EMDR targeting of the specific themes and images can help to eliminate the shame, disturbance, and possibly the "positive charge," of those images. In Chapter 4, *Applying EMDR Therapy to Sexual Health Targets*, Robert Miller shares a brief outline of his Feeling State Addiction Protocol along with some case examples. If necessary we can help our clients find more positive, judgment-free ways to experience some of those formerly distressing erotic feelings (whether dominance, submission, rebellion, connection etc.).

SUMMARY

Human sexual and reproductive anatomy is not as simple and binary as was once thought. Chromosomes, hormones, and cell receptors all influence which groups of organs tend to develop together. An estrogen-dominant androgen system, along with XX chromosomes, tends to result in the development of clitoris, labia, vagina, ovaries, Fallopian tubes, cervix, uterus, and so forth. A testosterone-dominant androgen system, along with XY chromosomes, tends to result in the development of penis, scrotum, testes, prostate, and so on. About 1% to 2% of the population has combinations of chromosomes, hormones, and gonads falling into the "intersex" category. Most healthy bodies have various levels of estrogen, progesterone, and testosterone, as well as a perineum, urethra, anus, and nipples. Some individuals may report discomfort with body parts; this discomfort can alert us to potential EMDR targets.

Unprotected sexual activity can result in STIs. Pregnancy prevention and the option for abortion remain concerns for many sexually active individuals. Experiences with STIs and unwanted pregnancies can lead to shame; this shame can unearth possible EMDR targets.

Since the 1940s there have been many scientists, biologists, sociologists, and psychologists researching human sexuality (e.g., Kinsey, Kaplan, Basson). Jannsen and Bancroft are recent researchers, formulating the Dual Control Model of desire and arousal. The brain system coordinates the SES and the SIS. Interest and desire for sexual activity correlates with one's "sexual accelerator" being engaged. Active "sexual brakes" correlate with a disinterest and/or rejection of sexual activity. Many things can press on someone's sexual brakes, including a history of trauma or arguments with partners (all possible EMDR targets).

Spontaneous desire occurs when someone notices an interest in sexual activity arising, unrelated to anything sexual in the mind or environment. Responsive desire can occur when one person, with full consent, engages their partner with sexually relevant or erotic stimulation, resulting in that partner becoming interested in sexual activity.

Arousal nonconcordance is when someone reports incongruous sexual arousal and interest. For instance, a trauma survivor may ashamedly report having had an erection and/or orgasm during unwanted sexual activity, and affirm they did not want the activity at all. Bodies often respond to sexually relevant stimuli regardless of actual interest or desire; therefore, sexual trauma victims should never be blamed or made to feel that "they wanted it." Lubrication also varies greatly according to many factors—no one should be judged about their amount of lubrication. Manufactured or natural lubricants can bridge the gap between sexual interest and comfort. Any of these reported situations (unwanted arousal, lubrication shame) might benefit from EMDR therapy.

Most folks can benefit from identifying a preferred sexual personality style (Sexual Trancer, Partner Engager, and/or Role Enactor) for themselves. Differences in partner style may be behind some sexual incompatibilities.

Erotic and/or Sexual Arousal Templates form from birth to present. Helping our clients explore and understand these templates can lead to possible EMDR targets if shame or discomfort is reported.

REFERENCES

American College of Obstetricians and Gynecologists. (2007, April). http://www.acog.org/about_acog/news_room/news_releases/2007/acog_advises_against_cosmetic_vaginal_procedures

Bancroft, J., Graham, C. A., Janssen, E., & Sanders, S. A. (2009). The dual control model: Current status and future directions. *Journal of Sex Research, 46*(2–3), 121–142. https://doi.org/10.1080/00224490902747222

Bancroft, J., & Janssen, E. (2000). The dual control model of male sexual response: A theoretical approach to centrally mediated erectile dysfunction. *Neuroscience and Biobehavioral Reviews, 24*(5), 571–579. https://doi.org/10.1016/s0149-7634(00)00024-5

Basson, R. (2000). The female sexual response: A different model. *Journal of Sex & Marital Therapy, 26*(1), 51–65. https://doi.org/10.1080/009262300278641

Boston Women's Health Book Collective. (2001). *Our bodies, ourselves*. Simon and Schuster.
Buehler, S. (2021). *What every mental health professional needs to know about sex, third edition*. Springer Publishing Company.
Carnes, P. (2001). *Out of the shadows: Understanding sexual addiction* (3rd ed.). Hazelden
Dodson, B. (1996). *Sex for one: The joy of self-loving*. Three River Press.
El-Hamamsy, D., Parmar, C., Shoop-Worrall, S., & Reid, F. M. (2021). Public understanding of female genital anatomy and pelvic organ prolapse (POP); A questionnaire-based pilot study. *International Urogynecology Journal*. Advance online publication. https://doi.org/10.1007/s00192-021-04727-9
Geddes, L. (2021, May). Most Britons cannot name all parts of the vulva, survey reveals. *The Guardian*. https://www.theguardian.com/lifeandstyle/2021/may/30/most-britons-cannot-name-parts-vulva-survey
Joannides, P. (2017). *Guide to getting it on, unzipped V.9.0*. Goofy Foot Press.
Kaplan, H. S. (1977). Hypoactive sexual desire. *Journal of Sex & Marital Therapy, 3*(1), 3–9. https://doi.org/10.1080/00926237708405343
Kinsey, A. C., Pomeroy, W. B., & Martin, C. E. (1948). *Sexual behavior in the human male*. Indiana University Press.
Kinsey, A. C., Pomeroy, W. B., Martin, C. E., & Gebhard, P. H. (1953). *Sexual behavior in the human female*. Indiana University Press.
Loulan, J. (1984). *Lesbian sex*. Spinster's Ink.
Masters, W. H., & Johnson, V. E. (1966). *Human sexual response*. Little, Brown.
Mayo Clinic Staff. (2021). *Kegel exercises: A how to guide for women*. Mayo Clinic. https://www.mayoclinic.org/healthy-lifestyle/womens-health/in-depth/kegel-exercises/art-20045283
McMahon, K. (2010) Sexual styles survey. Personal communication.
Morin, J. (1995). *The erotic mind: Unlocking the inner sources of sexual passion and fulfillment*. Harper Perennial.
Mosher, D. (1980). Three dimensions of depth of involvement in human sexual response. *Journal of Sex Research, 16*(1), 1–42. https://doi.org/10.1080/00224498009551060
Nagoski, E. (2015). *Come as you are*. Simon & Schuster.
Nagoski, E. (2019). *The come as you are workbook: A practical guide to the science of sex*. Simon & Schuster.
Nagoski, E. (n.d.). *Ten tips for making the most of responsive desire*. Nagoski Booklet.
Orenstein, P. (2016). *Girls and sex: Navigating the complicated new landscape*. Harper Collins Publisher.
Pauls, R. N. (2015). Anatomy of the clitoris and female sexual response. *Clinical anatomy (New York, N.Y.), 28*(3), 376–384. https://doi.org/10.1002/ca.22524
Resh, E. (2018). *Hormones, health, and love* [Presentation]. Brattleboro Retreat, Brattleboro, Vermont.
Tkacs, N., Herrmann, L., & Johnson, R. (2020). *Advanced physiology and pathophysiology* (1st ed.). Springer Publishing Company.
Toulson, A., & Landon, A. (2021a, May). *Gender, sex, and sexuality inclusion in anatomy & physiology education* [Conference Workshop]. Human Anatomy and Physiological Society.
Toulson, A., & Landon, A. (2021b, May). *Bio 218: Reproductive anatomy: Most important points* [Class handout]. Department of Biology, Holyoke Community College.

SUPPLEMENTAL MATERIALS FOR CLIENTS

SEXUAL STYLES SURVEY

Couples Therapy Inc., 125 Guest Street, Boston, Massachusetts

Following are characteristics that happen in sex. These can be thought of as preferred pathway of involvement. I want you to imagine your ideal sexual situation with your ideal sexual partner. Alternatively, imagine the kind of sex you'd like to have when you want sex to be "normal" or maximally satisfying for you. While many answers might fit, rank order them as (3) "most important," (2) "less important" or (1) "not important.

There are no right or wrong answers.

1. Setting: In the ideal setting, I'd like:
   ___ Privacy: Freedom from distraction. Temperature, lighting, and freedom from distraction may all be important.
   ___ Psychological: A good relationship.
   ___ Freedom: Playful, inventive, fantasy, drama.
2. Mood: Ideally, I'd like to feel:
   ___ Calm: Relaxed and serene. Relaxing and getting in the mood can be a necessary preliminary to concentrate on sexual stimulation.
   ___ Romantic: Loving toward my partner.
   ___ Good about myself: High self-esteem, playful.
3. Sexual technique: What we do ideally should be:
   ___ Slow: Familiar, slow-paced, nothing sudden or unexpected. Gentle, rhythmic sensation without abrupt alterations in tempo or pressure leads to a familiar sense of enjoyed pleasure.
   ___ Tender: A lot of kissing, eye contact, and full body contact.
   ___ Innovative: Full of variety, skillful in love making in all areas of sexuality and the ability to be sexually responsive.
4. Sexual style: I'd like sex that is:
   ___ Sensation-focused: Good sex is all about connecting with the sensations, being receptive to one's partner, and being in touch with your inner self. Passive, receptive concentration and surrender, rather than the active pursuit of the novel thrill or novel self-expression, are preferred.
   ___ Mutual: Good sex is all about affectionate sharing, cuddling, and mutual pleasuring.

___ Active: Expressive in action, sound, and facial expression. I don't have to guess that they are enjoying themselves. Novelty adds spice.
5. Role expectations: In the ideal, my partner is:
___ In tune: They are sensitive to where I'm at, and aren't jarring in the way they interact with me.
___ Affectionate: They demonstrate their love for me in word and deed.
___ Complementary: Good sex happens with partners who are complementary and work well together to turn up the heat.
6. Sex talk:
___ "Shhh": Unless I'm hurting them or need to provide important feedback, I'd prefer to let our bodies do the talking. Mention pleasurable sensations or feelings…that's okay.
___ Romantic endearments: I want to know how they feel about me. Intimate conversation may be a good seduction or may accompany the sex.
___ Arouse me: I like lusty or directive language, some might call it "dirty talk."
7. Fantasies:
___ Scriptless: My fantasies are often visual, sensory, or synesthetic. They don't have to have a plot, I can imagine a kiss, a touch, or an image and that's enough.
___ Romantic: I imagine my lover's face from precious moments, tender things we've done together, or the romance of our sex in my fantasies.
___ Novel: I like to imagine more innovative or daring fantasies, even if I wouldn't want to act them out in real life. "Let's pretend," is fun. Hey, it's just a fantasy, right?
8. Conception of sex:
___ An altered state: Great sex lets me escape the cares of my everyday life with the one I love. Or feeling ecstatically transported, floating on a sea of sensations.
___ Loving merger: Great sex for me reminds me of the love bond I feel. It is being deeply connected to my partner.
___ Ecstasy: Great sex is an adventure involving ecstatic expression and is "nonvolitional." It is so passionate that I'm swept away by it. Novel scripts or new props keeps things interesting.
9. Orgasm:
___ Absorbing: The best orgasms are intense sensations with a fading of my consciousness.
___ Flow: The best orgasms are like two people merging into one…we lose our individuality and become one in union with each other.
___ Intense: The best orgasms are dramatic, expressive, and nonvolitional. They sweep me away without any effort on my part.

Use the following scale (1–5; 1 = *Not true for me* and 5 = *True for me*) to indicate "how true" the following statements are. Write your answer before each statement.

10. ___The most important aspect of my mood when I get into sex is that I be relaxed and receptive.
11. ___ I believe that I would feel very excited having secret sex in a semi-public place.
12. ___Ideally all sexual techniques begin and build from kissing the partner's face and lips.
13. ___ I like to have sex at a time when I am sure that there will be no distractions to interrupt or interfere with my enjoyment.
14. ___When I'm feeling really good about myself, then I love to make love.
15. ___The setting in which I have sex is less important than the present feelings existing between me and my partner.
16. ___ I like my partner to stay with a sexual activity that is feeling good rather than skipping around from here to there.
17. ___ I use my imagination to increase my absorption into the sensory experience of sex.
18. ___When my heart is bursting with love, I know our sex will be bursting with pleasure.
19. ___ I pride myself in being quite accomplished in the techniques of oral sex.
20. ___To increase my excitement, I often imagine during sex that I am with another partner or in a more exotic setting.
21. ___Sometimes I imagine that my partner is pledging their love to me for life in the act of sexual intercourse.

Scoring

For questions 1 through 9, if the respondent most frequently ranks the first option (i.e. privacy, calm, etc.) as most important, then they likely fall under the "sexual trancer" category. If they most frequently rank the second option (i.e. psychological, romantic, tender, etc.) as most important, then they likely fall under the "partner engager" style. If they most frequently rank the third option (i.e. freedom, innovative, active, etc.) as most important, then they likely fall under the "role enactor" style.

For questions 10–21, the following "highly true" categories apply to sexual trancer, partner engager, role enactor.
Sexual trancer: 10, 13, 16, 17
Partner engager: 12, 15, 18, 21
Role enactor: 11, 14, 19, 20

Dual Control System

I have included here some helpful articles I wrote for my monthly newspaper column, *Sex Matters*, that can be photocopied and handed out to clients to further explain some of the concepts, particularly the *Dual Control System* and *Sexual Styles Survey*.

The Dual Control System of Desire and Response
By Stephanie Baird, LMHC

(Originally published August 2019 in the *Montague Reporter* newspaper monthly *Sex Matters* column.)

Over these last few weeks many of my clients have discussed issues of lower interest and desire in their usual sexual relationships/activities. Today I'd like to provide a refresher of sexual arousal and desire models and where we are in our cultural and scientific thinking about arousal and pleasure.

Some of you might be familiar with the 1950s and 1960s research and theorized models by Kinsey and Masters and Johnson. Those incredibly brave early pioneers, after interviewing thousands of folks and observing willing human subjects engaging in sexual activity in their labs, concluded that healthy sexual functioning involves this sequence: excitement, plateau, orgasm, resolution. Basically, a human experiences sexual stimulation, notices excitement developing (lubrication in vaginas, flushing of skin, erections of clitoris and penis, faster breathing, etc.) then plateauing of this arousal until an orgasm occurs, followed by the body returning to a pre-sexual restful state.

However, it was only a matter of time before researcher Helen Singer Kaplan exploded this linear trope into the more nuanced Triphasic Model: desire, arousal (excitement and plateau), and orgasm. **Desire,** duh, became a critical component (it wasn't just about a sunny spring day, there had to some *interest* on your part as well). Now that we finally got ***desire*** on board, sex and biology researchers could step back and see that our brains account for a great deal of our sexual interest and response abilities.

In the late 1990s Erick Janssen and John Bancroft at the Kinsey Institute developed the Dual Control Model of sexual response. This model consists of two parts: sexual excitation system (SES) and sexual inhibition system (SIS). Emily Nagoski, a treasure who is living, teaching, and researching in our lovely Pioneer Valley, has an entire chapter devoted to this in her sexual bible for women (and the people who love them): *Come as You Are* (2015).

Essentially, as she writes in her book, "your central nervous system (brain and spinal cord) is made up of a partnership of accelerator and brakes - like the pairing of your sympathetic nervous system ('accelerator') and your parasympathetic nervous system ('brake')...what is true for other aspects of the nervous system must also be true for the brain system that coordinates sex: a sexual accelerator and sexual brake," hence the SES and SIS.

The SIS actually has two brakes: an emergency brake that notices all the immediate dangers and turn offs in the environment such as your kid screaming in the next room or a grouchy text from your boss. There is also a second brake that emits more of a "chronic, low-level 'no thank you' signal associated with a 'fear of performance failure' like worrying about having an orgasm." Nagoski states that we don't necessarily need to differentiate what is happening with which brake, we just need to know that we all have these two brakes, and we all have sexual accelerators, as well. Some folks have a sensitive SES and/or a sensitive SIS, no matter what is happening in the environment. Because of this model, I now talk almost exclusively with my clients about their sexual accelerator and brakes.

This Dual Control Model paved the way for Rosemary Basson to develop her nonlinear, slightly circular model of emotional intimacy, sexual stimuli, and relationship satisfaction in 2001. This model includes elements like spontaneous desire (that warm sunny day that just happens to light up an erogenous zone), sexual motivation linked to emotional and physical satisfaction, and responsive desire (which is when you may not necessarily be burning for sexual interaction, but your partner is interested and applies all your favorite pleasurable courtship rituals and touches to get you interested).

Responsive desire is NOT about "giving in" (especially in this essential, long overdue zeitgeist of "enthusiastic and freely given consent") but rather about being receptive to sexual activity in the context of what you consider to be erotic, such as receiving a very skillful foot rub with knowing hands that then travel up your body.

Now that you know about the Dual Control Model as well as the inclusion of elements such as emotional intimacy and sexual responsiveness, we can think about what can help you turn off the brakes when you want, and turn on the accelerator. We live in a very hectic world of chauffeuring children, with often both parents working, or a single person working two or three serious jobs/hobbies, plus managing chores, errands, finances, and so on. (I don't know about you, but I find life here in the Pioneer Valley particularly intense. Folks not only have their work they do for income, but many folks volunteer, homestead, do activism, teach or take yoga, write, make music, or paint in their free time, plus find time for friends and travel!) So what can you do to tune into your brakes and accelerator?

Try to find quiet moments where you can pay attention to your Dual Control System. If you have a lot pressing on your brakes you may need to work pretty hard getting your mojo back. You might need to say NO to extra responsibilities and chores, or even regular ones. Has your work infringed too much via emails on the mobile, when you were supposed to be off the clock? Is your cell phone or computer sucking away all your free time? Perhaps scheduling periodic "mental/sexual health" afternoon or days off from work or social connectivity could help, or take yourself to a remote Airbnb or cabin.

Have you provided too much childcare lately? Ask for help with any kids you might have – can the grandparents, siblings, best friend, and so forth take them off your hands for an evening or day or two? Obsessed much with climate change and current politics? Make some phone calls to politicians and then get in bed with a vibrator and one-hand read. Is the bedroom too messy for your taste? Designate a couple hours to set the mood for your self, your most important date.

Now that you've let up on the brakes, you can start zooming that accelerator to 60 or even a 100 mph. Take some alone time (do you see a theme emerging?), put sensual music on, dig out that old erotic or romance book in the back of your closet, whether it be *Twilight* or an ancient *Herotica* book of feminist erotic stories. Get your wedding lingerie or banana hammock out, or peruse local or online retailers for something new and exciting. Take a nap, and take your time waking up from it. Try to recall some fantasies or outstanding sexual moments from your young adulthood, often a time of more expansive sexual exploration. Watch those sexy scenes from *Ghost* or *Sense8* (Season 1, episode 6, Netflix, thank you). Go to the beach and enjoy the flesh show. These are just a few ideas to get your accelerator going.

Lastly, I'd be remiss in addressing sexual health if I didn't throw in a nod to physical health, sleep, and nutrition. Most of us religiously get our teeth cleaned twice a year and keep up with annual physicals and eye exams, yet completely ignore sexual hygiene (unless there is an emergency like a possible pregnancy or STI). All of us could benefit from regularly checking on our sexual hygiene as well.

In conclusion, go forth and pay attention! Notice what grabs your erotic attention in the environment, and what stifles it. Then set about readjusting your exposures so that you can let up on those brakes and press that accelerator to 100 mph, at least from time to time.

Sexual Styles

The Dual Control System of Desire and Response
By Stephanie Baird, LMHC
(Originally published November 2019 in the *Montague Reporter* newspaper monthly *Sex Matters* column.)

This month I share a concept called "Sexual Styles" which can help you figure out your own sexual style, and possibly those of any partner(s). Most of you are probably familiar with personality tests and styles. The Myers-Briggs helps us nail down our level of introversion versus extroversion, thinking versus feeling, judging versus perceiving, and so on. The Enneagram helps us figure out a main personality style, whether "helper," "leader," "peacemaker," "individualist," and so forth. So why wouldn't we have unique sexual styles? Turns out, we likely gravitate to one of these three categories: "sexual trancer," "partner engager," and "role enactor."

Let's examine these styles in the categories of setting, mood, sexual techniques, style, role expectations, sex talk, fantasies, ideas of sex, and orgasms.

Sexual trancers are a bit like the introverts of the Meyers-Briggs. They tend to like privacy and freedom from distractions. They enjoy a calm, relaxed, and serene mood. They like slow pacing and repetitive movements, and can be passive, sensual, and inwardly oriented. They prefer less frequent talking during sex so that they might be absorbed more easily into sensations. Their own fantasies may revolve around about visual or sensory images.

The partner engager enjoys being psychologically engaged with their partner, preferably in what they consider a "good" relationship. They relish a romantic and loving mood, lots of kissing, eye contact, and full body contact. Affectionate sharing, mutual pleasuring, romantic endearments, and love songs can be important parts of their repertoire. They expect their partners to act lovingly toward them, enjoying a flowing, harmonious union with their partner. Their fantasies may include the face of their partner, memories of union with their partner, and other romantic images.

Role enactors are more like the extroverts of the Myers-Briggs and enjoy interactive sex. There is a tendency toward dramatic, possibly even slightly exhibitionist elements, bringing a very playful mood, pride in variety and skill of sexual techniques, and lots of active movement, sound, and facial expressions. Lusty sex talk, dramatic orgasms, novel situations, roleplays, and interest in ecstasy also show up in this style.

The Northampton Sex Therapy Associates developed a wonderful short survey that folks can take if they are interested. Your therapist can hand you a copy. More simply, as you read through the preceding categories, if one sticks out as your main jam, then you've probably identified where you fit.

Most folks, just like in the Myers-Briggs, demonstrate flexibility in their sexual personality style. You might mostly be a trancer, but if you have a role enactor partner, they bring out more playfulness and variety. Or perhaps your main style is partner engager, with a side of trancer. You need to feel connected and mutual with your partner, allowing some trance action for orgasm.

There is no right or wrong sexual style, like being an introvert is as completely valid as being an extrovert. Where trouble can brew is when you have, say, a trancer matched up to a role enactor. Those are pretty different styles, which means you both might have to work fairly hard to make sure everyone's needs are met. This could look like the role enactor coming up with an elaborate roleplay scenario, bringing in sex toys, props, blindfolds, and so on. The trancer may need to engage in this active style for some time to fulfill the emotional and sexual needs of the role enactor. Once fulfilled, the role enactor can more easily provide the distraction-free, sensual focused zone for the trancer to get into their sensations.

Also, just like in life, sexual opposites can attract. So instead of thinking, "we've got such a big river to cross," think about how fun it can be to build that sexual bridge. This is a great exercise in creative thinking, getting the juices flowing, coming up with ways for different styled folks to feel satiated, together.

Lastly, long-term couples can notice a waning sex life over time and might jump to a few dozen conclusions about this, when it could be as simple as different sexual styles. In the beginning of romance, folks easily cross all the bridges of differences, and can show high flexibility in moving back and forth in sexual style. However, as time goes on, and life gets in the way, folks tend to stratify back to their main style. A couple complaining of reduced sex life, or very different interests in sex frequency, might actually be grappling with very different styles. The role enactor isn't getting their curiosity piqued, and so has given up on sex. The partner eEngager hasn't felt emotionally connected to their partner in some time, so turns to Netflix instead. Learning about your own style and asking for your needs can go a long way in correcting the ship's course.

In short, it's never too late to identify your sexual style and start asking more for what turns you on!

3

Sex Therapy Frameworks and Sexual Problems, Dysfunctions, and Disorders

Wendy Stock, PhD

LEARNING OBJECTIVES

- EMDR clinicians will learn about modern sex therapy frameworks, including the *New View of Women's Sexual Problems.*
- EMDR clinicians will be provided with the Sexual History Questionnaire (by Jassy Casella Timberlake, LMFT) to obtain client sexual health information.
- EMDR clinicians will learn about the persistent orgasm gap and corrective psychoeducation.
- EMDR clinicians will learn about conditions for good and great sex.
- EMDR clinicians will understand that trauma treatment is important to complete before addressing sexual concerns.
- EMDR clinicians will learn about sensate focus.
- EMDR clinicians will learn about sexual problems reported in sex therapy (and affecting many individuals in general): desire disorders, arousal disorders (erectile disorders), orgasm disorders (pre-orgasmic, premature ejaculation), and genito-pelvic pain penetration disorder (vaginismus, dyspaurenia, etc.).

GENDER LANGUAGE

In this chapter the term "man" refers to individuals with a penis, testes, prostate, and so on, and/or socialized into a masculine gender (generally speaking, cismen). The term "woman" refers to individuals with a vulva, labia, clitoris, vagina, ovaries, and uterus, and/or socialized into a feminine gender (generally speaking, ciswomen). This particularly pertains to how researchers have categorized individuals in the studies mentioned, although individuals with different combinations of identities and genitals may experience many of the pleasures and difficulties explored in this chapter.

MODERN SEX THERAPY FRAMEWORKS

Introduction

How culture constructs sexuality profoundly impacts our understanding of sexual health and how we define sexual problems. It guides and often narrows what we look for as we assess individuals seeking treatment, and what areas we may overlook. Culturally determined conceptions of sexuality, if we are unaware of their limitations, potentially impede our ability to offer the most effective treatment to our therapy clients. As clinicians, it is incumbent on us to be aware of cultural lenses, and to select the best components from the range of different models of sexuality, building upon existing models with critical awareness. The field of sex therapy has undergone an exciting evolution as it has matured to encompass broader models that better describe sexuality across different populations and social contexts.

For many decades the prevailing dominant cultural model of human sexuality was based on a model that narrowly defines sexual functioning as an unvarying progression of physiological responses, and failure to experience this progression as sexual dysfunction and therefore mental illness. These traditional approaches developed with a heteronormative focus, holding the ability to "achieve" sexual intercourse as the main criterion of healthy sexual functioning.

Early approaches to sex therapy were based on a model of sexual arousal by William Masters and Virginia Johnson (1966) that proposed a four-stage model of sexual arousal: excitement, plateau, orgasm, and resolution. Masters and Johnson's work provided invaluable information about the human physiology of sexual arousal, including the role of the clitoris in female orgasm, previously largely overlooked. Their work provided the basis to contest the dominant and inaccurate view that women should always orgasm during penetrative sex, and that the inability to do so was a form of pathology. Unfortunately, in emphasizing sexual physiology, this model lent itself to medicalized approaches to solving sexual problems, to the exclusion of relational factors and social context.

To their credit, Masters and Johnson (1979) revised their treatment model to incorporate a relational view, defining the couple, rather than the individual, as the appropriate focus of therapy. However, as Perelman (2014) notes, couples-based sex therapy was seen as a short-term, problem-focused, and directive approach that often overlooked the context of overall relationship dynamics, power issues, and the social context in which sexual problems emerged.

Later, Helen Singer Kaplan (1979) proposed a three-stage model, adding a desire phase to arousal and orgasm. The addition of a desire phase encouraged consideration of physical and psychological factors that may affect desire for sex. The current diagnostic nomenclature for sexual dysfunctions (*Diagnostic and Statistical Manual of Mental Disorders* [*DSM-5*], American Psychiatric Association [APA], 2013) is based on these earlier models of sexual functioning (desire, arousal, and orgasm), and adds a category for sexual pain disorders.

Although these linear stage-based models may be descriptive for some individuals, they have been criticized for failing to account for the social and relational context in which sexual problems occur. This lack of context has vast implications for treatment of sexual problems. Several alternative approaches are discussed that provide contextual, multifaceted analyses of causes of sexual problems, and suggest effective directions to address them.

Evolution of Sex Therapy: Feminist Reconceptualization of Sexual Problems

Feminist sex therapy has led the field in recognition of the limitations of a biologically based approach to human sexuality. Tiefer (1988) critiqued sexual dysfunction nomenclature as omitting empirically based information on what people socialized as women ("women" in this historical context refers to individuals with clitorises and vulvas) consider important in their sexual lives, including intimacy, negotiation, and communication. Tiefer (1996, p. 53) recommended that feminist-informed sex therapy include "corrective genital physiology education, assertiveness training, body image reclamation, and masturbation education." Naomi McCormick (1994), another feminist sex therapist, recommended that therapists treat individuals and couples for deficits in tenderness, poor communication, sexual selfishness, disinterest in oral sex, and unwillingness to cuddle. A feminist approach to sex therapy uses existing scientific knowledge about biology, medical approaches, and empirically validated treatment techniques while adding the following ingredients: recognition and willingness to intervene to address gender inequality, power differentials in relationships, valuing emotional and subjective aspects of sexuality, recognition that traditional sex roles underlie sexual problems, and awareness of the role of sexual coercion, abuse, and trauma in causing sexual problems. Finally, awareness of the relational context of sexual dysfunction is inherent in a feminist approach to sex therapy.

Rosemary Basson (2002) introduced a circular model of the female sexual response cycle that emphasizes subjective experience. An important tenet in Basson's model is that a person's sexual response can be ignited at any phase in the cycle, and that not all sexual encounters begin with spontaneous sexual desire. Her model emphasizes that the relational context of the sexual encounter greatly influences motivations to have sex, and the ultimate outcome of a sexual interaction.

The New View of Women's Sexual Problems

The most prominent and organized challenge to the dominant paradigm of sexual dysfunction comes from the New View of Women's Sexual Problems, a collaboration of feminist academics, researchers, scholars, clinicians, and activists. Incorporating Basson's (2002) model and extending far beyond, sexual disorders (including but not limited to those people with clitorises) defined by the field of psychiatry as mental illness can alternatively be understood as problems tied to lack of information, lack of access to healthcare, powerlessness, relational issues, or the result of violent trauma. Sexual problems are seen as arising within a broader framework of cultural and relational factors. The competent clinician should take a history inclusive of all these issues.

Jassy Casella Timberlake's *The Sexual History Questionnaire* (NSTA, 2019), included at the end of this chapter, is one very comprehensive tool to use with any individual, regardless of genital configuration, to help determine difficulties and pleasures. The clinician can ask these questions verbally to clients, or send them home with the questionnaire if the client seems well regulated and motivated to answer on their own. If administered verbally, it could take one to several sessions.

The *New View of Women's Sexual Problems* offers a blueprint for a comprehensive assessment with inherent implications for treatment, depending on the information obtained. The utility of this model for assessment and intervention will become apparent in the following section, addressing the prevalence, frequency, and treatment of common sexual dysfunctions (http://www.newviewcampaign.org/manifesto3.asp) (Kachak & Tiefer, 2002).

The *New View* considers four main categories of causes of sexual problems:

I. ***Sexual Problems Due to Sociocultural, Political, or Economic Factors***
   A. Ignorance and anxiety due to inadequate sex education, lack of access to health services, or other social constraints (this includes lack of biology and gender vocabulary and information)
   B. Sexual avoidance or distress due to perceived inability to meet cultural norms regarding correct or ideal sexuality, including:
      1. Anxiety or shame about one's body, sexual attractiveness, or sexual responses
      2. Confusion or shame about one's sexual orientation or identity, or about sexual fantasies and desires
   C. Inhibitions due to conflict between the sexual norms of one's subculture or culture of origin and those of the dominant culture

D. Lack of interest, fatigue, or lack of time due to family and work obligations
II. *Sexual Problems Relating to Partner and Relationship* (e.g., issues with the partner [including dislike, betrayal, or medical status], desire discrepancies, poor sexual communication, decreased sexual interest due to life demands)
III. *Sexual Problems Due to Psychological Factors* (e.g., sexual aversion, mistrust, or inhibition of sexual pleasure due to past experiences of physical, sexual, or emotional abuse [and any resulting PTSD symptoms], general problems with attachment, rejection, cooperation, or entitlement, and depression or anxiety)
IV. *Sexual Problems Due to Medical Factors* (pain, or lack of physical response during sexual activity despite a supportive and safe interpersonal situation, adequate sexual knowledge, and positive sexual attitudes [e.g., local or systemic neurovascular, circulatory, endocrine medical conditions; sexually transmitted infectionss; pregnancy; drugs, medications, or medical treatments side effects])

All the complex facets in the development and maintenance of the sexual persona over a woman's lifetime are interrelated and relevant to the present state of a woman's sexual functioning or problem condition. Issues implicit in this classification scheme also include the following:

A. Current developmental stage
B. Childhood and adolescent conditioning experiences
   1. Religious and/or spiritual teachings and practices
   2. Gendered power relations
   3. Parental modeling of sexuality
   4. Sex education (formal and/or informal)
C. Previous experiences (positive and negative) with intimacy, love, attraction, and sexual activity

COMMON SEXUAL PROBLEMS REPORTED IN SEX THERAPY

The most recent demographically representative study (Laumann et al., 1999) in the United States found that 43% of women and 31% of men reported at least one sexual dysfunction.

Among subjects identified as women:
- 33% lacked interest in sex
- 24% were unable to orgasm
- 14% experienced pain during sex
- 21% reported trouble lubricating

Among subjects identified as men:
- 16% lacked interest in sex
- 8% were unable to orgasm
- 29% orgasmed too early
- 10% had trouble maintaining or achieving an erection

Gendered Orgasm Gap

The large gap in orgasm frequency between women and men in heterosexual sexual activity provides a good illustration of the influence of relational factors on sexual problems. Laumann et al. (1999) reported that, while 75% of heterosexual men reported having orgasms from partnered sex on a regular basis, only about 29% of women reported the same. Related research (Wade et al., 2005) found that among women, those with more knowledge of the clitoris experienced orgasm more frequently on their own, but possessing this information was *not* related to frequency of orgasm with partners.

The authors point out that this disparity exists in the context of "gender inequality and a social construction of sexuality…that privileges men's sexual pleasure over women's, such that orgasm for women is pleasing, but ultimately incidental" (Wade et al., 2005). Women may not feel empowered or entitled to act on their sexual self-knowledge or to ask for the stimulation that they need for fear of being seen as unfeminine, too demanding, and less desirable to their male partners. The authors continue, "our findings are directly relevant to other means of safeguarding health, such as setting sexual boundaries and using condoms." The authors clearly demonstrate that gender inequality directly affects not only women's ability to claim their full sexual pleasure with male partners, but their safety from exposure to sexual disease and sexual violence. Sexual dysfunction should never be considered apart from social context.

A number of studies have shown that large percentages of women fake orgasm. Herbenick et al. (2019) reported that 58.8% of female participants (mostly heterosexual) reported faking an orgasm at some point in time. When the authors looked at women who *continue* to fake orgasms, these women indicated that they were embarrassed to talk explicitly about sex with a partner. The authors noted that the youngest age bracket (women 18–24 years old) were significantly more likely to say they did not know how to ask for what they wanted.

The situational and relational factors identified make a strong case for offering corrective sexual education, addressing sex role expectations, improving sexual communication, addressing relationship issues concerning sexual initiation, timing, power issues in couples, sharing of familial workload, examining unrealistic expectations, and learning to make sexual interactions more about connection than performance.

> **Case Study 3.1: Sara, Only Orgasmic on Her Own**

Sara, a 33-year-old heterosexual ciswoman, is in treatment for anxiety and depression, but recently introduced a sexual issue that she wants to address. In her previous sexual relationships, she has never had an orgasm with any partner. However, she is easily able to orgasm on her own during masturbation. She reports typically becoming sexually aroused during partner sex, and sometimes feels that she is close to orgasm. At that point, she becomes self-conscious and "fakes" having an orgasm. Her stated concerns included: embarrassment that she is "taking too long" to orgasm, worries that her partner is becoming bored or tired, worries that she'll be "too much trouble" or "too demanding" as a partner, and fears that her partner may lose interest in her, and that she could lose the relationship. She has never told any previous partner that she didn't have orgasms, having felt trapped if her "lie" were revealed, which would have a negative impact on trust in these relationships.

Therapy to date has included normalizing the challenges for many women in reaching orgasm with partners (not receiving effective stimulation for sufficient duration, not feeling comfortable providing direct feedback to a partner, gender socialization to put others' needs first). Boundary and self-esteem issues have also been addressed as part of Sara's therapy. Now in a new and promising relationship, Sara has felt empowered to discuss this issue with her new partner *before* they have engaged in sexual contact. She has decided that she deserves to have orgasms when she wants them with a partner, and that she wouldn't want to be with a partner who wasn't equally committed to her sexual pleasure. To his credit, the new partner has offered her reassurance that he will be open to her feedback, and will take as long as she needs. This rewarding outcome is not always guaranteed, but the most important achievement is Sara's changed valuing of herself, and her expectations of future partners.

CORRECTIVE SEXUAL EDUCATION: DEBUNKING SEXUAL MYTHS AND PROVIDING INFORMATION

Tiefer (1996) referred to the need for "corrective sexual education" in addressing sexual problems. Sex therapy almost invariably requires a psychoeducational component, sometimes during the assessment phase, and sometimes as treatment progresses. The myths discussed in the following are commonly held, and astoundingly impervious to the availability of more accurate information provided by science and readily accessible online. Providing accurate information can have a profound impact on presenting symptoms, and at times can ameliorate them, as described in the examples. Space prevents a thorough debunking of each myth.

Common and Persistent Sexual Myths

General Cultural Myths

People should be able to read their partner's physical signals during sex without any verbal communication.
Pornography accurately portrays sex.

Myths About Female Sexuality

All people with vaginas should be able to orgasm through penetrative sex.
Misunderstanding the significance of vaginal lubrication: It is commonly believed that the presence or absence of vaginal lubrication is an accurate indicator of female sexual arousal.
Sex is only good if you have an orgasm.
Douching is necessary to keep the vagina clean.
Painful sex is normal.

Myths About Male Sexuality (As Identified by Bernie Zilbergeld's *Male Sexuality* [1978])

People with penises should not have certain feelings (e.g., vulnerability, sadness).

In sex, as elsewhere, it is performance that counts.
The man must take charge of and orchestrate sex.
The man is always ready and always wants to have sex.
All physical contact must lead to sex.
Sex equals intercourse.
Sex requires an erection.
Sexual intercourse is always a linear progression on increasing excitement terminated only by orgasm.
Sex is natural and spontaneous.

> **Case Study 3.2: Alexis, Lubrication Is *Not* a Valid Measure of Sexual Arousal!**

Alexis, a ciswoman, is being seen in treatment for lack of sexual desire with her cismale fiancé. Relationship issues had already been successfully addressed (equalizing relative contribution to household chores among them). With further assessment, it became apparent that Alexis has a healthy interest in sex, and masturbates on average three times weekly. However, she often makes excuses to avoid having sex with her partner, although she does experience pleasure and orgasm when she "gets past the initial part," as she put it. What became apparent was that both partners were relying on the state of her vaginal lubrication to determine how and when to initiate intercourse. As Masters and Johnson (1970) put it, "lubrication signifies only the capacity for penetration, not the desire."

On some occasions, Alexis was profusely lubricated but was not feeling ready for penetrative sex. Both partners assumed that she was, and what resulted was sometimes painful cramping when the penis hit the cervix in her essentially unaroused vaginal barrel (not elongated with the uterus being pulled back and out of the way). An unaroused vaginal barrel is about 3 inches in depth; an aroused vaginal barrel is approximately 6 inches in depth. Lubrication is not a good independent measure of female arousal, yet it is often used as such. Alexis did not feel empowered to ask to slow things down, as she assumed that she was aroused, even if not subjectively aware of it.

On other occasions, Alexis was feeling aroused but wasn't lubricated at all. Her partner kept stimulating her very dry vaginal tissues manually - the fragile mucous membrane is easily abraded with extended rubbing and friction. This became so irritating physically and experientially that Alexis would sometimes preempt further stimulation by initiating intercourse, which caused further irritation that sometimes became painful.

This example is included here because this scenario is encountered frequently in sex therapy. Sharing the following information proved quite helpful in Alexis's treatment: Vaginas may lubricate more, less, or not at all during different phases of their menstrual cycle, when using oral contraception, or when using certain medications (antihistamines dry out *all* mucous membranes; diuretics can have the same effect). Lubrication is a misleading measure of sexual arousal. When in doubt, the female partner should be asked and should be encouraged to trust her subjective sense of her body. When sex is desired, lubrication can be applied *proactively* – it makes stimulation feel more pleasurable and less irritating from the onset and does not need to imply a lack of responsivity in the female partner, nor a lack of skill in the other partner (frequent misapprehensions in this situation).

Another myth at play in Alexis's case was the belief that it is normal for sex to sometimes hurt, accepting this as a precondition for having sex. This led to her avoiding sex completely, or initiating painful intercourse to "get it over with." This case also illustrates the relevance of the New View of Women's Sexual Problems model (described earlier) in identifying multiple factors that may apply to women's sexual problems: inadequate sex education, lack of vocabulary to describe subjective or physical experience, lack of information about human sexual biology, anxiety about one's sexual responses, lack of time and energy due to family and work obligations, ignorance or inhibition about communicating sexual preferences or pacing of sexual activity, and loss of interest over conflicts over commonplace issues.

Corrective Sexual Education: Sexual Anatomy and Physiology

Understanding one's own sexual response and having the means to verbalize preferences are often greatly facilitated by sharing materials on sexual anatomy and physiology with sex therapy clients. The illustrations provided by Suzann Gage in *A New View of a Woman's Body* (1981) dramatically increase accurate and empowering education. Chapter 3 of her book, titled *The Clitoris: A Feminist Perspective* (open access https://wiki.lereset.org/_media/ateliers:nvwb_clitoris_suzann_gage.pdf) redefines the clitoris as a much more substantial sexual organ that includes a complex of connected erectile tissue underlying the skin, in contrast to the popular understanding of the clitoris as only the head of the clitoris (see Figures 3.1 and 3.2). This chapter contains illuminating illustrations of a non-aroused and aroused clitoris, comparing these to the equivalent in the penis, with striking similarity. Sharing these illustrations with accompanying explanation often paves the way for better communication in couples of any gender combination. For clients to see that their sexual arousal is physiologically real often results in a radical change in feeling more entitled to pursue their own sexual pleasure.

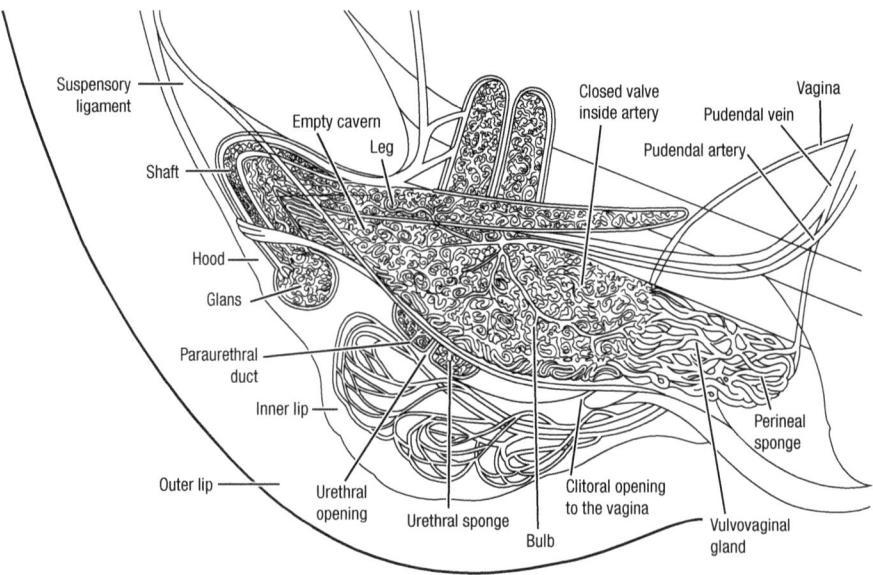

FIGURE 3.1 Cross-section of the nonerect clitoris.

Source: Adapted from Federation of Feminist Women's Health Centers. (1981). *A new view of a woman's body*. Feminist Health Press.

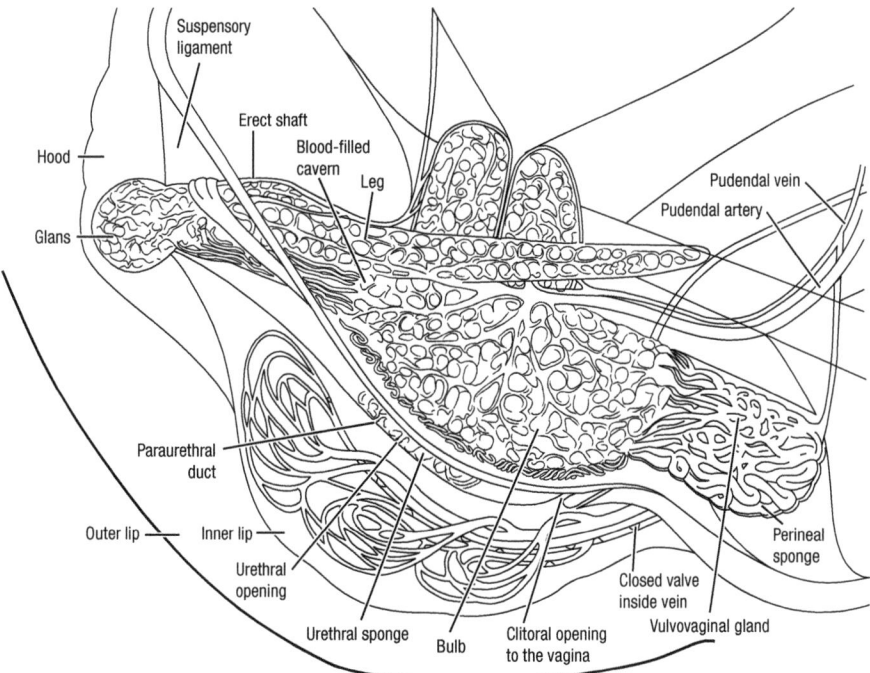

FIGURE 3.2 Cross-section of the clitoris during sexual arousal.

Source: Adapted from Federation of Feminist Women's Health Centers. (1981). *A new view of a woman's body.* Feminist Health Press.

CONDITIONS FOR GOOD SEX

Dr. Bernie Zilbergeld, in his book *The New Male Sexuality* (1978), suggests that knowing our conditions for good and great sex is essential to optimizing our sexual enjoyment. The converse is also true: When people are unaware of the importance of having conditions or prerequisites, they are at risk for disappointment, and even sexual problems or dysfunctions. Simply introducing this concept to clients in sex therapy often has a profound impact, resulting in clients' feeling entitled to assert their conditions for when they engage sexually. Examples of these conditions include feeling physically and emotionally safe, trusting, and intimate with your partner; physically comfortable and capable;aroused; able to relax; alert; positive about the environment; and an absence of performance pressures from either self or partner.

> **Case Study 3.3: Maddie, Conditions for Good Sex**

Maddie rarely turned down her partner's initiations for sex, but she reported frequently being distracted by self-consciousness and unable to respond fully during sexual interactions. Some of her distracted thinking was about having had a hard day at work, and not having had time to unwind. Easily addressed in therapy, Maddie now felt comfortable taking more time to unwind. More prominent were Maddie's worries about her body (perspiration, vaginal odor) especially when her partner engaged in oral sex. Maddie shared that she specifically worried excessively about her vaginal odor, although her partner had been reassuring and engaged, even when they had sex after Maddie's gym workout. She felt that she should not insist on taking a shower first, because her partner didn't seem to mind. Reinforcing Maddie's right to have her own conditions for comfort, and therefore respond sexually, allowed her to speak up about these conditions. Maddie became more engaged, present, and comfortable, enjoying her sexual encounters more fully.

SEX THERAPY WITH SEXUAL TRAUMA SURVIVORS

Rather than addressing this area at the end of a section on treatment of sexual dysfunctions, as if it were an unusual and separate issue, it is crucial to emphasize here that implementing treatment of sexual problems is unlikely to work in cases where there is unprocessed sexual trauma. Given the relatively high frequency in the general population of childhood sexual abuse and sexual assault, we know that these experiences put people at higher risk of having mental health sequelae. This population is over-represented in the clinical population, which also applies to those seeking sex therapy. Common presentation includes sexual interaction triggering memories of abuse, states of dissociation ranging from feeling present but disconnected, and/or mild depersonalization (sensation of watching oneself as if from outside one's body). A brief loss of awareness during a sexual encounter can be common.

Some survivors of childhood sexual abuse report the ability to feel initial sexual arousal, but as they approach high arousal and potential orgasm, sexual arousal dissipates suddenly. Some of these individuals experience a fear of loss of control of their bodies.

For most survivors of sexual assault and abuse, the trauma must be addressed therapeutically before anything is done in sex therapy. Even with a supportive partner, the individual with unprocessed trauma will not be able to respond well to sex therapy interventions. Sex therapists may refer these clients for EMDR

Therapy; therefore, it is helpful to be familiar with the information throughout this chapter (and book) in the joint goal of improving client sexual health.

Trauma Processing *First* With Sexual Trauma Survivors: Two Approaches

The following is a very brief description of two well-known approaches to the treatment of trauma. A longer discussion of these approaches, and others not included here, would exceed the scope of this chapter. It is helpful to provide clients information about these approaches. Several handouts available via open access online are referred to in this next section. As this book is geared toward EMDR clinicians, the EMDR therapy section here is very brief. It is useful to know about trauma-focused cognitive behavioral therapy (TF-CBT), as some of our clients may request this therapy as well.

Trauma-Focused Cognitive Behavioral Therapy

TF-CBT shares a great deal of common features with other empirically validated cognitive processing approaches to trauma, including those developed by Herman (1992), Christine Courtois's work on treatment of complex trauma (2004), and Edna Foa et al.'s (2008) model of Prolonged Exposure Therapy. The cognitive processing approach is based on the idea that when trauma is not fully processed, the trauma remains in active memory, more easily triggered by trauma-associated cues, and remains a drain on mental energy for the client (Ehlers & Clark, 2000). The memories follow an intrusion-avoidance pattern, but the exposure is never long enough to process or desensitize the traumatic memory. TF-CBT involves a trust relationship with the therapist and trains the client in emotional regulation techniques, thus creating a stable base to support the active processing of the traumatic memory. Writing and other expressive techniques provide the brain an opportunity to integrate the narrative and affective components of the traumatic memory.

What Is TF-CBT? (Psychology Tools, n.d.-b) is an information sheet describing the key principles of TF-CBT and is available at https://www.psychologytools.com/resource/what-is-tf-cbt/. It outlines the differences between trauma and post-traumatic stress disorder (PTSD), describing some of the key components of cognitive-behavioral therapy (CBT) for PTSD.

CBT is a collaborative form of therapy: the client and therapist first form a trusting working relationship.

Components of TF-CBT:

Grounding and Stabilization—Relaxation and/or other techniques
Work With Memories—Talking, writing, drawing, and so forth

Work With Beliefs—Making sense of what the client thought at the time of the trauma and questioning what is a fair and rational way to think about themselves and their current situation (Grey et al., 2002)

Reclaiming Your Life (sometimes referred to as the "Resilience Phase" of trauma therapy)—PTSD often has the effect of stealing people's lives; it is common after trauma to start avoiding things that cause emotional discomfort, but this can have the effect of shrinking their world. Effective therapy is directed at taking back the things that the client used to enjoy, and building a new life that they can value.

Eye Movement Desensitization and Reprocessing

Eye movement desensitization and reprocessing (EMDR) therapy is a distinct therapeutic approach that uses bilateral stimulation (i.e., eye movements) to aid the integration (processing) of distressing and/or traumatic information. EMDR therapy is commonly used to treat PTSD, recommended by the American Psychological Association and the National Institute for Health and Care Excellence (NICE; UK) as an effective treatment. PTSD is the subject of the majority of EMDR research (Shapiro, 2001; Solomon & Shapiro, 2008). EMDR therapy is increasingly being used to treat other conditions in which disturbing memories occur such as anxiety and depression. *What Is EMDR?* (Psychology Tools, n.d.-a) is a one-page information sheet describing the key principles of EMDRA available at https://www.psychologytools.com/resource/what-is-emdr/. It is helpful to use this as a handout for clients who may want information before choosing between EMDR and TF-CBT. Listed in the following are the main points covered in this handout:

The theory behind EMDR therapy is that many psychological difficulties are the result of distressing life experiences that have not been stored in memory properly and are unprocessed or blocked. These traumatic memories may need help to become processed, and EMDR therapy is one method.

Normal memories are stored by a part of the brain called the hippocampus. The hippocampus is like a librarian that catalogues (processes) events and stores them in the right place. However, some traumatic events (such as accidents, abuse, disasters, or violence) are so overwhelming that the hippocampus does not do its job properly. When this happens, trauma memories are stored in their raw, unprocessed, form. These trauma memories are easily triggered, leading them to replay and cause distress over and over again.

Treatment of Sexual Problems in Sexual Trauma Survivors: After Trauma Processing

Once the treatment of trauma processing has occurred, clients are in a better position to work directly on the effects of trauma on their sexuality. Wendy Maltz, MSW, has written and created excellent self-help resources for survivors of sexual trauma. These can be used in conjunction with a trauma therapist, individually and/or with their partners in sex therapy. Her materials are available on her website, healthysex.com, and include the books *Incest and Sexuality* (Maltz & Holman, 1987) and *The Sexual Healing Journey* (Maltz, 2012), and the videos *Partners in Healing* and *Relearning Touch*. Full versions of both videos are available on her website. As described on Maltz's website, *The Sexual Healing Journey* helps survivors to identify the sexual effects of their abuse, create a positive meaning for sex, develop a healthy sexual self-concept, gain control over upsetting reactions to touch and sex, improve partner intimacy, incorporate non-demand, sensual touch with sex, and address sexual functioning concerns.

Maltz's approach also addresses helping survivors heal from having unwanted sexual fantasies. This can include the survivor taking themselves through a repatterning of the process of sexual socialization (e.g., engaging in non-demanding and consensual touch with a partner) and developing fantasies that do not involve unwanted sex. Maltz emphasizes the importance of sexual communication and boundary setting in her work with survivors.

TREATMENT OF COMMON SEXUAL DYSFUNCTIONS

Sensate Focus, the Foundation of Sex Therapy Interventions

The brilliance of the sensate focus technique, developed by Masters and Johnson (Linschoten et al., 2016), fulfills both a diagnostic function and also a therapeutic intervention that allows improvement of communication deficits in couples. Utilizing this technique before addressing a specific presenting sexual dysfunction is crucial in laying a groundwork of constructive communication and sensual, non-demand touching. This method often serves to alleviate some of the contributing factors of performance pressure and poor communication patterns.

In the beginning stages of sensate focus, couples are encouraged to touch each other's bodies and feel for sexual sensations but refrain from touching breasts or genitals or engaging in intercourse or direct genital touching.

The primary benefits of this approach are:

Introducing sensual touching and deeper connection: In our culture, sex often becomes narrowly focused on genitals, and the rest of the body is ignored. The sensate focus exercise helps to remind us to re-introduce sensual touching as a pleasurable end, as well as a practice that can help awaken us to a deeper and more gratifying sexual experience with our partners. The exercises work to build gradual desire for full genital sexual involvement. As the couple becomes more skilled at giving and receiving verbal feedback and being present in the moment (may take several sessions), they are then encouraged to touch breasts and external genitals, and then eventually to include intercourse or penetrative sexual activity.

Communication deficits assessed and improved: The ubiquitous myth that verbal communication should not be needed during sexual interactions is a major factor in sexual dissatisfaction and sexual dysfunctions. Many individuals believe that providing feedback during sex is unromantic and takes away from the desired mood. Individuals socialized as women often fear being too "bossy" in bed, fearing disapproval from their partners should they speak up. Ongoing communication in real time is learned, increasing the ability to provide supportive, gentle feedback about the exact level of touch that will work for the recipient.

Diagnostic function: Sensate focus also provides crucial diagnostic information to the therapist, a window in therapy to explore and develop methods of working with barriers to intimacy, rather than trying to ignore or "bypass" negative feelings. Ignoring one's feelings and pretending to feel comfortable prevents true intimacy.

Goals of Sensate Focus as Presented to Clients (Stock, n.d., Unpublished Handout)

- To learn ways to touch each other in a sensual, pleasing manner, not dependent an expectation or demand for sexual arousal or sexual "performance" for oneself or for one's partner
- To practice communicating to your partner your preferences in being touched, in a direct, clear, and constructive manner
- To fully recognize any barriers to physical and emotional intimacy

Sensate Focus Exercise Instructions (Stock, n.d., Unpublished Handout)

Timing/scheduling: Collaboratively schedule 1 hour for each sensate focus session. Sex and sex therapy homework often takes a back seat to most other activities, including the laundry. Scheduling time for a sex therapy date is the best way to ensure that it will happen, and is a valuable approach after therapy is over to maintain changes that you have/will make. Try to space these sessions during the week, rather than trying to squeeze them in under pressure on the day before your next therapy appointment.

Setting/environment: The partner who initiates the session is responsible for creating a comfortable environment—room temperature, lighting, beverage, for example. You are encouraged to try using massage lotion (almond oil or commercial massage lotion) in consultation with your partner. Some people prefer the feel of talcum powder or cornstarch powder, rather than liquid emollients. You may wish to use a large towel to protect your sheets.

Make certain that your cell phones are off and that you will not be interrupted. If you share your home with others, you may choose to let them know that you are spending an hour of "we" time. This is also excellent role-modeling behavior for maintaining a healthy couple relationship.

Take turns (alternating who gets to go first and last) with one partner being the "giver" and the other the "receiver" for 30 minutes each. Make sure that you allow your partner to touch the front and back of your body during your turn as receiver. Although you may experience sexual arousal at times during the sensate focus exercise, sexual arousal is not the goal of this exercise, and it is not intended as a prelude to sexual engagement.

During your turn as receiver, you are only responsible for relaxing and focusing on your sensations, and telling your partner, at the time, three things that feel good about how they are touching you. You also need to tell your partner at least one thing that doesn't feel good, but phrased in terms of what you would like them to do to make it feel better (please move your touching up/down, right/left, harder/softer, to a different location, etc.).

During your turn as giver, try touching your partner in different ways. Breasts and genitals are "off-limits." Use different parts of your hands, different pressures, long, short, circular stroking, and so forth. Do pay attention to your partner's verbal feedback. Also, try to be aware of how you feel in the giver role. Remember that no one is a mind reader, and that it is your partner's responsibility to verbally guide you if they want something different from what you are doing.

DIAGNOSES AND TREATMENT APPROACHES FOR SPECIFIC SEXUAL DYSFUNCTIONS

The following sections are very brief, condensed descriptions of standard cognitive behavioral approaches to treatment of sexual dysfunctions. Crucially, these treatment protocols must be understood and implemented with the requirement of having already conducted the broader, contextual assessment practices described earlier in this chapter. Sexual dysfunctions are embedded in social and relational contexts, including those with a history of sexual trauma. The focus in the following is primarily on treatment techniques, predicated on completion of a thorough assessment. Using these methods presupposes that treatment of other conditions has occurred (unprocessed sexual trauma, severe depression, etc.) that could interfere with treatment of sexual problems.

Additionally, while many of the titles of these disorders are gendered, it is understood that transgender individuals that possess pertaining genitalia (e.g., a transmale who possesses a clitoris), or intersex folks with different combinations, may also experience these issues.

Desire Disorders: Hypoactive Sexual Desire Disorder

Sexual desire, or drive, includes interest in sexual stimuli, wishing for sexual activity, planning for sexual activity, or feeling frustrated when sexual activity does not occur.

The *DSM-5* (APA, 2013) defines hypoactive sexual desire disorder (HSDD) as persistent or recurrently deficient sexual or erotic thoughts, fantasies, and desire for sexual activity that has persisted for a minimum of 6 months, and causes significant distress.

The *DSM-5* has controversially combined desire and arousal diagnoses for people with vaginas. It has been argued that this amalgamation of these two diagnoses is not supported by empirical findings (Althof et al., 2017). For purposes of this chapter, desire and arousal disorders will be considered separately.

Many people reporting low desire function quite well sexually by all objective criteria, yet they have no subjective experience of sexual desire. Individuals presenting for treatment of low sexual desire can be characterized as "wanting to want" sex. Low desire can be either global or situational. Some clients have sexual desire but do not want to sexually engage with their partner, but still masturbate regularly. Others do not experience any sexual urges, reporting few or no sexual thoughts or fantasies. Still others may identify as asexual and need permission to embrace this identity.

Many factors can influence a lower desire and *must* be addressed before implementing specific techniques addressed at increasing sexual desire. Some factors include hormonal influences (e.g., age related/postmenopausal decrease in estrogen or testosterone, elevated prolactin during nursing that can dramatically decrease desire), medication side effects, medical conditions or treatments, and/or substance abuse. Cultural background can play a role (sexual norms often socialize women to believe that desiring sex is sinful, resulting in guilt and shame). History of untreated trauma or abuse can result in the client having intrusive thoughts or "flashbacks" during sexual activity. Relationship conflict and/or poor or absent communication can also impede desire and interest.

Cognitive behavioral treatment for clients with low sexual desire generally focus on a "priming" effect of increasing the frequency of sexual thoughts, fantasies, and awareness of sexual stimuli via a Desire Diary, Desire Checklist, priming the pump (seek out erotic material), fantasy time-outs during the day, scheduling sex, and so on.

Relational Factors in Creating Sexual Desire

Relationship factors impact sexual desire and affect willingness to participate in sex. The prevalence rate of low sexual desire in ciswomen is high, reaching 43% (Kingsberg & Rezaee, 2013). Desire is often embedded in a relational context, and it is important to attend to the underlying motivational forces that trigger it.

Basson's (2002) non-linear model of sexual response, discussed earlier, is circular, incorporates the need for intimacy, and acknowledges that desire can be responsive or spontaneous, and may occur either before or after arousal.

Arousal Disorders

Female Sexual Arousal Disorder

Female sexual arousal disorder (FSAD; considered separately from hypoactive sexual desire here) is described as absent or reduced sexual excitement or pleasure in most sexual encounters, absent or reduced internal or external "sexual cues," and absent or reduced genital or non-genital sensations during sexual activity in all or mostly all sexual encounters. These symptoms must cause clinically significant distress and have persisted for a minimum of 6 months.

FSAD has some unique features from HSDD. Sometimes FSAD co-occurs with reduced or absent sexual desire, but in other cases, it exists as a separate entity. For example, a client may report that they are quite interested in having sexual interaction, or that they attempted to masturbate, but that despite sufficient stimulation, there is diminished or no genital arousal response. This can be frustrating for the individual who is interested and willing to become aroused.

Meston and Stanton (2017) reviewed existing research on FSAD, summarized here. Contributing factors to FSAD overlap with those that can also contribute to female HSDD: biological (e.g., medical health, hormones, and medications) and psychological factors (e.g., stress, relationships, comorbid mental illness, history of sexual abuse). Inhibitors of sexual arousal can also include negative body image, fear of negative consequences for sexual activity (e.g., bad reputation, pregnancy), or feeling used by a sexual partner.

Implications for treatment of FSAD include attention to psychological and historical factors that may impact the ability to be aroused. The factors mentioned within the discussion of HSDD would be applicable for treatment of arousal deficits in women as well. Help the client assess whether they are receiving effective and sufficient stimulation to allow their bodies to become sexually aroused. Genital self-exploration, self-touch and partner-touch psychoeducation and practice, and sensate focus exercises are often helpful.

In the instance of decreased or no lubrication, proactively applying lubrication to the external inner labia and clitoral area at the beginning of sexual activity can make a dramatic difference in the experience of pleasurable sensation from touch. Topical lubricants do not in themselves create sexual arousal, but instead may facilitate and optimize the possibility of experiencing arousal. Lubrication can be very helpful for postmenopausal clients who may generate less lubrication and experience atrophy of vaginal tissues and epithelial density (rendering the vaginal tissue more subject to abrasion and microscopic tears).

Hormonal (off-label use of the testosterone patch, estrogen treatment) and non-hormonal therapies (the antidepressant bupropion) have been used to treat both reduced desire and arousal in clients (reviewed by Meston & Stanton, 2017). Comparable drugs to the PDE5 inhibitors (Viagra, Cialis, Levitra) can increase vaginal engorgement and vaginal blood flow, but not increase subjective sexual arousal.

As with treatment of low desire, psychological treatments for FSAD include psychoeducation about factors that can inhibit desire, couples' interventions (e.g., scheduling time for physical and emotional intimacy), communication training, cognitive restructuring of dysfunctional beliefs (e.g., a good sexual experience does not always end with an orgasm), sexual fantasy training, and sensate focus exercises. Treatment may also include identifying distracting, negative thoughts and learning to let go of these during sexual activity. These might include myths and misconceptions about sex, negative emotions, performance anxiety, and body image concerns. Cognitive restructuring can help people identify their fears and dysfunctional beliefs.

Erectile Disorder

It was once thought that erectile dysfunction (ED) was predominantly due to psychogenic causes. More recent studies have indicated that neurologic, vascular, and hormonal abnormalities are involved in a considerable percentage of cases of erectile dysfunction. It is now recognized that both organic and psychogenic factors can contribute to ED to different degrees for an individual client (LoPiccolo & Stock, 1986).

Medical conditions and medications may contribute to erectile issues. However, even with a mild organic impairment, if psychological, behavioral and technique difficulties are eliminated by sex therapy, the client may be able to attain a full erection.

The introduction of Viagra (sildenafil) in 1998 and other similar medications, all phosphodiesterase-5 (PDE5) inhibitors, such as tadalafil (Cialis), and vardenafil (Levitra) that facilitate erection, revolutionized the treatment of ED. Even clients that have medical issues contributing to erectile difficulties often respond to these medications. However, Tiefer (1988) has raised the concern that medicalization of sexuality can obscure the effects of social contributions to peoples' sexual complaints, including rigid gender roles, unrelenting standards of performance, relationships of unequal power, and histories of sexual victimization. The ability to attain an erection does not address a lack of emotional connection, intimacy, or physical sensuality in a relationship.

Metz and McCarthy (2004) have written an excellent self-help book, *Coping With Erectile Dysfunction,* that offers a psychoeducational approach and guidelines that can be used by the male client independently, or in conjunction with sex therapy. Here are a few of the many points covered in this book that address the social, cultural, and relational factors associated with erectile problems.

1. By age 40, 90% of people with penises will have at least one erectile difficulty. This is a normal occurrence.
2. View the erectile difficulty as a situational problem; do not overreact and label yourself "impotent" or put yourself down as a "failure."
3. It is natural for erections to wax and wan during prolonged pleasuring.
4. You do not need a penis to satisfy a partner. Orgasms can be achieved manually, orally, with sex toys, or with rubbing.
5. Erections do not need to occur for ejaculation. Ejaculation can come from a flaccid penis.
6. If the penis is flaccid, give and receive sensuous, playful non-demand touching. The basis of sexual response is relaxation and sensuality.
7. A sexual experience is best measured by pleasure and satisfaction, not whether you had an erection, how hard it was, or whether everyone was orgasmic.

Orgasm Disorders

Female Orgasmic Disorder

As defined in the *DSM-5* (2013), female orgasmic disorder is characterized by difficulty experiencing orgasm and/or markedly reduced intensity of orgasmic sensations and must cause marked distress or interpersonal difficulty to be diagnosed. There is wide variation in the type and intensity of stimulation that elicits orgasm in women as well as the subjective experiences of orgasm. Female orgasmic disorder may be lifelong or acquired, generalized (occurring in all situations) or situational (occurring in select situations). An example of the situational type of the disorder is a woman who has orgasms through masturbation but not during partnered sexual activity.

Primary Female Orgasmic Disorder
Women with primary female orgasmic disorder have not previously experienced orgasm in any situation. Generally no medical conditions are associated with this lifelong absence of orgasm. This dysfunction can be due to a learning deficit, and some therapists, including this author (W. Stock), characterize these clients as "pre-orgasmic" rather than inorgasmic.

The most effective treatment to date for pre-orgasmic clients is a program of directed masturbation developed by LoPiccolo and Lobitz (1972). Masturbation has been shown to be the most probable method of producing an orgasm, as well as producing the most intense orgasm (Masters & Johnson, 1966). Learning to masturbate provides accurate proprioceptive feedback, enabling identification of the most effective sexually arousing stimulation techniques. Directed masturbation components includes self-exploration, body awareness, effective self-stimulation training, and the use of "orgasm triggers" (Heiman et al., 1976; LoPiccolo & Lobitz, 1972). The recent book *Come as You Are* (Nagoski, 2015) is very helpful and instructional for clients.

Secondary Female Orgasmic Disorder

A second type of orgasmic dysfunction, which perhaps includes an even larger group than those who have never experienced an orgasm, involves situational or secondary orgasmic dysfunction. Masters and Johnson (1970) use the term *secondary orgasmic dysfunction* to include (a) any woman who was previously able to achieve orgasm from some means of stimulation but who is currently rarely orgasmic, and also to describe (b) any woman who is currently able to attain orgasm only in response to restricted types of stimulation.

The latter category is sometimes seen in clients who have only learned to orgasm with the use of a vibrator, and want to learn how to have orgasms with other forms of stimulation. The label of *secondary inorgasmia* has also been applied to clients with a wide range of sexual functioning, including those who experience orgasm only with strong interfemoral pressure or while lying face-down in bed.

For dependence on vibratory stimulation, the client can go "cold turkey" from using the vibrator, as the intense stimulation provided by vibrators exceeds what is possible from self or partner stimulation. The period of withdrawal is thought to help the brain "reset" to being able to experience less intense stimulation as pleasurable. During this period of withdrawal, employing the directed masturbation treatment program described previously can help the woman client begin to discover other ways of touching herself that can be effective, as her nervous system learns to be able to tune in to less intense stimulation.

The treatment for women who are dependent on only one form of stimulation to orgasm and who want to broaden their repertoire of effective stimulation can follow this procedure as well. It is common for masturbation in positions that allow for greater ease of partner access may feel awkward or unnatural at first, but most clients are able to learn new patterns of arousal.

Many women require clitoral stimulation to reach orgasm, and many do not receive adequate clitoral stimulation to reach orgasm in their sexual relationships, as discussed earlier in this chapter. Inadequate or ineffective stimulation is a rule-out prior to diagnosing female orgasmic disorder. Only a relatively small number of people with vaginas report that they consistently experience orgasm during intercourse. Psychoeducation can help normalize clitoral orgasms.

De-emphasizing goal orientation regarding wanting to have an orgasm in every sexual encounter has been stressed in the sex therapy literature. However, ciswomen as a group have long undersold themselves in many heterosexual relationships by not insisting on adequate stimulation and not putting their sexual pleasure on equal standing with that of their partners. For this reason, the instruction to de-emphasize having orgasm may need to be tempered with the encouragement to feel entitled to the fullest measure of sexual pleasure and satisfaction that is desired by these clients.

Premature Ejaculation

The cause of premature, or early ejaculation, is not well understood. It should be noted that what defines this dysfunction is culturally relative. Many clients hold themselves to unrealistic standards for how long they believe they should last before ejaculation during intercourse. It is important to assess how the client is defining this problem when this is the presenting complaint. For some, anxiety may contribute to worsening this tendency, and for others, having gone a long time without orgasmic release may also contribute.

It is helpful to normalize this condition as existing on a normal continuum of latency to orgasmic threshold. The basic treatment resets the brain to accommodate to a longer period of intensity of stimulation without triggering the orgasmic reflex. Metz and McCarthy (2003) have written an excellent self-help book, *Coping With Premature Ejaculation,* which offers a psychoeducational approach and guidelines that can be used by the client independently, or in conjunction with sex therapy. The major points covered in their book that address the social, cultural, and relational factors associated with erectile problems include the following: premature ejaculation is very common among men (30%), and that with treatment, most clients can learn better control; traditional do-it-yourself techniques (numbing cream, focus on non-sexual thoughts) are often ineffective; the most effective technique is the stop/start technique done first with self-stimulation, then during partner sex (described in their book); realistic expectations are crucial—contrary to cismale bragging and media myths, intercourse seldom lasts longer than 10 minutes, and sex need not end when ejaculation occurs; enjoy and share intimacy, pleasure, orgasm, and afterplay with a partner. There are many more points in the book.

Delayed Ejaculation

Inhibited ejaculation has received very little attention in the therapeutic literature. As initially reported by Masters and Johnson (1970), this remains a relatively rare dysfunction, and the etiology still remains unclear. This dysfunction may be global or situational, with most of these clients being able to ejaculate during masturbation, sometimes with partner stimulation, but most commonly, not during penetrative sexual activity.

Clinical case studies suggest a variety of psychological factors, but there is virtually no supporting empirical research. Inhibited ejaculation can result from physiologic conditions such as multiple sclerosis. Similarly, several medications, including antihypertensives, sedatives, anti-anxiety, and anti-psychotic agents, may have the side effect of preventing ejaculation.

This author (W. Stock) has treated several cases of inhibited ejaculation during sexual interaction with a partner that occurred following a devastating betrayal of trust by a partner. In these cases, addressing the emotional trauma and loss of trust in therapy resulted in remission of inhibited ejaculation. Reducing performance anxiety and increasing physical stimulation remain the major treatment elements for inhibited ejaculation (LoPiccolo, 1977).

Sexual Pain Disorders: Genito-Pelvic Pain Penetration Disorder

Genito-pelvic pain penetration disorder (GPPPD) is a new diagnosis for sexual pain disorders in the *DSM-5* and combines the diagnoses of vaginismus and dyspareunia in the previous version of the *DSM*. GPPPD subsumes a number of diagnoses, including vulvodynia, vaginismus, and non-coital sexual pain disorder.

Vaginismus and dyspareunia may co-exist, or may occur independently of each other, as described in the following. For this reason, these two dysfunctions are discussed separately.

1. Combination of vaginismus and dyspareunia: A medical condition may exist that causes vaginal pain and, when penetration is attempted, the association of pain from penetration can result in a secondary pattern of involuntary, reflexive spastic contraction of the vaginal musculature that renders penetration even more painful or impossible, resulting in a combination of both disorders.
2. Vaginismus alone: A client may exhibit the involuntary spastic contraction of vaginal musculature without any organic pathology that renders penetration difficult or impossible.
3. Dyspareunia alone: A client may have a medical condition that causes pain with genital touch and/or penetration, but does not exhibit spastic contraction of the vaginal musculature. Penetrative activity may be painful but not complicated by tightening of the vaginal opening.

Vaginismus

The term *vaginismus* refers to spastic contraction of the circumvaginal musculature (pubococcygeus or PC muscle), such that the penis, or other objects, cannot be admitted to the vagina without great difficulty and great pain. Vaginismus is distinguished from *dyspareunia,* which refers to pain during coitus from any source other than vaginismus. Vaginismus is sometimes situationspecific. For example, it may be possible for a woman to insert a tampon, but not be able to tolerate a pelvic examination, or be unable to tolerate intercourse or other penetrative activity, in any combination of these presentations. Many women with vaginismus are easily responsive and orgasmic with masturbation and non-penetrative couple activities. It has been suggested that without the imperative of heterosexual intercourse, that vaginismus would be a non-issue. However, if vaginismus prevents regular Pap testing, this could be a life-threatening condition, as early detection of abnormal cervical cells is highly effective in preventing cervical cancer. A gynecologic exam, to the degree possible, is recommended to eliminate the possibility of a co-existing medical condition that requires treatment.

Factors associated with vaginismus include the following:

1. Negative learning history: A history of initial painful penetration that results in subsequent involuntary contraction of the PC muscle during subsequent attempts. Many women have unsuccessfully tried to overcome this condition by attempting to engage in intercourse to overcome the symptom. They often mistakenly think that they need to physically stretch the vaginal opening.
2. History of sexual trauma (rape, childhood sexual abuse)
3. Sexual shame and guilt
4. Fear of pregnancy, fear of contracting sexually transmitted infections
5. Ignorance of sexual anatomy and sexual response: Attempted penetration without sufficient arousal and/or lubrication, for example
6. History of medical conditions that have caused painful penetration in the past (yeast infections, urinary tract infections)
7. Painful childbirth or difficult healing experience from episiotomy or tearing of surrounding tissues: Fear of pain may persist even if conditions have resolved.

If a careful history and pelvic exam have substantiated the diagnosis of vaginismic response to sexual activity, as opposed to dyspareunia, the client may be appropriately treated using sex therapy techniques. The effective treatment element in resolution of vaginismus is a combination of relaxation training, learning to voluntarily contract and relax the PC muscle, and gradual introduction of progressively sized dilators performed under the woman's control at home. The goal of this treatment is to create new learning association between penetration and no pain, rather than continuing to further engrain the previous association between penetration and pain. This technique has nothing to do with stretching the vaginal opening. Instead, it is based on the client learning to relax the PC muscle enough to accommodate an object, gradually, by tensing and relaxing the PC muscle around the dilator, and never forcing an object into the vagina if at all painful. With each tense and relax contraction, the PC muscle relaxes more to be able to accommodate further insertion of the dilator. If there is any pain or discomfort, the client is instructed to stop the exercise, relax via deep breathing, and try once more or on a different day.

This progressive dilation program is extremely effective if the client and partner follow it, without rushing progress to larger dilators, finger insertion, and entry of the penis. Ultimately, the couple (if heterosexual) can then try penile penetration. This best introduced with the client in superior position, so that she can control the pace and depth of penetration. Other factors, including rape, incest, or other sexual trauma, or couple systems issues, may require further therapeutic attention addressing the issues raised by these events, if these emerge during treatment.

Dyspareunia

Dyspareunia refers to pain from genital touch that may include painful penetration, although may not include vaginismus (involuntary contraction of the PC muscle). Medical factors associated with dyspareunia include treated or untreated vaginal infection, history of urinary tract infections associated with spastic urethra or sensitivity at the urethral opening, inflammatory dermatitis, surgical or post-delivery scarring, endometriosis, vulvodynia/vestibulodynia, interstitial cystitis, pelvic floor dysfunction, inadequate vaginal lubrication, estrogen deficiency, or sequalae of medical treatments such as pelvic radiation.

Untreated or persistent yeast or bacterial vaginosis infections can result in intense stinging and burning during and especially after intercourse. Endometriosis can fluctuate during the menstrual cycle, worsening when endometrial tissue enlarges due to higher estrogen during the cycle. Ideally, the client may be able to localize the pain and describe when it is more apparent, hopefully keeping track with a written log.

Childbirth scarring can affect the perineal area, as well as internal scarring from ligament tearing that has healed with scar tissue. Not always obvious during a gynecologic exam, this can become apparent during sexual arousal, when the internal erectile tissue expands and the uterus is normally pulled upward to elongate the vaginal barrel. Adhesions from scar tissue can pull on adjacent tissue during sexual arousal, as scar tissue is not elastic. Education of the client about this possibility can empower them be able to report in concrete terms where and when the pain occurs, and may help avoid the symptoms as being dismissed as entirely psychosomatic. It is crucial for the client to have had adequate assessment, diagnosis, and treatment of medical issues associated with dyspareunia.

Seemingly idiopathic cases may relate to a history of genital pain, and sometimes a history of abuse or sexual trauma.

Treatment of dyspareunia may include (Mindyra, 2021) cognitive behavioral therapy (e.g., relaxation), physical therapy (including psychoeducation on anatomy and the protective role of voluntary muscle contraction), botulinum toxin type A injections (which reduce muscle hyperactivity), prescribed topical treatments, and surgical treatments as a last resort (removing sensitive or painful areas).

SUMMARY

Humans can experience many pleasures, and many difficulties, with sexual activity. The sex therapy field continues to evolve, taking into account the diverse experiences across gender. The New View of Women's Sexual Problems is a more recent and very comprehensive approach assessing factors impacting all genders, including lack of information; lack of access; lack of interest, energy, or time; and erotophobic attitudes, and so on. *The Sexual History Questionnaire* (NSTA, 2019) is one tool to help obtain a comprehensive client sexual health history.

There is a persistent gendered orgasm gap (individuals with clitorises report fewer orgasms overall than individuals with penises). Correcting myths, psychoeducation, and prioritizing sexual pleasure for people with clitorises can help reduce this gap. There are many conditions for good or great sex, for all genders. It is helpful to know what they are for oneself, and communicate needs to others.

For any client seeking sex therapy that also has a history of trauma, it is usually important and more productive to treat the trauma first. Sex therapists may refer these clients for EMDR therapy.

Sensate focus is an important and helpful tool that sex therapists often prescribe to help clients

increase awareness of sensation and communication with their partner.

Clients seeking sex therapy may report symptoms that indicate any of these diagnoses: desire disorders, arousal disorders (erectile disorders), orgasm disorders (pre-orgasmic, premature ejaculation), and genito-pelvic pain penetration disorder (vaginismus or dyspareunia). Sex therapists are trained to treat these disorders. Understanding the broader cultural context in which humans develop their sexual selves is critical to considering a full picture of a particular client's sexual functioning. EMDR clinicians may help sex therapists adjunctly with the processing of any disturbing, traumatic, or difficult material getting in the way of improved sexual functioning.

REFERENCES

Althof, S., Meston, C. M., Perelman, M. A., Handy, A. B., Kilimnik, C. D., & Stanton, A. M. (2017). Opinion paper: On the diagnosis/classification of sexual arousal concerns in women. *Journal of Sexual Medicine, 14*(11), 1365–1371. https://doi.org/10.1016/j.jsxm.2017.08.013

American Psychiatric Association. (2013). *Diagnostic and statistical manual of mental disorders*. (5th ed.). American Psychiatric Publishing.

Basson, R. (2002). Women's sexual desire – disordered or misunderstood? *Journal of Sex Marital Therapy, 28*(Suppl 1), 17–28. https://doi.org/10.1080/00926230252851168

Courtois, C. A. (2004). Complex trauma, complex reactions: Assessment and treatment. *Psychotherapy: Theory, Research, Practice, and Training, 41*, 412-425.

Ehlers, A., & Clark, D. M. (2000). A cognitive model of posttraumatic stress disorder. *Behaviour Research and Therapy, 38*, 319–345. https://doi.org/10.1016/s0005-7967(99)00123-0

Foa, E. B., Keane, T. M., Friedman, M. J., & Cohen, J. A. (Eds.). (2008). *Effective treatments for PTSD: Practice guidelines from the International Society for Traumatic Stress Studies* (2nd ed.). The Guilford Press.

Gage, S. (1981). Chapter 3, The clitoris: A feminist perspective. In *A new view of a woman's body: A fully illustrated guide*. The Federation of Feminist Women's Centers, S. Gage (Illustrator). https://wiki.lereset.org/_media/ateliers:nvwb_clitoris_suzann_gage.pdf

Grey, N., Young, K., & Holmes, E. (2002). Cognitive restructuring within reliving: A treatment for peritraumatic emotional "hotspots" in posttraumatic stress disorder. *Behavioural and Cognitive Psychotherapy, 30*, 37–56. https://doi.org/10.1017/S1352465802001054

Heiman, J., LoPiccolo, L., & LoPiccolo, J. (1976). *Becoming orgasmic: A sexual growth program for women*. Prentice-Hall.

Herbenick, D., Eastman-Mueller, H., Fu, T. C., Dodge, B., Ponander, K., & Sanders, S. A. (2019). Women's sexual satisfaction, communication, and reasons for (no longer) faking orgasm: Findings from a U.S. probability sample. *Archives of Sexual Behavior, 48*(8), 2461–2472. https://doi.org/10.1007/s10508-019-01493-0

Herman, J. L. (1992). Complex PTSD: A syndrome in survivors of prolonged and repeated trauma. *Journal of Traumatic Stress, 3*, 377–391. https://doi.org/10.1002/jts.2490050305

Kachak, E., & Tiefer, L. (Eds.). (2002). *A new view of women's sexual problems*. Haworth Press. [manifesto on pp. 1–8, also available online: http://www.newviewcampaign.org/manifesto3.asp].

Kaplan, H. (1979). *Disorders of sexual desire*. Brunner/Mazel. New York.

Kingsberg, S. A., & Rezaee, R. L. (2013). Hypoactive sexual desire in women. *Menopause, 20*(12), 1284–1300.

Laumann, E., Paik, A., & Rosen, R. C. (1999). Sexual dysfunction in the United States: Prevalence and predictors. *JAMA: Journal of the American Medical Association, 281*(6), 537–544.

Linschoten, M., Weiner, L., & Avery-Clark, C. (2016). Sensate focus: A critical literature review. *Sexual and Relationship Therapy, 31*(2), 230–247. https://doi.org/10.1080/14681994.2015.1127909

LoPiccolo, J. (1977). Direct treatment of sexual dysfunction in the couple. In J. Money & H. Musaph (Eds.), *Handbook of Sexology*. Excerpta Medica.

LoPiccolo, J., & Lobitz, W. (1972). The role of masturbation in the treatment of orgasmic dysfunction. *Archives of Sexual Behavior, 2*, 163–171. https://doi.org/10.1007/BF01541865

LoPiccolo, J., & Stock, W. E. (1986). Treatment of sexual dysfunction. *Journal of Consulting and Clinical Psychology, 54*, 158–167. https://doi.org/10.1037/0022-006X.54.2.158

Maltz, W. (n.d.-a). *Relearning touch*. Retrieved September 15, 2021, from https://healthysex.com/booksdvdsposters/videos/relearning-touch/

Maltz, W. (n.d.-b). *Partners in healing*. Retrieved September 15, 2021, from https://healthysex.com/booksdvdsposters/videos/partners-in-healing/

Maltz, W. (2012). *The sexual healing journey: A guide for survivors of sexual abuse* (3rd ed.). William Morrow/HarperCollins.

Maltz, W., & Holman, B. (1987). *Incest and sexuality: A guide to understanding and healing*. Lexington Books.

Masters, W., & Johnson, V. (1966). *Human sexual response*. Little, Brown.

Masters, W., & Johnson, V. (1970). *Human sexual inadequacy*. Little, Brown.

Masters, W., Johnson, A., & Kolodny, L. (1979). *Textbook of sexual medicine*. Little, Brown.

McCormick, N. B. (1994). *Sexual salvation: Affirming women's sexual rights and pleasures*. Praeger.

Meston, C., & Stanton, A. (2017). Evaluation of female sexual interest/arousal disorder. In W. IsHak (Ed.), *The textbook of clinical sexual medicine* (pp. 155–163). Springer.
Metz, M., & McCarthy, B. (2003). *Coping with premature ejaculation: Overcome PE, please your partner, and have great sex*. New Harbinger Publications.
Metz, M., & McCarthy, B. (2004). *Coping with erectile dysfunction: How to regain confidence and enjoy great sex*. New Harbinger Publications.
Mindyra. (2021). *Female genito-pelvic pain/penetration disorder (GPPPD) in adults*. Mindyra Health Corporation. https://www.mindyra.com/solutions/adults/femalegenito-pelvicpain/penetration
Nagoski, E. (2015). *Come as you are*. Simon & Schuster.
Perelman, M. (2014). The history of sexual medicine. In D.L. Tolman & L.M. Diamond (Eds), *APA handbook of sexuality and psychology: Vol. 2. Contextual approaches* (pp. 137–179). American Psychological Association.
Psychology Tools. (n.d.-a). *What is EMDR?* https://www.psychologytools.com/resource/what-is-emdr/
Psychology Tools. (n.d.-b). *What is trauma-focused cognitive behavioral therapy (TF-CBT)?* https://www.psychologytools.com/resource/what-is-tf-cbt/
Shapiro, F. (2001). *Eye movement desensitization and reprocessing: Basic principles, protocols, and procedures* (2nd ed.). Guilford Press.
Solomon, R. M., & Shapiro, F. (2008). EMDR and the adaptive information processing model: Potential mechanisms of change. *Journal of EMDR Practice and Research, 2*(4), 315–325.
Stock, W. (n.d.). *Sensate focus instructions* (unpublished handout).
Tiefer, L. (1988). A feminist perspective on sexology and sexuality. In M. Gergen (Ed.), *Feminist thought and the structure of knowledge* (pp. 16–26). NYU Press.
Tiefer, L. (1996). Toward a feminist sex therapy. *Women & Therapy, 19*(4), 53–64.
Timberlake, J. C. (2019). *The sexual history questionnaire*. NSTA.
Wade, L. D., Kremer, E. C., & Brown, J. (2005). The incidental orgasm: The presence of clitoral knowledge and the absence of orgasm for women. *Women & Health, 42*(1), 117–138. https://doi.org/10.1300/J013v42n01_07
Zilbergeld, B. (1978). *Male sexuality: A guide to sexual fulfillment*. Little, Brown & Company.

SUPPLEMENTAL MATERIALS FOR CLINICIANS

SEXUAL HISTORY QUESTIONNAIRE

Northampton Sex Therapy, LLC

40 Main Street, Suite 103
Florence MA 01062 / 413-587-0095
Northamptonsextherapy.com

Client Name:
Date(s) of Administration:

CURRENT CONCERN

What prompted you to come at this point for therapy?
Who initiated seeking therapy?
Have you seen therapists previously? What were your experiences with these professionals?

DESIRED OUTCOME

What is your primary goal for our work together?
If therapy is successful, what will you be able to do that you are unable to do now?
How will this change anything in your current life, relationship, personality, or partner's personality?
What significance does the problem have with respect to your own sexual functioning? How does the problem affect your partner's sexual functioning?

HISTORY OF CONCERN

When did the problem first occur? What was happening in your life at that time?
(If there is more than one problem, or both/all partners have a problem): Which problem do you recall as having developed first?

Is there any situation in which the problem improves?
When does the problem occur? Is there anything that makes it worse?

SEXUAL HISTORY

Contact with other children:

As a child, did you engage in sexual play or exploration with other children? Describe where and how you did this.
How often did you do this?
Who initiated these games? What role(s) did you play?
How did you feel about doing this?
Were you ever caught doing this? What happened?
What was your major source for information about sex?
In what ways has your religion and family background influenced your attitudes toward sex? Were you allowed to ask questions?
What was the age of your first sexual feeling (in whatever way you define that)?

MASTURBATION

At what age did you first experiment with masturbation? How old were you when you first masturbated? Where were you and what did you do?
With what frequency did you masturbate in your teens?
How did you learn about masturbation?
How did you feel about masturbation?
What techniques have you used for masturbation?
How often do you currently masturbate?
Are you able to talk with your partner about self-pleasuring/masturbation?

UNWELCOME SEXUAL CONTACT/ABUSIVE BEHAVIORS

As a child, did anyone ever touch you, or make you touch them, in a way that made you uncomfortable either at the time or looking back on it now?
Did anyone ever make sexual comments to you or comment on your body in a way that made you uncomfortable, then or now?
Did you have any sexual contact with adolescents or adults? Were you forced or coerced to have sex against your will?
Did you ever sexually touch other children your own age in a way that was upsetting to them at the time? Were you aware that what you were doing might be upsetting?
What words or label do you use to describe these experiences?
Did you ever tell anyone else about any of these experiences? What happened when you did?

Was there ever hitting, biting, pushing, shoving, slapping, or other physical aggression toward you, siblings, or a parent in your home? Could you describe this?

Were there any upsetting experiences related to sex as a child that we have not discussed? If so, could you describe them?

PUBERTY AND ADOLESCENCE (AGES 10–20)

Body changes for adolescents assigned female at birth:

When did you first notice your breasts beginning to develop? Were you the first person to notice? How did it come to your attention?

Did you experience breast development earlier, later, or about the same as most of your friends?

How did you feel about your developing breasts? How did others react?

Did you have erotic dreams as an adolescent? If yes, was there a theme to them? When did you begin to menstruate? Describe the circumstances when it first occurred.

Had you been taught about menstruation in advance? By whom?

Was this information shared with one or more family members? With whom?

Was it discussed among your friends? What were your feelings about the possibility of beginning to menstruate? Were you earlier, later, or about the same as most of your friends?

Did you develop a regular menstrual cycle? How long did this take? Have you had any menstrual difficulties?

Have you had sex during your period, or during the period of a partner who menstruates? How do you feel about this?

How did you feel when you first learned that some people have nocturnal emissions ("wet dreams")?

Body changes for adolescents assigned male at birth:

How old were you when your voice began to change? How did you feel about it? How long did it take to settle into your adult range?

How old were you when you had your first nocturnal emission ("wet dream")? How did you react? Had you been taught about these in advance? By whom?

Was this information shared with one or more family members? With whom? Did you take steps to conceal the evidence of your wet dreams?

Did you have any problems with the developments of puberty?

How did you feel when you first learned that some people have menstrual periods?

Have you ever had sex with someone who menstruates while they were having their period?

How do you feel about this idea?

Body changes for all:

How and when did your body change during puberty?
How did you feel about these changes?
Were these changes what you expected or hoped for?
How did you feel about your height, weight, hair, skin?
How are your feelings about your body connected to your race, ethnicity, culture, and so on? Did you engage in attempts to change or control your weight while you were growing up?
How did you feel about this? How was your family involved in noticing, commenting on, or trying to control your weight?
Did the body changes you experienced during adolescence bring up any concerns for you about your gender identity or gender presentation?

ADOLESCENT DATING BEHAVIOR

How would you describe your junior/senior high school social life? Were most of your friends male, female, or other genders?
At what age did you start to notice the sexual development of your peers? How did you feel about it?
At what age did you start to date? In groups? On single dates? Did you date same sex partners, different sex partners, or a variety? Did your parents allow dating or did you have to take steps to conceal it?
How did you feel about the dating behavior of your peers?
Did you date many different people or did you usually have a steady relationship with one person at a time? How old were you when you had your first steady relationship? How old was your partner, and what was their gender?
How did your social life change when you left home or went to college?

ADOLESCENT GENDER JOURNEY

How did your sense of your gender change, stabilize, or evolve during adolescence?
Did you talk to anyone about the thoughts and feelings you were having about your gender? How did they respond?
How did you cope with any negative or confused feelings you had about your gender during this time? Did you seek any medical or counseling support? What was that experience like?
Did your behaviors and gender presentation during adolescence match with the expectations those around you had for someone of the gender assigned to you? If yes, what was that like for you? If no, what was that like for you?
Were you ever targeted for harassment or violence because of your gender or gender presentation in adolescence?

Did anyone ever suggest that the adults in your life should try to change or affirm your gender presentation and/or gender identity? What happened?

FOR SEXUAL AND GENDER MINORITY CLIENTS

At what age did you first begin to identify yourself as potentially "different" in terms of your sexuality or gender?
At what age did you become aware of others who might be like you?
At what age did you acknowledge that you might be [your sexual orientation], or [your gender]? At what age did you decide to tell someone else? Whom did you choose to tell first? How did they respond? What was that like for you?
Can you talk about what the process of coming out to yourself and others was like during adolescence? Who knew and who did not know?
How did your close friends respond if and when they knew?
How did people in your school environment respond if and when they knew? Were you ever the victim of intimidation or violence at school? Who could you talk to about this?
Who else was supportive of you during this time?
How was your family life affected by your sexual or gender identity?
Were you able to date and engage in sexual activity with partners of your preferred gender(s)?
How were you able to express your sexual or gender identity at this time? What was it like to live in your community as a sexual or gender minority?
What else should I know about your experiences with sexuality and gender as an adolescent?

ADULT GENDER JOURNEY

How has your sense of your gender changed, stabilized, or evolved during adulthood?
Have you talked to anyone about the thoughts and feelings you were having about your gender? How did they respond?
How have you coped with any negative or confused feelings you have/had about your gender during adulthood? Did you seek any medical or counseling support? What was that experience like?
Have your behaviors and gender presentation during adulthood matched with the expectations those around you had for someone of the gender assigned to you? If yes, what was that like for you? If no, what was that like for you?
Have you ever been targeted for harassment or violence because of your gender or gender presentation in adulthood?
Did anyone ever suggest that you should try to change or affirm your gender presentation and/or gender identity? What happened?

At this time, do you have any desire to change anything about your lived gender identity or your gender presentation? What, if anything, do you think you might do about that?

UNWELCOME SEXUAL CONTACT/ABUSIVE BEHAVIORS

As an adolescent, did anyone ever touch you, or make you touch them, in a way that made you uncomfortable either at the time or looking back on it now?
Did anyone ever make sexual comments to you or comment on your body in a way that made you uncomfortable, then or now?
Did you have any sexual contact that you did not want at the time?
Were you forced or coerced to have sex against your will?
Did you ever feel taken advantage of sexually?
Did you ever sexually touch other adolescents in a way which was upsetting to them at the time?
Were you aware that what you were doing might be upsetting?
What words or labels do you use to describe these experiences?
Did you ever tell anyone else about any of these experiences? What happened when you did?
Was there ever hitting, biting, pushing, shoving, slapping, or other physical aggression toward you from an intimate partner? Could you describe this?
Were there any upsetting experiences related to sex as an adolescent that we have not discussed? If so, could you describe them?

ADULTHOOD (AGE 20 TO PRESENT)

Current attitudes toward sex:

How would you describe your attitude toward sex and your own sexuality at present?
What specific aspects of sex are enjoyable to you?
What aspects do you dislike or find unpleasant?
Is there anything about your current sexual life that causes you to feel guilty or distressed? What are your beliefs about the purpose of sex?
How important is sexual pleasure?
How important is procreation?
What is the importance of sex in your life?

What is your current attitude toward each of the following:

- Your genitals, your partner's(') genitals
- Menstruation
- Vaginal secretions
- Semen
- Masturbation

- Fellatio ("blowjobs")
- Cunnilingus ("eating pussy")
- Foreplay
- Penetrative sex
- Anal penetration or intercourse
- Sexual fantasy
- Adult films/pornography
- Erotic literature
- Sex toys
- Nudity
- Bondage and discipline, dominance and submission, sadism, and masochism

FANTASY

Have your fantasies changed significantly over the course of your adult life? How frequently do you engage in sexual fantasy currently?
What kinds of fantasies are most frequent for you at this time?
Are you comfortable with the content of your fantasies?
Who can you share your sexual fantasies with?

MENOPAUSE

Type of hormone supplement used, if any: _____
For how long? Was it prescribed or over the counter?
What are any concerns you may have about being pre-/peri-/post-menopausal?

ORGASM

What have been your experiences with orgasm?
Alone?
With a partner?
Would time seem wasted without an orgasm with a partner?

BODY IMAGE

How did and how do you feel about your body? Please talk about how you felt as a child, growing up, as a young adult, and now.
How would you *like* to feel about your body?
Does the way you feel about your body impact your enjoyment of sex?

PAINFUL SEX

Have you ever experienced pain during sex play?

If yes, please describe the nature of that pain.
What have you done to address this issue?

HISTORY OF SEXUAL EXPERIENCES AND RELATIONSHIPS

Describe the history of your sexual relationships. Talk about the number of partners, what sexual activities you have experienced, and the issues and conflicts that have emerged for you in intimate relationships. If you have had a "type" please describe that type:

IF CURRENTLY PARTNERED

How many emotional partners do you have? How many sexual partners? How do you define the boundaries of your current relationship(s)?
What label(s) do you use to describe the relationship(s)?
If you are in a current relationship, how often do you and your partner(s) have affectionate non-sexual contact? Is that enough for you? For your partner(s)?
How attractive do you think you are on a scale of 1 to 10? _____
How attracted are you to your partner(s) on a scale of 1 to 10? _____
How attracted do you think your partner(s) is/are to you?
How do you feel about your own body?
If you are in a relationship, how do you feel about your partner(s)' body(ies)? How do you imagine your partner(s) feel(s) about your body?
How are these feelings communicated?
Are you ever criticized or shamed by a partner about your body?
Does anyone in your life try to control how your body looks?
How comfortable are you with your sexual orientation?
Have you ever thought you might like to have a relationship or sexual contact with someone of another gender?
Have you discussed this with anyone?
Is it something you have seriously considered acting on?
Have any of your partners experienced such feelings?
How has this affected the relationship?
How much conflict is there in your relationship(s)? How well do you each deal with conflict?
What kinds of stressors are you experiencing currently in your lives that might affect your sexual or emotional relationship(s)?
If you are currently in a long-standing relationship, how has sex changed over the course of the relationship?
Why do you think it has changed?
How do you and your partner(s) feel about this?
If you are currently in a long-standing relationship, have you ever been sexually involved with another person outside of the boundaries of the relationship(s)?

How many times? For how long?

How did you feel about this?

Did your partner(s) know about the outside relationship?

What effect has this activity had on your relationship(s)?

What was the purpose or meaning of the outside sexual activity?

Has/have your partner(s) ever been sexually involved with another person outside the boundaries of the relationship?

Did you know about it at the time? How did you feel about this?

What effect has this activity had on your relationship(s)?

What was the purpose or meaning of the outside sexual activity?

Describe any feelings you may have about having sexual contact with your present or possible sexual partner(s).

Describe your present sexual interactions, such as penetrative sex or masturbation, turn ons, your present pattern for sexual pleasure, frequency of sexual interactions, your current number of partners, and so on. (Do partners cuddle, hug, spoon, kiss hello/goodbye. Who initiates what kinds of touch?)

Do you feel you most often "give your best" when having sex with your partner(s)?

Are you proud of the way you express your feelings toward your partner(s) at this time? If not, what's missing in your opinion?

Do you WANT your partner(s) during sex or just "want sex"?

Do you WANT to be aroused and involved sexually?

What would you like from an ideal sexual partner, or your current partner? What would you be willing to give to such a partner?

Do you tell your partner what pleases you most sexually? What displeases you?

What do you want most in the way of attitude, behaviors, and so on from your partner that they do not provide you now?

What attitudes or behaviors do you receive from your partner that you value the most?

What attracts, excites, and stimulates you sexually? Describe the situation you find most desirable and stimulating for being sexual?

What trait, behavior, or habit does your partner have which tends to diminish your sexual feeling for them?

Are you interested in sexual practices that include power and pain play, that is, dominance/submission/bondage?

Do you look at pornography? If so, with what frequency? Do you use pornography to masturbate? What kinds of pornography do you enjoy?

Specific sexual acts:

Do you or your partner have sex with more than one person at a time? If yes, do you usually do so together, or separately?

Do you ever use sex toys during your sexual activity? What kind, and how do you use them? How often?

Do you read erotic or pornographic books or magazines, or watch adult erotic or pornographic videos?
How often?
Is/are your partner(s) aware of this? How do they feel about it?
Do you ever share these materials with your partner(s)?
Do you visit adult websites? How often?
What activities do you engage in online?
Is/are your partner(s) aware of this?
How do they feel about it?
How do you feel about your partner's(') use of erotic or pornographic materials or adult websites?
Do you or your partner(s) ever prefer to dress in certain clothing (such as clothing of another gender or costumes) or materials (such as rubber or leather) for the purposes of sexual enhancement?
Who else knows about this?
How does this affect the relationship?
Do you engage in activities that you would describe as "kinky" or ? What activities? Describe them. How often do you engage in them? bondage and discipline, dominance and submission, sadism, and masochism
How do you feel about this activity?
Is/are your partner(s) aware of this? How do they feel about it?
Do they engage in these activities with you?
Have you ever engaged in sexual activities for money, including exotic dancing, posing for photos, engaging in sexual acts, working a phone sex line, engaging in online sexual activities?
For how long? How often?
Describe what activities you engaged in.
How do you feel about this activity?
Is your partner aware of this? How do they feel about it?
Have you ever paid money for sexual activities or services, including hiring an escort, hiring a sex worker or prostitute, "erotic massage with release," purchasing subscriptions to adult websites, phone sex lines, paying for bondage and discipline, dominance and dubmission, sadism and masochism activities?
How often? How do you feel about this activity?
Is your partner aware of this? How do they feel about it?
Are there other specific activities I have not asked about that are an important part of your sexual life?

ALCOHOL/SUBSTANCE USE

How often and how much do you (and does your partner) drink/use?
Do either you or your partner smoke? How much?

Do you use recreational drugs? What kinds, how much, and how often? Have you ever had a blackout or memory loss while drinking/using?

SEXUAL HEALTH

Are you currently seeing a body worker, e.g., chiropractor, acupuncturist, physical therapist?
If yes, please describe the nature of your physical discomfort:
Do you have any pre-existing medical conditions that may affect your sexuality (e.g., diabetes, hypertension, heart disease)? Are you currently taking any prescribed medications (such as for hypertension, diabetes, depression, anxiety, or cardiovascular disease)? If yes, list: _____
What medications or drugs, including over the counter drugs and herbal supplements, do you use?
How has HIV/AIDS or other sexually transmitted infections impacted your sexual activity?
Do you know about safer sex practices? To what extent do you engage in safer sex? Why or why not?
Have you or your partner(s) ever experienced an unwanted pregnancy? What happened?
How was the decision made about what to do?
How do you feel about that?
Do you have any worries or concerns about your sexual health and well-being as an adult?
Who can you go to for information or feedback?
Do you have any disabilities or other physical or mental conditions that affect your ability to function sexually?
Do you require assistance from a partner or caregiver in order to participate in sexual activity with yourself or a partner?
Are you able to get assistance when you need it?
Do you have sufficient privacy and adaptive equipment for the sexual activities you want to engage in?
Are you noticing any effects of aging on your body and your sexual activity?

Any other information:

Describe anything else related to your past or present experiences. Include anything that may be important for me to know, so that I may assist you in reaching your sexual goals.

4

Applying EMDR Therapy to Sexual Health Targets

Stephanie Baird, LMHC

LEARNING OBJECTIVES

- EMDR clinicians are provided an overview of the EMDR therapy basic protocol Phases 1–8 as it relates to sexual health.
- EMDR clinicians obtain an overview of helpful resources for sexual health, including new resources such as the *Bubble Boundary* and Nancy Simon's *Self-Compassion Container* (available at the end of this chapter, formatted for photocopying).
- EMDR clinicians learn about positive and negative sexuality-related cognitions.
- EMDR past and present targets relating to sexual trauma/abuse, molestation, sexual disgust, orgasmic and other sexual difficulties are explored.
- The most helpful excerpts from the EMDR Protocol for Sexual Dysfunction (previously published in Springer Publishing's *EMDR Scripted Protocol: Special Populations* [Pillai-Friedman, 2009]) are provided.
- Numerous EMDR therapy and sexual health case studies are provided to illustrate this integration.
- "Out of control" sexual behaviors are discussed and Robert Miller, PhD, provides information and case studies regarding his *The Feeling-State Addiction Protocol*.

- EMDR clinicians learn about resources to assist in managing potential complex dissociative symptoms.

THE STANDARD EMDR THERAPY PROTOCOL AND SEXUAL HEALTH

Introduction

Now that current basic sexual health and sex therapy information has been provided, we can more fully explore and integrate sexual health with EMDR therapy. Since this book is directed to EMDR trained clinicians, I will briefly summarize the eight phases, discussing how sexual health can be addressed and integrated at each phase. Please refer to your training manuals, texts, and books by Francine Shapiro, Andrew Leeds, Marilyn Luber, and others for much more detailed explanations of the eight phases, including issues that may arise. These authors and several others have written extensively on the phases.

Sabitha Pillai-Friedman has developed the wonderfully specific and extensive *EMDR Sexual Dysfunction Protocol* for addressing reported sexual dysfunction. Previously published in Luber's *Eye Movement Desensitization and Reprocessing (EMDR) Scripted Protocols: Special Populations* (2009), please go to the Supplementary Files page offered as a companion to this book at https://connect.springerpub.com/content/book/978-0-8261-8676-8. Pillai-Friedman's 3-Pronged Protocol addresses sexual trauma in the past, present, and future. Most often, clients report feeling decreased reactivity and increased feelings of confidence after processing past sexual traumas. The current triggers offer clients a chance to process on-going reactivity to everyday triggers that compromise sexual functioning. At this point, the client has reached a point of neutrality when all negative responses to past and present events have been processed (Pillai-Friedman, 2009).

Some of her important points are integrated throughout this section.

Guidelines for Working With Clients While Processing Issues of Sexual Dysfunction

These helpful guidelines are from Pillai-Friedman's EMDR Sexual Dysfunction Protocol.

> Clients undergoing EMDR treatment for sexual dysfunction may often feel anxious and vulnerable during their sessions. This may be because the act of processing certain sexual events may trigger physical arousal that may lead to feelings of embarrassment and anxiety. It is important for the practitioner to establish a comfortable and safe relationship with the client before beginning EMDR treatment. There are certain guidelines that an EMDR practitioner needs to follow during the use of this protocol. Since the physical

proximity of the practitioner may activate arousal or anxiety, it is important to use a longer cord for the EMDR (theratappers) or headphones and maintain some physical distance from the clients during EMDR sessions. It is also useful for the practitioner to maintain a uniformly professional and neutral voice during the session. It may also help to prepare clients by letting them know that he or she may experience some arousal during the EMDR session and that it is normal. (Pillai-Friedman, 2009)

Phase 1: Client History and Treatment Planning

Phase 1 can often be accomplished during the intake session(s) and involves obtaining basic background information and assessing for readiness and timeliness of EMDR. I use a checklist with each client where I assess for any interfering medical conditions, major life or work transitions or issues, as well as administer the Dissociative Experiences Scale or the Adolescent-Dissociative Experiences Scale (Bernstein & Putnam, 1986; Frischholz et al., 1990) to check for any symptoms of dissociation. I also provide clients with Luber's *Handbook for EMDR Clients* (2001). This booklet explains EMDR therapy thoroughly, in layperson's terms, and has a section for the client to complete, including the top 10 positive and top 10 negative memories. These memories can be geared toward sexual history. The client may also opt to complete any difficult questions in session with you, to avoid triggering distress outside of the session.

Additionally, if a client mentions a sexuality-related concern when they contact you, you may want to introduce the Sexual History Questionnaire at this time (shared in Chapter 3). Depending on the client's history, this questionnaire can take anywhere from a partial session to several sessions to complete. However, many relevant EMDR targets may emerge as you progress through the categories, informing your treatment plan. Be sure to check for verbally informed consent to administer this very detailed and possibly invasively perceived questionnaire, assuring your client that they can skip questions or wait until more rapport has been established, if so desired. Depending on their comfort level and regulation skills, another option is having your client complete this questionnaire on their own, possibly saving more time.

As you take your client's history, look for any dysfunctional behaviors and symptoms that the client wishes to address. You will ultimately make a timeline for disturbing events and behaviors, past and present, which will form the outline for your EMDR work. Because therapeutic rapport has not yet been established, be careful with how much detail you gather regarding EMDR targets. During these initial meetings I write a list of targets that emerge, keeping this list very superficial with the "headlines" and ages of these targets. Take caution in activating emotional dysregulation during this phase, as EMDR resourcing has yet to occur. You can also ask about any positive sexual experiences for comparison.

Once further rapport and resourcing has been established, you can consider using the "Float-Back Technique" to look for any difficult to identify earlier targets. Adapted from Watkins and Watkins's Affect Bridge (1998), the "Float-Back elicits connections with any relevant sensory data that is prominent for the client such as earlier thoughts or beliefs, sensations, affect, smells, tastes, sounds, and so forth. Use the most relevant Float-Back Technique for your client" (Pillai-Friedman, 2009).

For "earlier thoughts or beliefs about the self" concerning the incident, have them use the Float-Back:

- Say, "*Think of _____ (state the issue that you are working on). Now notice what thoughts or negative beliefs you have connected with this issue and just let your mind float back to an earlier time in your life when you had those thoughts or negative beliefs about yourself, allow those thoughts to flow into your consciousness easily, just let your mind float back and tell me the earliest scene that comes to mind*" (Pillai-Friedman, 2009)
  Pause
- Say, "*What comes to mind?*_____
  _____ Or use the Float-Back to elicit connections to earlier sensations,
- Say, "*Think of _____ (state the issue that you are working on). Now notice what sensations you are feeling and just let your mind float back to an earlier time in your life when you had those sensations, allow those thoughts to flow into your consciousness easily, just let your mind float back and tell me the earliest scene that comes to mind*" (Pillai-Friedman, 2009).
  Pause
- Say, "*What comes to mind?*"
  "From this point it is helpful to create a comprehensive plan with your client to be clear about the goals in treatment. The next step is to choose the first memory to work on. Usually, if it is appropriate, encourage the patient to choose the earliest memory that relates to the dysfunction or sexual problem and create a targeting sequence plan that consists of all the connections or incidents that the client remembers" (Pillai-Friedman, 2009).

As mentioned previously, the main impetus for this book is the lack of sexual health addressed with EMDR clients, many of whom seek treatment for what can be considered sexual health-related targets like sexual assault and molestation. If your client has contacted you with the seemingly straightforward request to "deal with sexual assault trauma," you have a major opportunity to give the client permission to look beyond the trauma into overall sexual functioning. This can easily be integrated into Phase 1 as you ask questions such as, "How has this sexual assault affected your current sexual functioning?" or "once we work through the sexual assault, with your permission I'd like to check in about your sexual health. I'd like to make sure you are as empowered as possible in embracing optimal sexual health."

Phase 2: Preparation and Resourcing

The clinician may need to address secondary gain issues. What does the client have to lose if the sexual dysfunction is resolved? During this phase it is also important to prepare clients for the possibility that they may become sexually aroused during the EMDR sessions. Clients need to know it is quite normal and that there is no need to feel guilty (or ashamed) as a result. Processing sexual trauma may also affect their sexual relationship with their partner between sessions. They experience an increase or decrease in desire or experience flashbacks during sex. These reactions are normal and will get resolved as progress is made through continued EMDR sessions. (Pillai-Friedman, 2009)

For all EMDR clients, it is critical to make sure they have adequate emotional, mental, and physical resources available as they journey through EMDR therapy. Spiritual resources may also be helpful for some clients (Chapter 10 has more information). I use another checklist for this task, taking the client through several or all of these guided imagery exercises to help establish and/or intensify relaxation and coping skills.

Here is my checklist of resources I use to establish regulation and soothing. This list is by no means exhaustive as new resourcing continues to be developed.

1. ***Calm Place*** (instructed during EMDR Basic Training). Make sure you use the word "calm" or "soothing" to help your client develop this place, as the word "safe" can be triggering, especially for sexual assault/abuse survivors abused by attachment and/or caregiver figures.

2. ***Container.*** There are several versions of this containment imagery exercise out there, all searchable via Google. The purpose of this exercise is to help the client learn to contain these disturbing events in one mental place between EMDR sessions, thereby reducing the amount of disturbance of these targets in their daily life. The container is NOT about sweeping material under the rug or forgetting about the past. It is a skill to help your client attain more facility regarding when they would like to work on the disturbing material. The version I enjoy utilizing contains these elements:
   a. Invite your client to visualize a container that is strong and big enough to hold all of the disturbing material (both the targets they may and may not know about). Clients often pick things like filing cabinets, bookshelves, chests or trunks, safes, oil drums, Tupperware containers, dumpsters, and so forth.
   b. Provide slow to medium Bilateral Stimulation (BLS) while your client visualizes representations of the disturbing material going into the container. Have the client imagine this material as things like "file folders" of information, closed "books," pieces of paper, or liquid or smoke going into the container.

c. Have your client describe the container once more, now with all the material inside.
d. Invite your client to place a valve or slot that allows for one target/event to be removed, without disturbing the remaining contents.
e. Have your client notice a sign that says "to be opened when it serves my healing."
f. Have your client notice what percentage of material went into the container (as close to 100% as possible is preferred) and what form the material inhabits (paper, smoke, photos, etc.).
g. Have your client notice any positive emotions resulting from containing this material (e.g., relief, hope). Notice the body sensations that accompany this emotion (e.g., looser shoulders, chest, abdomen).
h. Reinforce successfully containing the disturbing material by intensifying the positive emotion, body sensation, and container imagery with slow to medium BLS.

Variations: Your client might want to obtain a literal physical version of this container (i.e., a real Tupperware or glass jar) and place words/objects representing the disturbing events inside. If you notice that your client has a lot of anxiety or daily worries, you might help them develop a second container for such daily worries that they can empty worrisome thoughts into at night before bed. For clients seeking treatment for sexuality-related concerns, they might benefit from sexuality-specific container for these targets.

3. *Resource Development Installation* (RDI; instructed during EMDR Basic Training). This general open-ended resource is excellent for guiding clients to develop a "team of resources" or helpful concepts like courage, strength, empowerment, and/or connection.

4. *Bubble/Shield Boundary Resource*. I developed this resource in 2017 for the many clients that reported trouble dealing with toxic individuals or situations. I find this to also be helpful with clients navigating the dating world and coming into contact with people potentially attempting to cross their sexual boundaries.

The Steps (most of these will be verbalized to your client):
a. Sometimes we need to enter a situation that we anticipate may be emotionally charged or toxic, or we simply want to increase our boundaries. We can use imagery and BLS to help.
b. Think of an image of a boundary around you, perhaps a bubble, shield, and/or armor, which will help protect you from negativity and toxicity. It might be invisible, or made of metal. Whatever you imagine is fine.
c. Image: _____.
d. I'll now apply BLS while you continue to describe the boundary with as much detail as possible. *(Slow to medium BLS now, and whenever BLS is indicated)*

Chapter 4   Applying EMDR Therapy to Sexual Health Targets

e. You may still want positive things to pass through this bubble/shield and find their way to your mind/body. *What mechanism* would allow positive things (compliments, good energy, etc.) to pass through? Perhaps a screen that only filters positive or neutral things through the shield?
f. Now describe your boundary again, with as much detail as you can, including the screen device. *(BLS on)*
g. Repeat after me, *"I am strengthening my boundaries."* *(BLS off)*
h. How do you feel, now that we have strengthened your boundary with this (bubble/shield/ armor)? _____ (what emotion?)
i. *(BLS on)* Once more, recall the image of developing and installing your _____. Become aware of the emotion of _____ and notice in your body where there are sensations that accompany this emotion. *(BLS off)*
What is the sensation _____ and its location _____?
j. *(BLS on)* As you see yourself strengthening your boundaries you become aware of the sensation of _____ in your _____ that tells you are experiencing feeling _____. Please repeat after me: _____ *in my* _____ *tells me I am experiencing* _____.
Now take a few slower, deeper breaths, experiencing the _____ *(power, protection, security, confidence, etc.)* that comes from increasing your boundaries and protection. *(BLS off)*
k. For added strength you can have your client bring up a low lever toxic situation (e.g., staff meeting with a toxic boss) and practice holding the boundary in place, using BLS.
l. Practice daily or as needed. The client can also do a drawing or collage of their boundary.

5. *The Self-Compassion* Container* (Developed by Nancy Simons, LMHC, 2018).

Originally developed for Sand Tray Therapy, Simons (EMDRIA-approved consultant) has also adapted her resource for EMDR therapy. Simons says, "The Self-Compassion Container exercise is a manifestation of our inner landscape, a landscape that holds the qualities of self-kindness, acceptance and shared humanity (Kristen Neff's components of self-compassion) … guiding us to wellness" (Simons, personal communication, May 5, 2021). I find this resource very helpful for our clients who have survived sexual trauma and frequently mention shame.
*First provide clients with psychoeducation on self-compassion.

Self-Compassion Guided Visualization Script

- Using guided visualization, we will develop a Self-Compassion Container. I will have you bring to mind a new container and then we will

design the inside space of the container. This container will be used to hold any negative thoughts, feelings, and body images that are connected to your trauma history and still trouble you today. We are designing a container that has the three qualities of self-compassion: *self-kindness, mindful awareness,* and *common humanity.*
- Use whatever technique (e.g., calm place) you prefer to guide your client into a settled place with present awareness.
- Take a few moments and begin to see what image appears for you when think about a self-compassion container. _____
_____
- The inside of the container is very important. Let's design the space so that you can see all the qualities of your self-compassion: self-kindness, mindfulness, and common humanity.
- For *self-kindness* I would like you to imagine an interior environment that can hold difficult thoughts and feelings in a gentle, caring, and supportive way. Sometimes people think about having special material like velvet or sand or cotton balls. Just think about self-kindness and notice what image comes up for you. When you see what that is, and without opening your eyes, tell me what you see.
- Let's develop an image for the quality of mindful awareness. Can you think of an image that will help you connect to your own ability to be mindful, that quality that allows you to just notice negative thoughts and feelings without getting stuck on them? Sometimes people think of this like puffy clouds in the sky floating by or a carousel going around. Just notice what comes to mind for you now. Stay with the image and without opening your eyes tell me what you notice.
- Now let's develop an image for the quality of common humanity. This is the ability to recognize that it is human nature to feel pain and that we are just like everyone else when we feel pain and that all people feel pain even if they don't always show it. Some ideas that other people have used are a picture of the globe or a web of light. Just notice what comes to mind for you now. Stay with the image and without opening your eyes tell me what you notice.
- (*Can apply slow BLS*) Try imagining that container resting within you; it could be in any part of your body; your head, your heart, your belly, your hands or even your feet. Tell me what you notice now.... (*End BLS*)
- Let's practice using the container. Think of a difficult experience that happened recently that on a scale of 0 to 10 is no greater than a 3. _____
- What is the negative belief about yourself that goes along with that experience? _____
- What are the negative emotions that go along with that experience? _____
- What do you feel in your body in relation to that experience? _____

Chapter 4   Applying EMDR Therapy to Sexual Health Targets

- Now, think about your container of self-compassion. (*Therapist can read a complete description to the client.*) I want you to imagine putting into this container any of the distress you just described to me. It can go in any way you want.
- (*Can apply medium BLS*) Take a moment to see what it feels like to offer this distress self-compassion; notice what is like to offer this distress an environment of self-kindness, a space to accept distress rather than always working so hard to push it away or avoid it. Notice how you are giving yourself a moment to see that this suffering that you have, no matter how big or small it is, makes you human. (*End BLS*)
- We will continue to use this Self-Compassion Container throughout the course of your EMDR treatment.
- Discuss what came up during this exercise. Sometimes people notice judgmental thoughts or self-doubt. You can encourage them to go back and notice those thoughts also belong in the container. Part of self-compassion is acceptance of what is—even the difficult thoughts that may emerge as you practice the Self-Compassion Container exercise.

6. *The Spiral.* This imagery resource, often learned in EMDR Basic Training, can quickly reduce body disturbance and is especially helpful if your client is reporting a disturbing sensation (either unwanted arousal or pain) in the genitals or other sexuality-related organs.
   The Steps:
   - When something is bugging/disturbing you, notice where you feel it in your body.
   - This is a form of energy. Notice the movement and imagine it as a spiral.
   - Is it spinning clockwise or counterclockwise?
   - Now make it spin in the opposite direction (can have the client hold theratappers and use slow BLS).

7. *The Lightstream.* This imagery technique was developed by Francine Shapiro and is often included in EMDR Basic Training. The Lightstream is helpful for calming body disturbances and pain, including sexuality-related disturbances (Shapiro, 2012).

Phase 3: Assessment

Once it has been established that your client can handle varying levels of emotional disturbance, finalize the timeline of EMDR targets, if you have not yet done so. This is a great opportunity to quickly go through the "headlines," particularly those related to sexual health, and determine your first target for EMDR processing, preferably the earliest target on the list. Always make sure your client knows they can ask for a time-out or not continue EMDR in a particular session, or any other session. This reminder of their being in charge is a great opportunity to help reinforce boundaries, consent, autonomy and agency.

- Once the target has been chosen, ask your client for the worst *image* associated with the target. If they indicate shame or embarrassment, particularly if due to a sexual nature, assure them that they can keep the image in their minds without revealing it to you (also known as "blind to the therapist").
- Next, help them determine a *negative cognition* (NC) about themselves that relates to this image. Possible sexual health related NCs are listed in a following section.
- Ask them for a positive cognition (PC) they would rather have about themselves regarding this event. Often these PCs can be directly opposite to the NCs. Possible sexual health related PCs are listed the section that follows.
- Have them bring up the image, then rate the Validity of Cognition (VOC) of this PC using the 1 to 7 Likert scale you learned about in your EMDR training.
- Have them bring up the image and NC, and ask about any *emotions* coming up now.
- Ask them to rate the current intensity of disturbance using the 11-point Subjective Units of Disturbance (SUD) scale you learned about in your EMDR training.
- Ask them where in their *bodies* are they experiencing those emotions.

Phase 4: Desensitization

Desensitization of the target occurs in this phase. Ask the client to bring up the image and the NCs, and notice where they feel this in their body. Provide 25 to 45 fast BLS sets. After each set ask them to take a breath, let it go, and report to you what they are noticing. Continue with as many sets as necessary until no new material arises.

If the client discloses or demonstrates embarrassment at the content of material (possible with sexuality-related content), they can be encouraged to report body sensations or emotions, keeping the details to themselves. Also reassure your client of your own comfort level (hopefully very capable) in hearing potentially troubling sexual material.

Once no new material comes up, check the SUDs. The SUDs should be a zero or an ecologically sound 1 in order to allow moving to the next phase. Francine Shapiro (2018) and others have written exhaustive books and articles detailing issues that may arise in Desensitization (such as looping or getting "stuck," potentially requiring cognitive interweaves), as well as all other phases. If you are noticing a lack of confidence in performing these phases, please consult the expert texts and seek additional EMDR therapy training and/or consultation.

Phase 5: Installation

This phase involves installing the PC to a 7 on the Likert scale (completely true). Ask your client if the PC they chose in Phase 3 continues to feel accurate and relevant, or if they would like to revise this statement. Once you have the final statement, ask them to hold the PC with the original image and rate how true the PC feels right now. Have your client hold these two things together in their minds and provide around 25 sets of BLS. Check the VOC after each set. Once this number is a 7, move to the Body Scan.

Again, there are many expert texts to consult if the PC is not quite reaching 7 due to blocking beliefs and so on. This phase is an incredibly important part of EMDR therapy. Installation strengthens the client's association of the formerly disturbing target with a newer, positive view of themselves. While desensitization can be likened to tearing down an old house, installation can be likened to raising an entirely new foundation and framing out the building. "The PC is (ideally) chosen on the basis of its ability to generalize and reshape the perspective of the greatest amount of dysfunctional material, as well as empower the client for present and future occurrences" (Shapiro, 1998). This statement works exceptionally well when applied to sexual health: "The (sexual health) PC is chosen on the basis of its ability to generalize and reshape the perspective of the greatest amount of dysfunctional [sexual health] material, as well as empower the client for present and future (positive sexual health)" (Shapiro, 1998) ["sexual health" is my addition].

Phase 6: Body Scan

Once the target is at a zero or 1, and the PC is at a 7 (fully installed), this step involves having the client bring up the original image and PC and scanning their body for any body sensation. If your client reports any disturbing or uncomfortable body sensation or tension, provide medium to fast BLS sets until these sensations resolve. If your client reports pleasant or even neutral body sensations (e.g., calmness, lightness), you can choose to provide slow BLS and ask the client to take slower deeper breaths to help reinforce this potentially hard-won calmer state. If possible, I like to spend 1 to 3 minutes reinforcing this calm state at the end of a successful EMDR session.

Phase 7: Closure

As your session draws to a close, hopefully your client has progressed all the way through the EMDR target, with a resolved Body Scan and back to "emotional equilibrium" (Shapiro, 2002). However, if the target is incomplete, you will need to help your client contain the activated material and reach equilibrium again. I typically do this by having the client use the "container" to contain any activated material, finishing with the "calm place" to fully equilibrate the client. If this is your client's first EMDR target experience, make sure they are aware that their mind/body may continue to process material after the session (generally a positive thing) and to note any relevant information for the next session (i.e., "taking a snapshot" for next time).

If you and your client are working on sexual health-related targets, you might also encourage your client to pay attention and notice what is changing with their Dual Control sexual brake and accelerator system as they undergo treatment. You can encourage them to keep a journal and notice what environmental, physical, emotional, or mental elements press on their brakes and their accelerators. This can be particularly helpful advice for clients who have felt distant or cut off from their sense of sexuality.

Phase 8: Re-evaluation

When the client returns for the next session, begin this phase by re-accessing "previously reprocessed targets" and review their responses to determine if "treatment effects have remained" (Shapiro, 2018). Again, refer to the many EMDR texts and books for more information about this phase. EMDR Future Templates are often included in this phase and will be explored in detail in Chapter 5.

In terms of sexual health, you can continue to encourage your client to notice what impacts their sexual brakes and accelerators between sessions as they journey toward a more empowered and positive relationship with their sexuality.

Current Sexual Difficulties Due to Anticipatory Anxiety (From the Sexual Dysfunction EMDR Protocol)

"The next part of the protocol for sexual dysfunction is to be used to address current on-going sexual difficulties due to anticipatory anxiety. For instance, someone who suffers from premature ejaculation may have developed so much anxiety due to their past failures that the anticipatory anxiety may predispose them to continued failure. Similarly, someone who may have suffered from (vaginal) sexual pain may continue to experience pain even after the physiological pain has been successfully treated medically. They may experience phantom pain and experience anticipatory anxiety that may compromise their sexual function. This cycle of defeat can be broken with EMDR" (Pillai-Friedman, 2009).

- Say, "*Describe what happens when you anticipate working with the _____ (state the issue that the client has been working on). Sometimes, people find it helpful to think of it as a movie. Please explain what happens in minute detail what happens before, during, and after you experience the sexual difficulty. Also, it is important to include the responses of your partner as well. For instance, _____ (state what actually happens or give an example) your partner sighs and turns away with disappointment or your partner gets up and leaves the room with an expression of irritation*" (Pillai-Friedman, 2009).____

- Say, *"Let's work with the part of the movie that causes you the most anxiety. We can use that as a target for EMDR work. What part causes you the most anxiety?"*

Proceed with standard EMDR and/or the remainder of the Sexual Dysfunction Protocol.

SEXUAL HEALTH EMDR POSITIVE COGNITIONS AND NEGATIVE COGNITIONS

This section explores possible PCs and NCs related to sexuality and sexual health concerns (see Box 4.1). All three established categories of cognitions contain opportunities for acknowledging and globalizing sexual concerns to life concerns. Mark Nickerson (2017) and others recently noted that a fourth category of "Connection" may be relevant for any given client, particularly those that may come from a more plural or collectivist cultural or familial background.

It is generally recommended in EMDR therapy to assist clients in choosing the most life-generalizable cognition pertaining to the target. For instance, if your client states "I was too dumb to see the red flags" (about a potential abuser), we would help them arrive at the more general "I'm not capable."

Box 4.1 Sexual Health Cognitions

POSSIBLE SEXUAL HEALTH NCs:

- *Safety/vulnerability:* I'm not safe // I'm powerless // I'm vulnerable
- *Responsibility (I did something wrong):* I should have done something // I'm weak // I'm guilty // My body betrayed me
- *Responsibility (I am defective—self-worth/empowerment):* I'm not worthy // I'm not good enough // I'm bad, stupid // I don't deserve pleasure/happiness // I can't be myself // I'm broken // I'm not worthy of respect and care // I'm dirty, disgusting
- *Control/choices:* I have no control // I have no choice // I can't ask for what I want
- *Connectedness and belonging (Nickerson, 2017):* I'm all alone, isolated, not normal (compared to the "dominant social norm")

(Continued)

> **Box 4.1 Sexual Health Cognitions *(Continued)***

POSSIBLE SEXUAL HEALTH PCS:

- *Safety/vulnerability:* I'm safe now // I have some power // I can protect myself
- *Responsibility (capable):* I did the best I could // I can trust myself and my judgment // It is not my fault // My body's biology works normally
- *Responsibility (self-worth/empowerment):* I am worthy // I am good enough/a good person // I am capable // I deserve pleasure/happiness // I can be myself // I'm healthy as I am // I'm worthy of respect and care // I'm innocent, clean, whole
- *Control/choices:* I am now in control // I have choices // I can ask for what I want
- *Connectedness and belonging:* I'm connected to others // I'm supported/cared for by others / I belong

EMDR "PAST" TARGETS RELATING TO SEXUAL HEALTH

As mentioned throughout this book, most of us are very familiar with clients seeking EMDR for sexual assault-related trauma (i.e., sexual assault of body parts, penetrative rape, and molestation). Here is a non-exhaustive list of some other targets that can be related to sexual health:

- Sexual harassment, stalking, or other demeaning acts
- Other coercive sexual experiences (e.g., being forced to watch pornography or exposed to unwanted sexual material)
- Perpetrator acts
- Demeaning/controlling behavior from a partner, particularly regarding one's attire of choice or jealousy-related comments
- Discovery of affairs and related images and evidence
- Physically painful sexual experiences
- Medical issues related to sexual health (e.g., surgeries, bodily changes)
- LGBTQI identity-related targets
- Harmful religious attitudes toward sexuality, orientation, and/or gender

EMDR "PRESENT" TARGETS RELATING TO SEXUAL HEALTH

Clients may also contact your office due to current and recurring sexual difficulties with little to no trauma history. Here is a non-exhaustive list of some common complaints that might be expressed.

- Lack of sexual interest with self or partner (if medical issues have been ruled out, then this is possibly related to erotophobic/anti-pleasure socialization, too many sexual brakes, and/or discovery of a partner's affair)
- Negative association with particular sexual acts (e.g., oral sex, vaginal/penile, cuddling/hugging, being approached/embraced from behind)
- Harmful and judgmental attitudes from family or religious environment
- Sexual disgust

EMDR THERAPY AND SEXUAL HEALTH CASE STUDIES

These three EMDR therapy case composites illustrate the helpfulness of holding a sexual health lens alongside an EMDR Therapy lens. Names and identifying features here and throughout the book have been changed and/or combined to ensure anonymity, and details from many cases have been combined to create "composites."

> **Case Study 4.1: Bianca, Blocked by Past Sexual Trauma and Repressiveness**

Bianca, a 24-year old White, bisexual, cisfemale graduate student grew up in a religious, sexually repressive family. She sought EMDR Therapy for PTSD symptoms related to two prior sexual assaults, including one at an organized event. She also reported a prior relationship with a controlling partner, which occurred after the sexual assaults. She noted some continued nightmares, interfering thoughts, and avoidance of certain places where she could potentially run into the assailants. She enjoyed performing artistically in a variety of settings, and identified as a progressive feminist who wished to embrace positive sexuality and explore a variety of sexual experiences.

At the time of treatment Bianca had a very supportive cismale partner Jose, who was completely respectful of her sexual autonomy, always asking for consent and available to process any PTSD symptoms that might occur due to sex-related activities. She noted that her partner frequently gave her oral sex, which she enjoyed, and that she wanted to return the favor, but felt this to be inappropriate for her feminist identity, religious upbringing, and prior trauma history. She felt dirty and ashamed whenever she attempted to provide oral sex.

At this point in her life, she had experienced "sexualization" and struggled with her parents' negative view of her "sexual identity," from the Our

Whole Lives (OWL) Circles of Sexuality. Within the 4-D Wheel framework she noted ample mental intrusions from her religious upbringing and feminist orientation, preventing her from enjoying the giving of sexual pleasure to her partner. All of these preoccupations and trauma-related symptoms completely dampened her sexual accelerators, which were initially in full gear at the start of the relationship with Jose. Indeed, the resurging PTSD symptoms were engaging her sexual brakes.

Bianca's negative cognitions related to the sexual assaults and controlling ex-partner included: "I'm alone, helpless, vulnerable, not capable." The positive cognitions she installed included: "I'm supported, connected, capable, strong, and have choices." She tended to experience physical disturbance in her chest or throat. After we spent several sessions clearing the prior sexual assault targets, she began to experience her relationship with her partner Jose as the equal, mutual, supportive, and loving relationship it was. We also targeted and processed the unhealthy messages from her family and society that sex was dirty, pinpointing images from conversations with parents prohibiting her from engaging in sexual activity.

Once we cleared out the negative familial and societal messages, we then targeted the negative self-talk and somatic upsetness (tightness in throat) that would occur after the few times of giving oral sex to her partner. Bianca noted that while giving oral sex, she felt okay about herself and enjoyed pleasuring her partner. But when it was over, and she had time to process, the negative thinking and somatic symptoms would begin.

We considered using an EMDR Future Template to get through any residual negativity toward giving her partner oral sex. By this time, she had reconciled both the feminist and religious notions of giving oral sex to be oppressive or shameful, and did not need a Future Template as she had successfully enjoyed an encounter, retaining positive feelings even days later. As using a Future Template on this subject could potentially feel awkward or embarrassing, I would have suggested this option: Bianca imagining herself post-oral sex, feeling comfortable, equal, and at ease, especially since she has enjoyed being the recipient often.

Case Study 4.2: Evelyn, Wishing to Try Dating

Evelyn, an older teenage Latinx transfemale (male to female), mainly attracted to masculine individuals, had experienced considerable sexualization from a trusted family member (including several specific humiliating molestations). Evelyn had also witnessed family violence and received bullying and other predatory behaviors. We spent many sessions processing

Chapter 4   Applying EMDR Therapy to Sexual Health Targets   117

these disturbing targets. Her negative cognitions included "I'm trapped, disgusting, not in control, not safe, only good for sex," and so on. She predominantly experienced the physical disturbance in her stomach. The positive cognitions we were able to install included "I'm fine as I am, I'm safe, I'm worthy, I can act, I have control and agency," and finally, "I'm a normal, sexual, healthy human."

Once we progressed two thirds through the long list of targets (about twenty-five events), she noted a developing interest in dating, imagining what it might be like to simply "hold someone's hand or experience a hug." Although it is preferable to wait until all targets are cleared prior to commencing future template work, since she reported a crush interest, she wanted to take a break from target work and improve her currently negative and fearful reaction to any form of intimacy.

Our first Future Template simply addressed effectively communicating physical boundaries (yeses and nos) to said "crush." She noted immediate anxiety, not surprising since we had not yet finished the target timeline, yet was able to get to neutral. We were then able to install the PC of "I can learn to act and set boundaries." Next we installed a future template of being hugged from behind (related to a prior traumatic event), with the PCs of "I can choose," and "I can receive healthy affection."

After installing these templates Evelyn reported being able to speak openly to her crush, establish boundaries, and enjoy simple affection such as hugging and snuggling. We then continued on with our timeline of EMDR targets.

Case Study 4.3: Nancy, Too Depressed to Be Sexual

Nancy presented with "relationship issues" and depression. She was a Black 27-year-old heterosexual cisfemale working in retail. She noted that her boyfriend wanted sex much more frequently than she did. One of her goals was to increase her frequency of sexual contact with her boyfriend. I provided psycho-education about sexual brakes, sexual accelerators, and information around identifying and asking for sexual pleasure. We hypothesized that accessing her sexual accelerators might prove much easier once any trauma was resolved and her sexual brakes were no longer in constant play.

Upon further assessment, she revealed her first sexual encounter was unwanted and nonconsensual. Her trauma history included school bullying, as well as a previous boyfriend cheating on her. She also reported experiencing racially motivated microaggressions such as being called names and receiving inappropriate sexual comments directed at her appearance. She noted confusion about what it meant to Black and female. Her negative cognitions included "I'm useless, not good enough, powerless, not in control." Her positive cognitions included "I'm good enough, worth it, strong, in control." She reported experiencing the disturbance of these targets mainly in her chest, sometimes as high as her heart or lower in her stomach.

As we cleared these EMDR targets, we noticed the relationship between her untreated trauma, confusion about the sexual mixed messages she has received as a Black woman, and lack of interest in sexual intimacy with her current partner. A great deal of sexual health psychoeducation was provided throughout treatment about general sexual health, self-advocating, female pleasure, the rights for Black women to pursue and enjoy pleasure, and boundaries.

We worked through a future template on "effectively enjoying an intimate encounter with your boyfriend." Her first response to this template was "interested and open," vastly different from her prior experiences. We were able to strengthen this with BLS and install the PC of "I'm strong, in control, powerful and have a right to sexual pleasure." She noted that a challenge that could arise might be stress interfering with her interest in intimacy (too many sexual brakes). She was able to come up with ways to deal with potential stress and experience relaxation once again, increasing her PC back to a 7.

"OUT OF CONTROL" SEXUAL BEHAVIORS

Introduction

Much discussion has been made of the term "sexual addiction" over recent years, particularly in relation to prevalently available internet porn. The current sexual health thinking eschews the term of *addiction,* preferring *out of control* sexual behavior.

Additionally, the governing body of sexuality education and counseling, the American Association of Sexuality Educators, Counselors and Therapists (AASECT), recently issued a historic statement in 2016 asserting that

> *AASECT recognizes that people may experience significant physical, psychological, spiritual, and sexual health consequences related to their sexual urges, thoughts, or behaviors. 1) AASECT does not find sufficient empirical evidence to support the classification of sex addiction or porn addiction as a mental health disorder, and 2) does not find the sexual addiction training, treatment methods and educational pedagogies to be adequately informed by accurate human sexuality knowledge. Therefore,*

it is the position of AASECT that linking problems related to sexual urges, thoughts, or behaviors related to a porn/sexual addiction process cannot be advanced by AAESCT as a standard practice of practice for sexuality education delivery, counseling, or therapy.

Obviously, whether someone's sexual behavior is "out of control" is completely subjective. However, it is generally agreed that any behavior interfering regularly with daily functioning and relationships might be designated "out of control."

It is very important with clients who present stating "I have an addiction" to truly assess to see if the behavior is as problematic and interfering as the client may present. Indeed, some clients may cry with relief to unburden themselves of what they deem as out of control (e.g., "excessive" porn viewing, multiple and frequent extramarital affairs, unwanted visits to strip clubs or sex workers, constant sexting) and are ready to receive any help necessary to get it "back under control."

However, these behaviors may be the result of deeper underlying problems such as relationship dissatisfaction/unhappiness/discord, or loneliness. Additionally, even as therapist and client work together to get the behavior more "under control," it is important to keep in mind that these behaviors may hold some erotic templates that are integral to the client. The goal is not necessarily to completely eliminate the behavior (unlike heroin addiction). Depending on the circumstances and client, it may be more appropriate to uncover the useful and positive elements of the feeling states and related erotic templates, helping the client reshape their behavior toward something they themselves deem more healthy and helpful.

If the client and EMDR therapist determine that the client's life would greatly improve if the particular problematic behavior is changed, then Robert Miller's Feeling-State Addiction Protocol is an excellent tool for shifting intrusive/negative behavior patterns. Anecdotally this is many local EMDR therapists' favorite tool (including myself) for helping with this shift. Another tool (not included in this text) is A. J. Popky's DeTUR (Desensitization of Triggers and Urge Reprocessing) protocol. DeTUR (2009) is an Adaptive Information Processing (AIP) model urge protocol to treat addictions and dysfunctional behaviors. Michael Hase's CravEx protocol (2009) can also help.

The Feeling-State Addiction Protocol (Robert Miller, 2010)

This section is written and provided by Dr. Robert Miller for this book.

The Feeling-State Addiction Protocol (FSAP) has been shown to be useful (Miller, 2004, 2010, 2012) for releasing people from the chains of the compulsion-causing memories that keep them locked into the past. The following is a short description of the Feeling-State Theory of Addictions identifying what role memories play in the formation of addiction and an explanation of how the FSAP eliminates compulsion-causing memories.

The psychological component of an addiction is the result of either the person's avoiding a negative feeling or seeking a positive feeling. Often the behavior is used alternatively for either the avoidance or the seeking of feelings, depending on the person's need at that moment. For example, a person may gamble to feel like a winner, or they may gamble to avoid feelings of anxiety. Treatment of the avoidance dynamic that causes addictions is targeted by processing the feelings and memories that the person is avoiding. Feeling-State treatment targets the intensely desired positive feeling that the person is seeking by performing the repetitive behavior.

A *feeling state* is a fixated memory that links a positive feeling with a behavior. Don's story is a good example of a behavioral problem caused by a Feeling State. Don would obsessively watch a video of a man receiving oral sex from a woman. Don stated that he identified with the man in the video. The feeling that Don identified when watching the video was the feeling of "acceptance." Don's Feeling State was composed of the feeling of "acceptance" linked with the fantasy of oral sex being performed on him. Whenever Don needed to experience the feeling of "acceptance," he would watch a video of a man receiving oral sex.

Don's story illustrates the Feeling-State Theory of the development of out of control behaviors—an intensely desired feeling becoming fixated with a behavior. Other types of behavioral problems such as gambling, pornography, and many other types of dopamine-rewarding behaviors can also have this intensely powerful psychological component, a Feeling-State memory, that makes the behavior difficult to resist doing.

The reason that the out of control behavior is difficult to resist is that the feeling the person is seeking is a normal, healthy feeling such as acceptance, belonging, or being desired. Everyone wants to experience these feelings. However, neglect or traumatic events can block a person from experiencing the desired feeling. The result is that the *need* to experience the feeling becomes more intense. Consequently, when there is an event in which the person experiences the intensely desired feeling, a Feeling-State memory is created linking the feeling with the behavior. From that point on, whenever the person wants to experience the feeling, they act out the behavior.

Once an Feeling-State memory is created, it doesn't go away. Feeling-State memories are similar to traumatic memories in that subsequent experiences do not change the Feeling-State memory. The person is drawn to do the behavior because the intensely desired feeling is linked with the behavior. When Don came to therapy, he was in a good relationship with a wife who loved him. However, Don still sought out his oral sex pornography whenever he needed to feel accepted. All the good experiences with his wife could not change the fixated Feeling-State memory linking the feeling of acceptance with oral sex.

The solution is to break the linkage between the feeling and the behavior. Once the link between feeling and behavior is broken, the person is no longer interested in doing the behavior. The critical part of the last sentence is "is no longer interested." Once the Feeling-State is broken, acting out the behavior no longer generates the desired feeling. It was never the behavior that the person wanted—only the feeling. Without the feeling attached to the behavior, the behavior is not exciting.

Case Study 4.4: Jerry Wants First-Time Sex, Every Time

Jerry self-reported a "sex addiction" in which he had to have "first time" sex with a different woman every time. Once he had sex with a woman, no matter how good the sexual experience, he still had to seek out another woman to satisfy this need. Jerry would cheat on his wife whenever she would go out of town, acting on his sexual urge. The last few years Jerry had started meeting with sex workers because it was easy for him to have "first time" sex.

Jerry's problematic sexual behaviors began in college when he was 20 years old. Jerry had wanted to have a relationship with a woman who, for over a year, had only wanted to be friends. Then they began a sexual relationship that lasted a few months. Because Jerry had been wanting to have sex with her for so long, the first time he had sex with her, it was "mind blowing." Jerry experienced an intense feeling of "acceptance" that he had wanted all his life but didn't get. The result was a Feeling-State memory linking the feeling of "acceptance" with a "first time" sexual encounter. From that point on, Jerry sought out women in order to experience the feeling of "acceptance" he had experienced when having "first time" sex.

Jerry's "first time" sex Feeling-State was treated by using the Feeling-State Addiction Protocol (FSAP). The FSAP uses the eye movement protocol of EMDR to break the linkage between the feeling and behavior. In the first session, Jerry was able to identify the feeling of acceptance as the feeling he was seeking. The memory of the sexual experience with the college woman was targeted using eye movements to process the memory. After three sets of eye movements, the linkage between the feeling of acceptance and the behavior of "first time" sex was broken. Once his Feeling-State memory was processed, Jerry's desire for "first time" sex was eliminated.

In the next session Jerry reported that not only did his desire cease regarding that sexual behavior, but processing the Feeling-State had had an impact in another area. Previously, whenever he was in the process of acting out his sexual urge he would begin looking at pornography. However, after processing the Feeling-State in the previous session, pornography was no longer interesting to him. In other words, Jerry was only interested in the pornography because it was leading to the feeling of acceptance he would experience when he acted out his sexual urge. Without the feeling of "acceptance" as a goal for the sexual acting-out behavior, the pornography was no longer exciting. Jerry's current life had been "run" by his 20-year-old self. Releasing Jerry from the chains of the Feeling-State allowed Jerry to seek the feeling of acceptance in healthier ways.

Jerry's therapeutic experience of a quick breaking of the Feeling-State memory is not unusual. The challenge for processing the Feeling-State is the identification of the feeling linked with the behavior. Usually, the feelings linked with sexual behaviors are easy to identify. Once identified, the Feeling-State is easy to process. After Jerry's Feeling-State of "first time" sex was broken, therapy focused on his underlying problems from childhood of why he so intensely needed to feel accepted.

As a result of eliminating the Feeling-State, Jerry did not have to contend with a whack-a-mole problem when he stopped acting out. The whack-a-mole problem occurs when a person attempts to control behavior. Controlling behavior does not eliminate the need for the feeling linked with the behavior. The person will seek other means to experience the feeling. Only breaking the link between the feeling and behavior frees the person to seek the desired feeling in a healthy manner. Processing the Feeling-State prevents both the whack-a-mole problem and relapse caused by a Feeling-State memory.

For a more complete understanding of the concepts and practice of the FSAP, see the articles cited in the following or the book *The Feeling-State Theory and Protocols for Behavioral and Substance Addictions*, 3rd Edition (Miller, 2021).

Feeling-State Addiction Protocol Summary

With Dr. Miller's permission, here is a summary of the FSAP. You may access his books about this protocol through his website at http://imagetransformationtherapy.com/

1. Obtain history, frequency, and context of addictive behavior.
2. Evaluate the person for having the coping skills to manage feelings if they are no longer using substances to cope. If not, do resource development before continuing. Install a Future Template if necessary.
3. Identify the specific aspect of the addictive behavior that has the most intensity associated with it. If the addiction is to a stimulant drug, then the rush/euphoria sensations are usually the first to be processed. However, if some other feeling is more intense, process that first.

The starting memory may be the first time or the most recent—whichever is most potent.
4. Identify the specific positive feeling (sensation + emotion + cognition) linked with the addictive behavior and its Positive Feeling-State (PFS) level (0–10).
5. Locate and identify any physical sensations created by the positive feelings.
6. The client visualizes performing the addictive behavior, feeling the positive feeling combined with the physical sensations.
7. Eye movements are performed until the PFS level drops to zero or 1.
8. Install Future Templates of how the person will live without having the feeling.
9. Between sessions, homework is given to evaluate the progress of therapy and to elicit any other feelings related to the addictive behavior.
10. In the next session, the addictive behavior is re-evaluated for both the feeling identified in the last session as well as identifying other positive feelings associated with the behavior.
11. Steps 3 to 9 are performed again as necessary.
12. Once the Feeling-States associated with the addictive behavior have been processed, the *negative beliefs underlying the Feeling-States are determined*, and the desired positive beliefs are chosen.
13. The negative feelings are processed and the positive beliefs are installed with the standard EMDR therapy protocol steps.
14. *The negative belief that was created as a result of the addictive behavior is identified*, and an alternate positive belief is chosen.
15. The negative beliefs are processed and the positive beliefs are installed.
16. Install Future Templates.

MANAGING POTENTIAL COMPLEX DISSOCIATIVE SYMPTOMS

There are many excellent books and resources providing guidance and suggestions for how to help our clients with dissociative diagnoses or symptoms such as emotional and/or cognitive decompensation, severe emotional dysregulation, numbing, and/or actively dissociating. As this book is focused on sexual health, please refer to these other sources for in-depth help. Some essential reference books include *The Haunted Self* (van der Hart et al., 2006), *EMDR and Dissociation: The Progressive Approach* (Gonzalez & Mosquera, 2012), *Looking Through the Eyes of Trauma And Dissociation: An Illustrated Guide for EMDR Therapists and Clients* (Paulsen, 2009), and *EMDR Toolbox: Theory and Treatment of Complex PTSD and Dissociation* (Knipe, 2019). Additionally, Farnsworth Lobestine and George Abbott in Massachusetts offer weekend long and/or monthly ongoing EMDR Therapy and Dissociation/Ego State workshops and trainings.

It cannot be emphasized enough that due to the societal shame and continuing erotophobic, punitive, and puritanical attitudes toward sexuality, for some clients addressing sexual health too soon (especially before dissociative and trauma symptoms are under control) can have deleterious effects.

Should you need to continue to work on stabilization and reduction of dissociation with your clients and are in need of immediate resources I highly recommend Schmidt's *Healing Circle* (Developmental Needs Meeting Strategy [DNMS]) and the *Conference Room/Meeting Place*.

The Developmental Needs Meeting System Healing Circle (Schmidt, 2009)

The Healing Circle is a remarkable resource that I use with most of my clients, whether or not they are exhibiting dissociative symptoms. This resource is particularly helpful for those clients who report little nurturing or protecting from caregivers while growing up. Using the scripts provided by Schmidt in her book *Developmental Needs Meeting Strategy* (2009) will help your client develop a Nurturing Adult Self, a Protecting Adult Self, and a Spiritual Adult Self. I especially love how these "selves" are gender-free and more based on universal qualities associated with protection, nurturance, and so forth. This is helpful for sexual health development, as most of us could have benefited from a positive protecting force, helping us understand boundaries and healthy sexual interaction, and a positive nurturing force, giving us validation and empowering appropriate information for us to nurture our own sexual gardens.

Conference Room/Meeting Place (Martin's and Fraser's "Dissociative Table")

The Conference Room AKA Meeting Place, developed extensively by both Martin (2012) and Fraser (1991, 2003), offers one of the best strategies for helping clients navigate and cope with dissociative symptoms. Please refer to their writings and books for details on how to develop a conference room with your client, and what to do once all your client's "parts" (both Apparently Normal Parts [ANP] and Emotional Parts [EP]) are present in the room.

It is very likely, particularly in the case of childhood sexual trauma survivors, that one or more EP may hold the sexual elements of the traumatic events. For example, a part may be an overly "sexualized" young child, or simply hold the sexual body sensation or negative emotion. When these parts come forward during conference room work, this is a great opportunity to provide psychoeducation to such EPs about healthy sexual development, following the PLISSIT (permission, limited information, specific suggestions, and intensive therapy) model of obtaining permission to speak about healthy sexual development. These young EPs can be encouraged to experience healthy development in a more appropriate manner. If you have age-appropriate sexual health development and boundary-related books in your office (e.g., *Your Body Belongs to You* [Spelman, 1997] or *Getting Smart About Your Private Parts* [Saltz, 2005]), you might consider inviting your client to read these books to the younger EPs within.

SUMMARY

In all eight phases of EMDR therapy sexual health can be introduced and explored. Sabina Pillai-Freidman's Sexual Dysfunction EMDR Protocol also has helpful information and ideas.

In the EMDR Preparation Phase, many EMDR resources are especially relevant for sexual health-related material. Two new helpful resources include the Bubble Boundary (good for new uncertain situations or ongoing toxic situations) and the Self-Compassion Container (excellent for helping clients cope with feelings of shame, a commonly reported emotion related to sexual trauma).

There is an endless list, unfortunately, of possible sexual health-related past and present targets. Many positive and negative cognitions, while generally used globally regarding a client, can apply more specifically to sexual health as well.

"Out of control" sexual behaviors can be addressed with EMDR therapy interventions such as DeTUR or CravX. This chapter includes information and case examples from Robert Miller about his FSAP in particular.

Clients may manifest complex dissociative responses and symptoms. If this occurs, more resourcing, particularly the DNMS Healing Circle and Conference Room/MeetingPlace, can be beneficial.

REFERENCES

Bernstein, E. M., & Putnam, F. W. (1986). Development, reliability, and validity of a dissociation scale. *Journal of Nervous and Mental Disease, 174*(12), 727–735. https://doi.org/10.1097/00005053-198612000-00004

Fraser, G. A. (1991). The dissociative table technique: A strategy for working with ego states and dissociative disorders and ego-state therapy. *Dissociation, 4*(4), 205–213.

Fraser, G. A. (2003). Fraser's "Dissociative table technique" revisited, revised: A strategy for working with ego states in dissociative disorders and ego-state therapy. *Journal of Trauma and Dissociation, 4*(4), 5–28. https://doi.org/10.1300/J229v04n04_02

Frischholz, E. J., Braun, B. G., Sachs, R. G., Hopkins, L., Shaeff, D. M., Lewis, J., & Leavitt, F. (1990). The dissociative experiences scale: Further replication and validation. *Dissociation: Progress in the Dissociative Disorders, 3*(3), 151–153.

Gonzalez, A., & Mosquera, D. (2012). *EMDR and dissociation: The progressive approach, first edition, revised*. Itradis.

Hase, M. (2009). CravEx: An EMDR approach to treat substance abuse and addiction. In M. Luber (Ed.), *Eye movement desensitization and reprocessing (EMDR) scripted protocols: Special populations* (pp. 467–488). Springer Publishing.

Knipe, J. (2019). *EMDR toolbox: Theory and treatment of complex PTSD and dissociation* (2nd ed.). Springer Publishing.

Leeds, A. (2016). *A guide to the standard EMDR therapy protocols for clinicians, supervisors, and consultants* (2nd ed.). Springer Publishing.

Luber, M. (2001). *Handbook for EMDR clients*. Trauma Recovery EMDR Humanitarian Assistance Programs.

Martin, K. M. (2012). How to use Fraser's dissociative table technique to access and work with emotional parts of the personality. *Journal of EMDR Practice and Research, 6*(4). https://doi.org/10.1891/1933-3196.6.4.179

Miller, R. (2021). *The feeling-state theory and protocols for behavioral and substance addictions* (4th ed.). ImTT Press.

Miller, R. M. (2004). *The Feeling-state theory of compulsions and cravings and decreasing compulsions and cravings using an eye movement protocol* [Doctoral dissertation]. Pacifica Graduate Institute.

Miller, R. M. (2010). The feeling-state theory of impulse-control disorders and the impulse-control protocol. *Traumatology, 16*(3), 2–10. https://doi.org/10.1177/1534765610365912

Miller, R. M. (2012). Treatment of behavioral addictions utilizing the feeling-state addiction protocol: A multiple baseline study. *Journal of EMDR Practice and Research, 6*(4), 159–169. https://doi.org/10.1891/1933-3196.6.4.159

Nickerson, M. (2017). *Cultural competence and healing culturally-based trauma with EMDR therapy.* Springer Publishing.

Paulsen, S. (2009). *Looking through the eyes of trauma and dissociation: An illustrated guide for EMDR therapists and clients.* Bainbridge Institute for Integrative Psychology.

Pillai-Friedman, S. (2009). Sexual dysfunction EMDR protocol. In M. Luber (Ed.), *Eye movement desensitization and reprocessing (EMDR) scripted protocols: Special populations* (pp. 151–166). Springer Publishing.

Popky, A. J. (2009). The desensitization of triggers and urge reprocessing (DeTUR) protocol. In M. Luber (Ed.), *Eye movement desensitization and reprocessing (EMDR) scripted protocols: Special populations* (pp. 489–511). Springer Publishing.

Saltz, G. (2005). *Getting smart about your private parts.* Dutton Books for Young Readers.

Schmidt, S. J. (2009). *The developmental needs meeting strategy: An ego state therapy for healing adults with childhood trauma and attachment wounds.* DNMS Institute, LLC.

Shapiro, F. (1998). *EMDR: The breakthrough "eye movement" therapy for overcoming anxiety, stress, and trauma.* Basic Books.

Shapiro, F. (2002). *EMDR as an integrative psychotherapy approach.* Mental Research Institute.

Shapiro, F. (2012). *Getting past your past: Take control of your life with self help techniques from EMDR therapy.* Rodale.

Shapiro, F. (2018). *Eye movement desensitization and reprocessing (EMDR) therapy, third edition: Basic principles, protocols, and procedures.* Guilford.

Simons, N. (2018). *Self-compassion container script* (personal communication May, 2021).

Spelman, C. M. (1997). *Your body belongs to you.* Albert Whitman Company.

Van der Hart, O., Nijenhuis, E. R. S., & Steele, K. (2006). *The haunted self: Structural dissociation and the treatment of chronic traumatization.* W.W. Norton and Company.

Watkins, J., G., & Watkins, H. H. (1998). *Ego states: Theory and therapy.* W. W. Norton.

Bubble/Shield Boundary Resource

The steps (most of these will be verbalized to your client):

a. Sometimes we need to enter a situation that we anticipate may be emotionally charged or toxic, or we simply want to increase our boundaries. We can use imagery and Bilateral Stimulation (BLS) to help.
b. Think of an image of a boundary around you, perhaps a bubble, shield, and/or armor, which will help protect you from negativity and toxicity. It might be invisible, or made of metal. Whatever you imagine is fine.
c. Image: _____
   _____.
d. I'll now apply BLS while you continue to describe the boundary with as much detail as possible. *(slow to medium BLS now, and whenever BLS is indicated)*
e. You may still want positive things to pass through this bubble/shield and find their way to your mind/body. *What mechanism* would allow positive things (compliments, good energy, etc.) to pass through? Perhaps a screen that only filters positive or neutral things through the shield?
f. Now describe your boundary again, with as much detail as you can, including the screen device. *(BLS on)*
g. Repeat after me, "*I am strengthening my boundaries.*" *(BLS off)*
h. How do you feel, now that we have strengthened your boundary with this (bubble/shield/ armor)? _____ (what emotion?)
i. *(BLS on)* Once more, recall the image of developing and installing your _____. Become aware of the emotion of _____ and notice in your body where there are sensations that accompany this emotion. *(BLS off)*
   What is the sensation _____ and its location _____?
j. *(BLS on)* As you see yourself strengthening your boundaries you become aware of the sensation of _____ in your _____ that tells you are experiencing feeling _____. Please repeat after me: _____ in my _____ tells me I am experiencing _____. Now take a few slower, deeper breaths, experiencing the _____ *(power, protection, security, confidence, etc.)* that comes from increasing your boundaries and protection. *(BLS off)*
k. For added strength you can have your client bring up a low lever toxic situation (e.g., staff meeting with a toxic boss) and practice holding the boundary in place, using BLS.
l. Practice daily or as needed. The client can also do a drawing or collage of their boundary.

The Self-Compassion* Container (Developed by Nancy Simons, LMHC [2018])

*First provide clients with psychoeducation on self-compassion.

Self-Compassion Guided Visualization Script

- Using guided visualization, we will develop a self-compassion container. I will have you bring to mind a new container and then we will design the inside space of the container. This container will be used to hold any negative thoughts, feelings, and body images that are connected to your trauma history and still trouble you today. We are designing a container that has the three qualities of self-compassion: *self-kindness, mindful awareness,* and *common humanity.*
- Use whatever technique (e.g., calm place) you prefer to guide your client into a settled place with present awareness.
- Take a few moments and begin to see what image appears for you when think about a self-compassion container. _____
  _____
- The inside of the container is very important. Let's design the space so that you can see all the qualities of your self-compassion: self-kindness, mindfulness, and common humanity.
- For *self-kindness* I would like you to imagine an interior environment that can hold difficult thoughts and feelings in a gentle, caring, and supportive way. Sometimes people think about having special material like velvet or sand or cotton balls. Just think about self-kindness and notice what image comes up for you. When you see what that is, and without opening your eyes, tell me what you see.
- Let's develop an image for the quality of *mindful awareness.* Can you think of an image that will help you connect to your own ability to be mindful, that quality that allows you to just notice negative thoughts and feelings without getting stuck on them? Sometimes people think of this like puffy clouds in the sky floating by or a carousel going around. Just notice what comes to mind for you now. Stay with the image and without opening your eyes tell me what you notice.
- Now let's develop an image for the quality of *common humanity.* This is the ability to recognize that it is human nature to feel pain, that we are just like everyone else when we feel pain, and that all people feel pain even if they don't always show it. Some ideas that other people have used are a picture of the globe or a web of light. Just notice what comes to mind for you now. Stay with the image and without opening your eyes tell me what you notice.

- (can apply slow BLS) Try imagining that container resting within you; it could be in any part of your body: your head, your heart, your belly, your hands, or even your feet. Tell me what you notice now.... (end BLS)
- Let's practice using the container. Think of a difficult experience that happened recently that on a scale of 0 to 10 is no greater than a 3. _____
- What is the negative belief about yourself that goes along with that experience? _____
- What are the negative emotions that go along with that experience? _____
- What do you feel in your body in relation to that experience? _____
- Now, think about your container of self-compassion. (The therapist can read a complete description to the client.) I want you to imagine putting into this container any of the distress you just described to me. It can go in any way you want.
- (can apply medium BLS) Take a moment to see what it feels like to offer this distress self-compassion; notice what is like to offer this distress an environment of self-kindness, a space to accept distress rather than always working so hard to push it away or avoid it. Notice how you are giving yourself a moment to see that this suffering that you have, no matter how big or small it is, makes you human. (end BLS)
- We will continue to use this self-compassion container throughout the course of your EMDR treatment.
- Discuss what came up during this exercise. Sometimes people notice judgmental thoughts or self-doubt. You can encourage them to go back and notice that thought also being in the container; part of self-compassion is acceptance of what is, even the difficult thoughts as you practice self compassion.

5

Sexual Health EMDR Future Templates and Resources, Body Image, and Pornography

Stephanie Baird, LMHC

LEARNING OBJECTIVES

- EMDR clinicians will review basic EMDR Future Template steps.
- EMDR clinicians will learn about the many possibilities of using EMDR Future Templates to improve sexual health, demonstrated with EMDR case studies.
- EMDR clinicians will learn about the potential interactions of self-esteem, body image, and social media on sexual health.
- An EMDR case study will demonstrate how to increase sexuality-related self-esteem with EMDR Future Templates.
- EMDR clinicians will learn about the potential impact of pornography on sexual health, demonstrated with EMDR case studies.
- EMDR clinicians will learn how to use the new EMDR resource—Strengthening a Confident and Joyful Sexual Self—with appropriate clients.
- EMDR clinicians will be briefed on helpful resources to share with clients for increasing sexual pleasure, as well as healthful maintenance exercises.

INTRODUCTION

As the thrust of this book is geared toward empowering the full sexual health of our clients, particularly sexual trauma survivors, this chapter critically focuses on those next steps of moving clients from symptom management and abatement to thriving sexual health. Using eye movement desensitization and reprocessing (EMDR) Future Templates is a relatively accessible and satisfying way to help our clients' address and embrace positive sexual health and is explained at length, illustrated with case studies. Additionally, as EMDR therapy continues to reduce PTSD-related symptoms, clients may mention (if they haven't already) sexuality-related concerns regarding self-esteem and body image. Ubiquitous social media comparisons and overexposure to pornography (for some individuals) can continue to negatively impact a possibly still delicate newfound sense of self-appreciation. We can use EMDR therapy to address the impact of social media and pornography on self-image, from isolating specific targets to identifying EMDR Future Templates. A new EMDR resource on Strengthening a Confident and Joyful Sexual Self provides another path for overcoming negative and limiting sexual beliefs by bringing empowered, joyful, and pleasure-focused sexuality into focus.

EMDR FUTURE TEMPLATES

EMDR Future and/or Positive Templates (Leeds, 2016; Shapiro, 2018) are incredible tools for helping our clients' minds/bodies continue with adaptive resolution and healing. These are best performed once all the relevant past and present EMDR targets have been processed. However, occasionally it is clinically appropriate and useful to initiate a Future Template prior to timeline completion. One example is where a client has an upcoming wedding or funeral they genuinely want to attend, but a childhood perpetrator may be in attendance (I have helped at least a dozen clients through this type of situation). However, this client has not yet processed all the relevant past targets related to the abuser. The Future Template (along with the Bubble/Shield Boundary) can help fortify your client through the event.

I have also found over the years that EMDR therapists often neglect or leave out Future Templates in clients' EMDR therapy. This is a grave disservice as Future Templates provide our clients the perfect opportunity for consolidating and applying their new, hard-won, positive-oriented neural networks toward possible future variations on what they have experienced. Lastly, if all the past and present EMDR targets have been processed, then installing Future Templates usually does not take very long, perhaps even just 5 or 10 minutes. This short time investment may be the icing on the cake to help our clients feel as confident and capable as possible.

Basic EMDR Future Template Script

We have worked on past experiences relating to your presenting problem as well as present situations triggering distress. Today, I'd like to suggest we work on how you will respond in the future to similar situations.

Desired Outcomes

Steps
1. Identify the future situation
   "I'd like you to imagine yourself effectively (doing) _____ _____."
   "You can run this scenario through a movie if you wish."
2. "What are you noticing?"
   Positive: Add Bilateral Stimulation (BLS) sets as long as additional positives are reported.
   Negative: Focus on body sensations and add BLS until negative sensations go away.
3. Install Positive Cognitive (PC) to Validity of Cognition (VOC) = 7 "Hold your PC with that situation. On a scale from 1 to 7, how true does it feel?" Install to 7 with BLS.

Problem-Solving Situations

1. Create a problem-solving situation.
   "I'd like you to think of a challenge you may experience in that situation."
2. "What are you noticing?"
   Positive: Add BLS as long as additional positives are reported.
   Negative: Focus on body sensations and add BLS until negative sensations go away.
3. Install PC to VOC = 7 "Hold your PC with that situation. On a scale from 1 to 7, how true does it feel?" Install to 7 with BLS.

POSSIBLE SEXUAL HEALTH EMDR FUTURE TEMPLATES

Here are some possible sexual health related EMDR Future Templates. The possibilities are endless.

- Client wants to become sexually intimate, but is fearful of being vulnerable to the point of avoiding internet dating sites, or places to meet potential sexual partners.

- Client wants to resume sexual intimacy with their partner, but still notes some anxiety and skittishness.
- Client is nervous or anxious about saying yes or no to specific sexual activities.
- Client is nervous about discussing sexually transmitted infections (STIs) and contraceptive status with a potential sexual partner.
- Client is nervous about coming out as lesbian, gay, bisexual, transgender, or queer (LGBTQ) to family, friends, and/or at work.
- Client is nervous about gender transition and "passing" in different scenarios.
- Client is nervous about some aspects of future gender transition surgeries.
- Client is nervous about bringing up sex-related concerns/fantasies/wishes/needs to a partner.
- Many others...

Case Studies of Sexual Health EMDR Future Templates

Case Study 5.1: Jaime, Transmale Struggling With Physical Contact

Jaime is a 17-year-old biracial (Latinx and White) transmale who wants to snuggle with a romantic interest, and feel relaxed and calm while doing so. While a great many of the EMDR targets had been processed (most having to do with childhood molestation by a peripheral caregiver), there were still a few EMDR targets to go. However, as James was noting a strong immediate interest in "Jack," he requested that we pause the EMDR timeline and work on increasing his comfort with cuddling. Through this Future Template, James was able to imagine enjoying some cuddling, despite the remaining EMDR targets of similar themes. He returned the following week stating the EMDR Future Template was a success and that he enjoyed his first consensual cuddle.

- Jaime's Future Template statement: "Imagine yourself calmly and confidently hugging 'Jack.'"
- Jaime's positive cognition: "I am worthy and can choose positive touch."

Case Study 5.2: Athena, Post-Affair Physical Distance

Athena is a 59-year-old White, married cisfemale who could not imagine touching her husband after his affair. She stated several times that she wanted to remain married to him, forgive him, and enjoy touching him again, as they had had a gratifying and mutual physically connective relationship prior to the affair. They were also in marriage counseling while we used EMDR therapy to process the affair's many details and betrayals. We had successfully processed most of the identified EMDR targets when Athena noted her wish to be able to touch her husband again. We created the EMDR Future Template, processing through it about two or three times until Athena reported eventually being able to hug and snuggle with "Steve."

- Athena's EMDR Future Template: "Imagine yourself calmly touching his body with interest."
- Athena's positive cognition: "I can enjoy touching and connecting."

Case Study 5.3: Adrian, Wants to be Playful During Sex

Adrian is a 45-year-old single Black self-identified "bottom" cisgender gay man who wants to be more active and playful during sex. Although not currently dating anyone, he noted that this ability was very important as he felt his confidence to date would increase as his sense of capability increased. A couple months after completing this EMDR Future Template, Adrian reported being able to talk more playfully with a new sexual partner.

- Adrian's EMDR Future Template: "Imagine yourself confidently and comfortably engaging in playful 'dirty talk' during a make-out session with a consenting and interested partner."
- Adrian's positive cognition: "I can capably interact playfully during sex."

Case Study 5.4: Kelly, Lingering PTSD Interfering With Sex

- Kelly was a 38-year-old cisfemale lacking sexual interest with a long-term cismale partner. During the intake process she disclosed a long-term teen dating violence relationship, with many instances of sexual violence, silencing, and "freezing" during sex. She was diagnosed with longstanding untreated PTSD. We processed her EMDR timeline of teen sexual violence. Kelly then wanted to "effectively receive touch and express reactions." Shortly after completing the EMDR Future Template Kelly noted initiating, engaging in, and enjoying pleasurable sexual activity with her boyfriend.

- Kelly's EMDR Future Template: "Imagine yourself effectively enjoying sexual activity with your partner."
- Kelly's positive cognition: "I can express myself."

Case Study 5.5: Jennifer, Erotophobic Background

Jennifer was a 32-year-old single, White, cisfemale molested once in youth, in a public sport setting, by a beloved community teacher. Her family of origin was very erotophobic (partly due to an oppressive anti-sex religious community) and never discussed anything sex-related. Although Jennifer went on to date a little bit here and there, she remained fearful of intimate possibilities and connections. She entered EMDR therapy to overcome this childhood sexual abuse as well as her anxiety around beginning romantic and/or sexual interactions such as conversing with a potential date, holding hands, and staying calm during an initial hug. A few months after completing this (and similar) EMDR Future Templates, Jennifer reported going on several dates with a patient and gentle man, progressively enjoying physical touch (hand-holding, hugging, kissing, full body touching) and eventually her first intercourse experiences (oral, penis–vagina). She found she enjoyed the body touching and kissing the most, and was able to continue experimenting with touch, articulating her likes and dislikes.

- Jennifer's EMDR Future Template: "Imagine yourself effectively meeting and talking to a man in public."
- Jennifer's positive cognition: "I can handle this."

Case Study 5.6: Donna, No More Trauma Symptoms, Sexually Avoidant

Donna was a 55-year-old White, married, cisfemale. Her very stable and positive marriage created favorable conditions where she finally felt safe to acknowledge and disclose childhood sexual abuse from a neighbor, cousin, and parish figure. We processed all the childhood sexual abuse EMDR targets, as well as middle school bullying mentioned later in treatment.

At timeline completion, she noted some lingering difficulty in giving and receiving pleasure to/from her husband. We then developed and processed a couple different EMDR Future Templates. She shortly reported enjoying several experiences of pleasure and touch with her husband.

Chapter 5 Sexual Health EMDR Future Templates 137

- Donna's first EMDR Future Template: "Imagine yourself effectively and joyfully receiving pleasurable touch from your husband."
- Donna's positive cognition: "I deserve pleasure and can receive pleasure."
- Donna's second EMDR Future Template: "Imagine yourself effectively and joyfully giving pleasurable touch to your husband."
- Donna's positive cognition: "It's healthy to give pleasure to someone I love. I can be a sexual being who enjoys giving pleasure, too."

The Future Template described in this section is different from the EMDR Future Template in the preceding examples. This template, created by Sabitha Pillai-Friedman (2009), is a small part of Pillai-Friedman's EMDR Protocol for Sexual Dysfunction, which is available as a Supplementary File to this book at https://connect.springerpub.com/content/book/978-0-8261-8676-8. I include this particular Future Template here to over-emphasize the usefulness of taking the time to install sex-positive paradigms and new neural networks.

Now that the past sexual trauma and triggers have been processed and current anticipatory anxiety has been treated through EMDR, positive sexual memories or sexual fantasies can be installed to ensure optimal sexual functioning in the patient's future sexual interactions. Positive sexual memories or sexual fantasies can be used to kindle positive sexual energy and desire, create positive anticipation about sexual activity, and avoid cognitive distraction that could interfere with sexual activity. If the client describes more than one positive sexual experience, more than one can be installed, (even) better for the client. (The installation of inner resource described in the following is inspired by the resource work of Popky, 2005.)

- Say, "*Now bring to mind a positive sexual experience. It can be an actual sexual experience you have had on your own or with a partner. It can also be a feeling you experienced when you felt positive about your sexuality. For instance, you walked into a party and received admiring glances or compliments from a potential sex partner. You can also bring to mind your favorite sexual fantasy that you use during masturbation or partnered sex.*"

- Say, "*What image represents the best part of your positive sexual experience?*"

- Say, "*When you bring the positive sexual image to mind, what would you like to believe about yourself now?*"_____

- Say, "*When you bring up that image of the positive sexual experience or fantasy and words that go with the image, what emotion(s) do you feel now?*"

- Say, "*Step into the image of the positive sexual experience or fantasy. Notice and experience the positive feelings, breathe in these feelings, move around in them, experience being successful. Notice what you see, feel, smell, and taste. Notice what it is like to feel the sexual energy and to function successfully. As you notice and experience those positive sexual feelings, touch your knuckle in this positive state until your positive state is most desirable. Increase pressure slightly to the same place on your knuckle as your positive feelings peak.*"

_____

- Say, "*Go with that.*" (Do BLS)
- *What do you notice?*"_____

Continue with the following:

- Say, "*As you listen to the positive words or sounds that you are saying to yourself and the positive words that others would be saying, adjust the auditory components: the volume, the tone, the tempo, the balance, and so forth, and, as the positive experience peaks, touch your anchor.*"_____
- Say, "*Go with that.*" (Do BLS)
- Say, "*What do you notice?*"_____
- Test the positive state by having the client touch their knuckle and notice the results. The client should report a positive experience. It is important for the client to have a strong, positive, sensory-based experience of having successfully achieved their goal anchored into their physiology. If this is not the case, repeat it with another memory or work to deepen the current memory.
- Say, "*Now touch your knuckle. What do you feel?*"

_____

- Say, "*Go with that.*" (Do BLS)
- Say, "*What do you notice?*"_____

Generally speaking, once all past and present EMDR targets have been addressed and processed, "the client is now ready to address the anticipatory anxiety and create a template for optimal functioning in the future. At the end of this EMDR (Sexual Dysfunction) protocol, clients usually report a marked decrease in reactivity related to their sexuality. Most clients also report a gradual change from negative anticipation of sexual events to positive anticipation. The EMDR treatment enables clients to participate in couple therapy and sex therapy with greater success" (Pillai-Friedman, 2009).

SELF-ESTEEM, BODY IMAGE, SOCIAL MEDIA, AND SEXUAL HEALTH

As the U.S. culture remains over-focused on appearances (as evidenced by many television ads and magazine covers in your local bookstore), many clients report struggles with body image. In particular, clients may note disturbances or embarrassment about weight, body shape or size (including breasts, vulvas, labia majora, penises, and testicles), hair type/presence or absence, "blemishes," scars, disfigurements, and so on. Many of my clients also report social media images having a negative impact on their self-esteem, feeling inadequate in person compared to other folks' posts, or to the visual "filters" available to alter their "selfies." Any or all of the negative self views may lead to avoidance of sexual engagement with others for fear of being seen as inadequate.

Some clients may genuinely have a diagnosis of body dysmorphic disorder where they obsess over and/or distort a self-perceived flaw that others would not notice. Other clients may have acquired an eating disorder diagnosis related to dislike of their body shape or weight. Any of these disturbances may impact a client's comfort and interest of their own or others' sexual health and sexuality. EMDR therapy certainly can be used to help treat traumatic and disturbing material related to these disorders, and possibly help disrupt obsessive and/or distorted thinking. As these specific diagnoses are outside the scope of this book, please seek additional resources and protocols if your clients need help in these areas (Beer, 2019; Forester, 2009; Seijo, 2019a; Seijo, 2019b; Zaccagnino, 2019).

Tina Fey's poignant essay in her book *Bossypants* (2011) called "All Girls Must Be Everything," brilliantly illustrates the modern cis- or transwoman's impossible appearance expectations. She describes all the things that can be wrong with a cis- or transwoman's appearance (e.g., "cankles…nipples too big or small…lunch lady arms…muffin top"). She then presents a list of the physical qualities every women must have (e.g., "blue eyes…full Spanish lips…hairless Asian skin…dance hall ass…long Swedish legs…the arms of Michelle Obama…"). I give photocopies of her short essay to clients who report body image struggles.

Cis- or transmen are not immune, as the proliferation of men's magazines over the last decade or so has also resulted in more pressure for men to become "metrosexual": grooming and working out in order to display hairless chests and eight-pack abs.

We are supposed to be satisfied if known transgender individuals, such as Laverne Cox or Caitlin Jenner, grace the cover of *People* magazine once a year. I *am* happy to note that as of this writing in June 2021, Elliot (formerly Ellen) Page made the news with the wonderful headline of "transgender joy" by showing pictures on Instagram of his new masculine chest (after top surgery removed the previous tissue).

Lastly, gender non-conforming or non-binary are generally not represented in the media. Happily for gender non-conforming folks, Demi Lovato recently came out as non-binary, using they/them pronouns. The more examples we all have (no matter our gender) of folks actively determining gender for themselves, the less we need to worry about our own gender presentation and all the trappings that often come with it. Representation matters.

It is helpful to note that many more magazines and catalogs now, compared to 10 or 20 years ago, feature more diverse bodies. My favorite body-positive catalogs that come through my mail or email include Lands' End, Old Navy, Athleta, Target, Anthropologie, Premme, Big Bud Press, and Summersalt swim wear (also featuring models with prosthetic legs or multi-colored skin). It is also now easier to find and "follow" many more body-positive folks on Instagram, Twitter, and so forth (e.g., Precious Lee, Lauren Nicole, Simone Charles), helping our neural networks get a good daily dose of realism and healthy self-love. I mention this to help inculcate hope that unrealistic expectations (perpetuated by every airbrushed and touched up model) seem to be slowly loosening their grip. However, lack of ubiquitous representation of different kinds of bodies, shapes, skin tone, gender expressions, and so on remain an overall problem.

Increasing Sexuality-Related Self-Esteem With EMDR Processing and Future Templates

Exploring clients' self body perceptions may, unfortunately, yield dozens of potential EMDR targets. You might also discover potential EMDR targets from any negative reports your clients provide from the "Strengthening a Confident and Joyful Sexual Resource" instruction (detailed later in this chapter) "to look in the mirror daily and write down everything they like." If they return to the next session stating they wrote down very little, or felt even too discouraged to attempt the exercise, then you have stumbled upon a cache of unprocessed material.

Case Study 5.7: Oliver, Negative Body Image Is Preventing Intimacy

Oliver is a 32-year-old Black heterosexual cisman-identified client seeking EMDR therapy due to prior childhood sexual abuse (groomed and molested by an after-school program facilitator), as well as lack of confidence regarding meeting and dating women. He also reported feeling distressed by his thinning hair, slight "belly," and shorter stature, stating that the number of tall Black men in sports and media does not help his self-image. Although he had experienced a handful of positive sexual encounters in his late teens and early twenties, he reported being mostly celibate by choice due to self-consciousness. EMDR therapy cleared his childhood sexual abuse targets fairly easily, leaving the remaining body image disturbances.

Oliver also noted that using Instagram reduced his self-esteem. Instead of feeling happy for his friends' adventures and activities, he often felt jealous of their perceived better looks. Once we weighed the pros and cons of cutting back on Instagram during our work, Oliver promptly deactivated his account and noted feeling a bit better almost immediately.

After making a list of the disliked body areas (thinning hair, belly, and height), we checked with float backs to see where the initial dislike originated. Targets related to Oliver's height originated in adolescence, when other peers grew taller than him, bragging about their height and wondering what happened to Oliver—"he was Black, after all." We processed those EMDR targets, then identified and processed current triggers (certain friends joking about height, saying too bad he'll never get into the NBA). His Negative Cognitions (NCs) tended to be "something is wrong with me" and "I'm not good enough." His PCs were "I am good enough and fine as I am."

We then installed EMDR Future Templates on how to assert himself with his friends, and how to see his height in a more positive light. Oliver's Future Template PC was "I am awesome the way I am." We also added an additional Resource and Development Installation (RDI) of shorter admirable and/or handsome men that included Martin Luther King, Gandhi, Prince, and Paul Simon. From there we used EMDR therapy similarly to target his belly and thinning hair dislike, focusing more on recent and present targets and triggers of seeing himself in the mirror and feeling invisible in certain settings.

Eventually we processed EMDR Future Templates on Oliver seeing himself effectively and confidently: (1) "meeting women," (2) enjoying clothed "hugging and kissing," and (3) comfortably "disrobing" with a potential romantic partner.

Soon after Oliver reported going on several dates with two different women he met online, and feeling comfortable to disrobe and enjoy sexual activity with one of the women.

IMPACT OF PORNOGRAPHY ON SEXUAL HEALTH

Introduction

Pornography has a complicated existence and is best understood in book-length examinations. Poll anyone on the street and you will get a wide array of emotional responses to the concept of pornography. Pornography is generally defined as showing sexually explicit content (photographs, film/videos, and/or writings in magazines and books, etc.) with the purpose of stimulating sexual excitement.

Some pornography can also include a supernormal stimulus nature of more violent or extreme pornography specifically designed to quickly shock recipients into having an intense physiological and/or emotional response, in some cases numbing said viewers over time to the extreme depictions of degradation.

Gloria Steinem argued in 1977 that if a ciswoman and a cisman engaging in sex were shown as having equal power, equal pleasure, and equal choice, and the imagery is egalitarian, non-coercive, and non-degrading, this should not be termed pornography, but "erotica."

At this point most people acknowledge that porn exists and will likely continue to exist in some form. Since humans could first make marks on walls and observe ourselves and each other, we have attempted to depict our sexuality, going back to images and sculptures of genitals in the Paleolithic and Mesolithic periods such as the Venus of Willendorf.

Many folks assume that most internet activity involves searching for porn. In reality, porn represents only 4% of the top million sites, and about 13% to 25% of web searches. One in three viewers of porn are woman-identified. Research shows there has been a decrease in child sexual abuse and adult rape over the years, possibly correlated to porn availability (statistics compiled by Kate Scalisi, "Sex Tech" webinar [2018], and Dr. Rosalyn Dischiavo, "Erotophobia" webinar [2020]).

Many sociologists, psychologists, evangelists, feminists, parents, lawyers, and justices have weighed in on what constitutes pornography versus something more "socially acceptable" that might land in the "erotic" category (e.g., the well-known *Fifty Shades of Grey* book series, as well as the "Bridgerton" Netflix series) versus straight-up pornography websites and magazines.

The SESTA law passed in 2018, while initially positive in the sense that it hoped to limit sex trafficking and slavery, also limits consensually working and paid sex workers, and even educational sexual health internet content that can now be labeled "obscene." Ultimately, the legalities of what can be outlawed and what is acceptable have remained complicated by varying perceptions of what the "average person" considers okay or not okay. Another troubling aspect of the porn industry overall is the lack of regulations overall.

Sex-positive activists have defined some working elements of ethical pornography as well as the concept of porn literacy. Ethical pornography (also sometimes called "feminist" or "fair trade" pornography) includes fair payment of the filmmakers and workers, is made in a safe environment where everyone is of consenting age and is respected, shows real (not faked) sexual pleasure (especially for female bodies), is created for all viewers (including ciswomen), is 100% consensual in every way, and shows diversity across body type, age, race, sexuality, and ability.

Rebekkah Rennick, in a Tapestry presentation on "Digital Sexuality and Youth" (2021), shared Responsible Sex Ed Institute's (affiliated with Planned Parenthood) *porn literacy* definition: "form of media that teaches individuals to think about, analyze, and evaluate the media they choose to consume and the media that is already around them, such as billboards and advertisements. Everything has a message, whether intentional or not. Knowing how, why, and for whom content was created can help youth (and adults) better understand what they see and hear and make healthy decisions."

Rennick noted that 89% of youth report the internet as their primary source of information and that "unwanted" exposures comprise 66% of youth exposure. Teaching our youth, our clients, and ourselves how to critique the images offered is becoming more and more essential for sexual health well-being. Indeed, there are real concerns and issues with most "mainstream" porn that is made by cismen for cismen. Much of this type of porn leaves out important elements like emotional intimacy, consent, using condoms, discussing sexually transmitted infection (STI) risks, and varying body types. And it often includes degradation of women, unrealistic behaviors, poor treatment, and poor financial reimbursement of the actors.

Boston University's professor and researcher Emily F. Rothman, via the Boston Public Health Commission, created a curriculum to teach youth porn literacy called "Start Strong" and presents some of this information in her TED Talk "How Porn Changes the Way Teens Think About Sex" (Rothman, 2019). This TED Talk as well as other resources on porn literacy and sex education programs like Our Whole Lives (OWL) can help clients and others in your life gain more accurate information on sexuality in general.

The Gottman Institute, a facility famous for researching and developing science-based approaches to healing and changing problematic relationship problems, published an "open letter to porn" on its website in 2016 (Gottman & Gottman, 2016).

It is worth reading this post in its entirety as they do not outright condemn porn, noting that when both members of a couple have an interest in viewing porn together, it can actually enhance communication about each person's likes and dislikes and even increase the woman's orgasm ratio.

However, the Gottmans do acknowledge many potential detrimental impacts of porn. Viewers can report lower self-esteem, inaccurate perception of relationship and sexuality information, possible decrease in intimacy between two people in a relationship (especially if one prefers engaging with porn versus a live human in the room), potential numbness to violence and degradation, and susceptibility to something called a "supernormal stimulus." Supernormal stimuli "are all around us" and include most things in advertising like "photoshopped" bodies, and even "junk food laden with unhealthy fats and sugars." The supernormal stimulus of porn can "lead to a lack of desire for sex with one's partner (which usually) is a normal sex stimulus" (Gottman & Gottman, 2016). Some men who report heavy adolescent porn use and masturbation later can then suffer from "porn-induced erectile dysfunction."

Clients have mentioned positive results from the Your Brain on Porn program (yourbrainonporn.com). Specifically, they report noticing improved sense of sexual health and abilities after 3 or 4 weeks of non-porn use. This program may be helpful for clients who report a daily constant use, interfering with daily and sexual functioning possibly due to overexposure to the "supernormal stimulus."

This is not to say that a client or individual must refrain from porn viewing for the rest of their life. Helping a client become more in charge of what and how often they view pornography can dramatically increase their sense of self and bring their sexual health into better balance.

Sex activists also highly encourage porn users pay for their porn, ensuring that consenting sex workers get paid a fair wage for their work. A few places for adults to look for ethical porn include makelovenotporn.com, Bellesa.co (porn by women), Ifeelmyself.com (focus on female pleasure), and spit.exposed ("queer porn for the pervacious"). Dan Savage hosts an annual porn film festival "for everyone" (humpfilmfest.com). David Ley (2016) has published a book on how to find ethical porn.

There is also a burgeoning audio porn market, possibly even more ethically minded, as there are no physical depictions. Some good audio options include tryQuinn.com (helping people feel comfortable in their bodies) and Dipseastories.com (celebrating healthy sex).

Pornography and EMDR Therapy

Indeed, if clients seek EMDR therapy for a self-reported so-called pornography *addiction*, then we can explore and potentially treat their unwanted behaviors (rephrasing them as *out of control*) through EMDR targeting and processing, including the Feeling State Addiction Protocol (Miller, 2010, 2012, 2021). Some questions to ask our clients include assessing how disruptive is it to daily life (relationships, work, etc.). We can also ask what is their preferred porn type and what it is doing for them. Some clients may prefer porn because masturbating to porn seems easier than engaging in partner sex, or that they enjoy the enthusiasm and eagerness often displayed. Others may report that they do not have to worry about performance anxiety, contraception, STIs, or negotiating another partner's sexual interests (Klein, 2010). And still others may note feeling inadequate with partners, overwhelmed with life responsibilities, or tired of boring and monotonous sex (Klein, 2010). Klein (2010) notes that the most common pathology regarding porn use is the secrecy, and that "rigidity around porn is rigidity." Certainly any kind of stressor that results in someone withdrawing from previously healthy and satisfying sexual relationships is worth exploring and may benefit from EMDR therapy, versus the actual porn use.

Indeed, the governing body of sexuality education and counseling, the American Association of Sexuality Educators, Counselors and Therapists (AASECT), issued a historic statement in 2016 asserting that

> *AASECT recognizes that people may experience significant physical, psychological, spiritual, and sexual health consequences related to their sexual urges, thoughts, or behaviors. 1) AASECT does not find sufficient empirical evidence to support the classification of sex addiction or porn*

addiction as a mental health disorder, and 2) does not find the sexual addiction training, treatment methods and educational pedagogies to be adequately informed by accurate human sexuality knowledge. Therefore, it is the position of AASECT that linking problems related to sexual urges, thoughts, or behaviors related to a porn/sexual addiction process cannot be advanced by AAESCT as a standard practice of practice for sexuality education delivery, counseling, or therapy.

Some clients may seek EMDR therapy because someone else exposed them to unwanted porn viewing. The EMDR therapy composites demonstrate how to process this type of trauma.

The more we all speak to our clients and each other about consent, healthy sexuality, positive relationships and well-being, the less we will be satisfied by the more exploitative types of porn foisted on us. Hopefully our clients can developed a balanced approach to porn and/or erotic imagery, using porn literacy strategies to find content that is appealing, inclusive, realistic, consensual, safe, and arousing, if they so desire.

EMDR Therapy and Porn Case Studies

These case composite examples focus on the disturbances that can particularly develop in children after being exposed to pornography—a "sexualization" typically falling within the covert sexual abuse category if no touching occurred.

Case Study 5.8: Akari, Unmonitored Access to Porn During Childhood

Akari, a 20-year-old self-identified queer Asian cisfemale college student, majoring in art, sought EMDR therapy for recent "negative sexual experiences that brought back memories of sex-related images and porn from childhood." She reported concurring recent depressive moments and episodes, and feeling overall down and disinterested, especially related to sexuality. Akari also noted having unmonitored internet access around ages 10 and 11, googling sexuality-related topics, and stumbling upon pornography. She recalled intense shame around her discoveries, to the extent that she felt "broken," no longer "innocent and pure" and had "thrown her life away."

As we developed the EMDR timeline, we ascertained 10 EMDR targets, four of which are mentioned here:

1. Age 10—An elderly man pushing her against a wall at a nursing home, reaching to touch her

2. Age 10—Being caught late at night searching the internet
3. Age 11—Watching a satire video and being caught by surprise to learn what "rape" actually was
4. Age 18—A friend taking advantage of her being drunk to touch her sexually, against her consent

Akari's NCs for the early pornography incidents were "I'm impure, disgusting, damaged, a bad person, dumb, and/or broken" as well as "I have no control" (for the early and recent sexual assault). Her PCs included "I'm normal, a good person." Regarding the sexual assaults, her PCs included "It's not my fault, I have choices now, I'm allowed to make mistakes, I'm learning, I can say no."

Akari was able to fully process through her EMDR target timeline, eventually bypassing a couple of later targets as her adaptive healing increased. As we approached the end of the target list she reported feeling more back "to normal" with improved interest in college, friends, and her art. She had started dating and noted that while she and her new partner were taking it slow, so far she was able to stay in the moment and enjoy physical touch and intimacy without any prior porn or assault images interfering. We also completed EMDR Future Templates on effectively "handling and enjoying" future sexual intimacy and activities (e.g., enjoying oral sex with her new partner).

Case Study 5.9: Martina, Child Exposed to Porn

Martina's mother brought her to EMDR therapy to process through prior sexual abuse from a caregiver's son. Martina, a female-identified Latina, currently age 9, was 5 years old when the 13-year-old son of her biological father's girlfriend "kissed and touched her, and showed her porn." Her parents had been divorced since she was 2 years old. At age 5, Martina showed inappropriate knowledge about sex soon after the incidents with the boy. A case was opened, investigated, and the boy was found guilty. Her father disappeared shortly after. Four years later Martina reported having "nightmares" and trouble hearing the words "sex," "penis" or other words with an "x" in them.

As Martina was very insightful and articulate, we developed a modified EMDR timeline of "yucky things" and were able to process through both the molestation from David (which included him wrapping his arms around her, preventing her from moving away from the porn on the computer screen), as well as the lingering vivid pornographic images she still remembered. Her NCs included "I'm trapped and disgusting." Her PCs included

"I'm free, I can just be a kid, I'm fine as a I am. Let adults deal with that stuff (sex)." Much psychoeducation, validation, and normalization of symptoms was provided as well. A few weeks later she reported no longer having nightmares or being bothered by the word "sex" or other words with an "x" in it.

EMDR RESOURCE: "STRENGTHENING A CONFIDENT AND JOYFUL SEXUAL SELF"

Introduction

Emily Nagoski's helpful TED Talk "Confident and Joyful Sexual Self" (2016) inspired the development of this EMDR resource. This EMDR resource is also influenced by the DNMS Healing Circle (Schmidt, 2009), EMDR Future Templates (Leeds, 2016; Shapiro, 2018), and is designed to be a slightly more boundaried and potentially less explicit version of the future template Sabitha Pillai-Friedman provides within her Sexual Dysfunction EMDR Protocol (2009).

The goal of this resource is to provide your clients with another opportunity to recognize and experience a positive sexual moment. Many humans in general, especially clients with trauma histories, do not spend much time prioritizing or focusing on their sexual health and pleasure. Experiencing this resource is a chance to slow down and allow one's neural networks to bathe in positive associations (whether from memory or fantasy).

If your client is unable to identify a positive sexual moment, that is okay, they can initially identify a positive moment from another area of life. Go through the resource two or three times, each time assisting your client in identifying something more closely approximating sexual content. Remember, this resource is appropriate for clients who actively wish to enhance a positive and joyful sexual self. If your client is not interested, do not proceed.

This resource is best facilitated toward the end of EMDR therapy when the client has reported a reduction in PTSD symptoms and/or triggers to sexual material. Ideally your client is expressing a wish to gain more confidence or get more in touch with their sexual needs. Hold off on this resource if your client is actively dissociating, continues to show trouble self-regulating, or unable to stay in the window of tolerance.

Good BLS options include the Butterfly Hug tapping, theratappers, and audio. These options allow the client to close their eyes and absorb into the experience. It is helpful to reiterate therapist/client boundaries before doing this resource. Remind the client that they are in charge of their body and can ask for a time out, report only what is comfortable, take as much distance physically as is allowable, or even move further from the video screen if this is through telehealth (but instruct them to keep their camera on).

Provide your client with the accompanying "Strengthening a Confident and Joyful Sexual Self" Client Worksheet ahead of time, instructing your client to follow the directions in the Preface daily between appointments. If your client has difficulty identifying and writing down their positive physical attributes, or seeing the "door to their sexual self," then more EMDR processing regarding body image and/or sexually related targets may be needed.

Anecdotally, some people who have experienced this resource reported the positive cognition automatically popping into their mind during sex. One person noted having an orgasm less than 2 minutes after the appearance of her positive cognition.

The Script for EMDR Clinicians

Preface

(You can read this slowly one or two sessions before planning to use the script. This is also in the client worksheet.)

"Confidence is knowing what is true about your body. Joy is loving what is true about your body" (Nagoski, 2016). Some things that can help body confidence:

1. Every day look at yourself in the mirror and write down everything you like.
2. For 2 minutes a day enter your calm place or think of a soothing activity, then see the door that opens to your authentic sexual self. "Shine a beacon of kindness and compassion through the door" (Nagoski, 2016).

The Script

I. Think of a time when you had a completely positive sexual encounter (with yourself or someone else). If no such encounter exists yet, you can

- think of a moment in your sexual or affectional fantasy life
- a different moment when you felt particularly confident (perhaps with work, sports/athletics, movement, or a creative activity such as drawing or music)
- or think of something positive you've seen or read that embodies the following skills or aspects

You felt:

1. Grounded and present
2. Affirmed and consenting
3. Open to new and positive ways of interacting (sexually or otherwise)
4. In touch with your needs
5. able to express your needs clearly
6. In touch with pleasant physical sensations and/or smells

7. Deserving of giving and/or receiving pleasure
8. Confident in your abilities
9. Desire to share this energy in some form (e.g., journaling, art, telling an appropriate friend or therapist, or transforming this energy into other areas)
10. And perhaps spiritually connected or in "flow"

II. Have you identified a *moment from your life*, either a physical moment, or from your mind?

Notice the physical sensations that go along with this. _____
What image, symbol, sensation, or concept can represent this positive moment? _____
Give it a simple cue word or phrase to remember it. _____
What is a positive cognition (PC) that we can put with this image? _____ (e.g., I'm worthy of pleasure. I'm safe as I pursue pleasure. I enjoy connection. I radiate joy.)
How true is this PC feeling right now on a scale from 1 to 7 (1 is "false," 7 is "true")? _____
Hold the PC _____ with the cue word _____.
Apply BLS.
How true is the PC now from 1 to 7? _____ (Continue to apply BLS sets until the PC gets to a 6 or 7).
What emotion are you noticing for yourself? _____ (looking for a positive emotion)
Where and how is that emotion in the body? _____ (looking for a positive sensation and the location)

III. Now let's go through each of the 10 skills I mentioned earlier. I'll have you hold the positive thought with the image and each skill. We will let each skill get strengthened, moving on to the next when you signal me. If a problem arises, let me know.
Now think of _____ image, _____ PC, notice any positive body sensation, and focus on…

1. Feeling grounded and present
2. Affirmed and consenting
3. Open to new and positive ways of sexually interacting
4. In touch with your needs
5. Able to express your needs clearly
6. In touch with pleasant physical sensations
7. Deserving of giving or receiving pleasure
8. Confident in your abilities

9. Desire to share this energy in some form (e.g., journaling, art, appropriately telling an friend or therapist, or transforming this energy into other domains)
10. Perhaps spiritually connected or in "flow"

How true is your PC now? _____ (ideally at a 7; if not at 7, inquire about any blocking beliefs and process).

IV. Now imagine or visualize a desired *future* encounter, whether with yourself or someone else. Take a moment to develop the setting, determine activities, and so on. How true is the PC _____ as you imagine this scenario? (Install to a 7 using BLS sets. Once the PC is at a 7, use slower BLS and have your client take some deeper, slower breaths, staying with the scenario for half a minute or so, breathing in the positive words and sensations.)

V. Optional: Ask client for a challenge that may arise in the desired future encounter.
When you think of this future encounter, are there any possible challenges that come to mind that may interfere with full enjoyment?
_____

Notice and eliminate any negative physical disturbances, or strengthen any positive physical sensations with BLS.
Install the PC to a 7.

VI. Further insight opportunity:
When you came up with this positive moment, what good things were happening in your life at the time to help set the stage?
_____

Case Study 5.10: Eliza Strengthens Her Confident and Joyful Sexual Self

Eliza, a late-30s cisfemale bicultural African American and Colombian (one parent was an immigrant from Colombia) married lesbian, had worked through all her prior EMDR targets (two were related to sexual assaults, three were related to family of origin denying her sexual orientation) and was now working on improving the quantity and quality of sexual interaction with her wife mainly through psychoeducation (both were completing the *Come as You Are Workbook*, 2019). Physical boundaries between therapist and client were reiterated. Eliza understood we could stop the resource at any time, and that she can report only what feels comfortable articulating.

Eliza was able to note some positive physical features for herself on the days between our appointments. She also reported using her calm place (a beach in Maine) to enter in a calm mindset and shine a beacon of kindness and compassion through it. As this was telehealth, the client worksheet had been emailed ahead of time. Eliza had printed it out and was ready to complete it as we progressed.

Eliza identified a positive sexual moment from a few years ago when she and her wife Chris were traveling. At one particular hotel in Georgia they experienced a great deal of sexual satisfaction and intense erotic connection, both very much feeling alive, free, and in flow. Eliza, very appropriately, did not go into detail, but affirmed that this was a positive sexual experience and chose to call it "Georgia hotel." The PC she chose to use was "I can capably and confidently enjoy giving and receiving pleasure." The PC started at a 5, and was able to increase to a 6.5 after two BLS rounds. She reported feeling confident and happy, noting that her sternum felt expansive and that she had butterflies in her stomach. We then combined the cue word ("Georgia hotel"), the PC ("I can capably and confidently enjoy giving and receiving pleasure"), and the 10 positive qualities. Eliza affirmed that each item strengthened, and reported that her PC was now at a 7.

For her future encounter, Eliza imagined a sexual encounter with Chris on a road trip at an upcoming hotel in New Hampshire. She reported easily being able to imagine details, sensations, and positive emotions. Her PC remained at a 7. As for a potential challenge, she wondered how this scenario would transpire if her wife was not interested in sex once they arrived at the hotel. We spent a few moments discussing various strategies, including conversations ahead of time to help set the tone and mood, and courting behavior Eliza might apply. We recognized that her wife often swims more in the "responsive desire" domain. As long as Chris consented to Eliza initiating courtship behaviors, there was a high chance Chris would be interested in engaging in sexual activity. Eliza reported initially feeling some tension in her sternum as we sorted through this challenge. After the strategizing we applied BLS. Eliza noted that the tension dissipated almost immediately and that once again she felt "good" butterflies in her stomach. Her PC of "I can capably and confidently enjoy giving and receiving pleasure" was once again at a 7.

Two weeks later Eliza reported that she and her wife indeed enjoyed a wonderful sexual experience in New Hampshire, and even continued with increased sexual activity returning home. They continued to work on communication and awareness regarding sexual needs, feeling positive about their mutual increase in interest and concern.

HELPFUL RESOURCES FOR IMPROVING SEXUAL PLEASURE

At last our society has reached a point were there are many professional and lay-person books and websites available to help individuals improve sexual pleasure, not just correct painful or traumatic experiences. I list all of the most recent and helpful resources in Chapter 11, Sexual Resources for EMDR Clinicians. As I would need another book to properly summarize all of the pleasure-enhancing recommendations and exercises available, I will simply mention four very helpful resources. There are a few continuities in all the books that mention sexual pleasure enhancement. These suggestions involve self-exploration and increasing comfort with one's body, open and honest communication with any partner(s), creating a sexy or positive context, with no pressure, and non-demand sexual time with partner(s)—not seeking immediate orgasm. Essentially, slowing down and smelling the roses; crucial reminders for our ever increasingly fast-paced world.

Kegels

Buehler's book on sex for mental health professionals (2021) includes several pleasure-enhancing techniques. Early in the book she shares "Kegels for Everyone" (p. 34) as a way for people with clitorises and vaginas to develop a "greater awareness of sexual sensation and arousal, as well as improved capacity for orgasm." Kegels can also "improve the quality of (penis) erection and increase ejaculatory timing." Kegels involve tightening and relaxing pelvic floor muscles, usually identified initially by stopping the "flow of urine" for folks with vaginas, or trying to stop gas from leaving the body, for folks with penises. "Slow Kegels" (also good for mindfulness) involve tensing the muscle group for three seconds, then fully relaxing for three seconds. Typically one performs about 10 of these squeezes for a full set, about five times a day. It is important to consult with a pelvic floor physical therapist or expert and vetted websites to ensure proper instruction. If done improperly (for instance, too much tightening, not enough relaxation), then you can make "the muscle too tight" (Buehler, 2021).

Mindfulness

Buehler (2021) and Ogden (2018) both mention the importance of breath and mindfulness in both getting in touch with and increasing pleasure. Buehler offers advice for the client to first pay attention to their breath (taking slightly slower breaths), then add in more focus (helping the mind follow the body), then finally link the mind and body. Once this is established, clients can tune into "what (they) are feeling and experiencing, (which) can increase arousal, emotional connection, and pleasure" (2021). Clients can say to themselves, "breathing in, I am aware of my (sexual) body, breathing out, I am aware of my (sexual) body" (Buehler, 2021). This practice can be particularly helpful during sex with another partner to help remain calm and present. Ogden (2018) discusses the neuroscience behind how "consciously regulating our own breathing (can) strengthen neuro networks that will change our automatic breathing rhythm to support excitement, arousal, and other sex-positive attributes."

Clitoral Orgasms

Nagoski's wrote her incredibly thorough and revolutionary book, *Come as You Are*, primarily because she was done with "living in a world where women are lied to about their bodies; where women are objects of sexual desire but not subjects of sexual pleasure, where sex is used as a weapon against women, and where women believe their bodies are broken" (2015). Thank goddess! For any person with a clitoris and vulva having difficulty with orgasm, they can find two very helpful exercises in the back of the book. Appendix 1 recommends and explains "therapeutic masturbation" to locate, understand, explore, and experience orgasm. The basic steps involving locating the clitoris, creating a sexy context (mentally, environmentally, etc.), touching all over the body, indirectly stimulating the clitoris, trying direct stimulation, and breathing. These steps are explained in much detail in her book (pp. 339–340).

Nagoski does not just stop there. Appendix 2 in *Come as You Are* (Nagoski, 2019) provides information about how to experience extended orgasm, aka ecstatic pleasure. This also involves breathing (notice the pattern throughout this section about breathing), building to orgasm very slowly and incrementally, backing away at each increase. For example, if orgasm is a 10 on a zero (no arousal) to 10 scale, then build to a 3, then back down, build to a 4, then back down, and eventually learn to hover around a 9. She recommends setting aside at least 45 minutes to an hour to explore this type of extended orgasm. Her instructions contain much more very relevant detail, so please consult her book for proper explanation.

Penile Erections

Many elements can impact penile erections. Buehler (2021) lists several straightforward strategies to help improve erections. Most of these strategies involve taking care of physical health by exercising, eating more healthfully, not smoking, having little or no alcohol, sleeping well, and keeping one's annual physical exam. Lack of exercise, poor sleep, excessive smoking and drinking can all impact the ability for oxygen to travel throughout the body and reach the penis. Avoid experimenting with any questionable products marketed toward penis enlargement or enhancement. They very rarely work and may cause discomfort, certainly in the lightening of one's wallet.

Metz and McCarthy's book *Coping with Erectile Dysfunction* (2004) continues to be a frequent reference among sex therapists, is highly informative and helpful, and contains many practical exercises to regain, retain, and enjoy erections. Much of their recommendations involve breathing (what a surprise) and also open and honest communication with oneself and one's partner(s).

The book *The Multi-Orgasmic Man* (Chia & Abrams, 2009), while written some time ago, thus reflecting some outdated gender ideas, contains exercises to help people with penises increase pleasure and separate ejaculation from orgasm, allowing for full body orgasms or several orgasms in one situation.

SUMMARY

The use of EMDR Future Templates is an important part of completing EMDR therapy and involves clients successfully imagining a desired future situation, behavior, or outcome. There are endless EMDR Future Template possibilities, but usually completing a handful tremendously helps our clients gain confidence. EMDR Future Templates are excellent tools in helping clients to address sexual health and improve sexual functioning. Pillai-Friedman's EMDR Protocol for Sexual Dysfunction has an excellent sexuality-related Future Template.

Self-esteem issues, poor body image or specific body concerns, social media, and pornography can all impact our clients' sexual health. Exploring these issues, locating and processing any relevant EMDR targets can greatly benefit our clients' sexual health and esteem.

The many case studies in this chapter illustrate the power of EMDR Future Templates to enhance both general and sexual health.

A new EMDR resource "Strengthening a Confident and Joyful Sexual Self" provides your clients with another opportunity to access, recognize, and experience a positive sexual moment (whether from their life or imagination). This resource is a chance to slow down and allow one's neural networks to bath in positive associations.

Many resources exist to help individuals increase their capacity for sexual pleasure. Most helpful exercises include Kegels, breathing, mindfulness, creating a sexy context (whether in one's mind or environment), good communication with oneself and partner(s), and non-demand sensual time. Taking care of one's physical body can also improve sexual response and pleasure.

REFERENCES

AASECT. (2016). *AASECT position on sex addiction.* https://www.aasect.org/position-sex-addiction

Beer, R. (2019). Protocol for EMDR therapy in the treatment of eating disorders. In M. Luber (Ed.), *Eye movement desensitization and reprocessing (EMDR) therapy scripted protocols and summary sheets: Treating eating disorders, chronic pain, and maladaptive self-care behaviors* (pp. 11–64). Springer Publishing.

Buehler, S. (2021). *What every mental health professional needs to know about sex, third edition*. Springer Publishing.

Chia, M., & Abrams, D. (2009). *The multi-orgasmic man: Sexual secrets every man should know*. Harper One.

Dischiavo, R. (2020). *Erotophobia and sex negativism in today's America* [Webinar]. Institute for Sexuality Education and Enlightenment.

Fey, T. (2011). *Bossypants*. Reagan Arthur Books.

Forester, D. (2009). Image is everything: The EMDR protocol in the treatment of body dysmorphia and poor body image. In R. Shapiro (Ed.), *EMDR solutions II* (pp. 165–174). W. W. Norton and Co.

Gottman, J., & Gottman, J. (2016, April 5). *An open letter to porn*. The Gottman Institute. https://www.gottman.com/blog/an-open-letter-on-porn/

Klein, M. (2010, April). *When sex gets complicated: Pornography, kink, cybersex, and other clinical challenges* [workshop]. AASECT, Florence, MA.

Leeds, A. (2016). *A guide to the standard EMDR therapy protocols for clinicians, supervisors, and consultants, second edition paperback*. Springer Publishing.

Ley, D. (2016). *Ethical porn for dicks: A man s guide to responsible viewing pleasure.* ThreeL Media.

Metz, M., & McCarthy, B. (2004). *Coping with erectile dysfunction: How to regain confidence and enjoy great sex*. New Harbinger Publications.

Miller, R. M. (2010). The feeling-state theory of impulse-control disorders and the impulse-control protocol. *Traumatology, 16*(3), 2–10.

Miller, R. M. (2012). Treatment of behavioral addictions utilizing the feeling-state addiction protocol: A multiple baseline study. *Journal of EMDR Practice and Research, 6*(4), 159–169.

Miller, R. M. (2021). *The feeling-state theory and protocols for behavioral and substance addictions* (3rd ed.). ImTT Press.

Nagoski, E. (2016, February). *Confidence and joy are the keys to a great sex life* [Video]. TED conferences. https://www.youtube.com/watch?v=HILY0wWBlBM

Nagoski, E. (2019). *Come as you are workbook: A practical guide to the science of sex*. Simon & Schuster.

Nagoski, E. (2021). *Come as you are: Revised and updated*. New York, NY: Simon & Schuster.

Ogden, G. (2018). *Expanding the practice of sex therapy: The neuro update edition, second edition*. Routledge.

Pillai-Friedman, S. (2009). Sexual dysfunction EMDR protocol. In M. Luber (Ed.) *Eye movement desensitization and reprocessing (EMDR) scripted protocols: Special populations* (pp. 151–166). Springer Publishing.

Popky, A. J. (2005). DeTUR, an urge reduction protocol for addictions and dysfunctional behaviors. In R. Shapiro. (Ed.), *EMDR solutions: Pathways to healing* (pp. 167–188). W. W. Norton.

Rennick, R. (2021). *Digital sexuality and youth* [Webinar]. Tapestry.

Responsible Sex Ed Institute. (n.d.). *Teaching porn literacy to youth*. Responsible Sex Ed Institute. Retrieved September 17, 2021, from https://responsiblesexedinstitute.org/rsei-blog/teaching-porn-literacy-to-youth/

Rothman, E. F. (2019, September). *How porn changes the way teens think about sex* [Video]. TED Conferences. https://www.youtube.com/watch?v=FhP0AfZdRZ4

Scalisi, K. (2018). *Intersections of sex and technology* [Webinar]. Institute for Sexuality Education and Enlightenment.

Schmidt, S. J. (2009). *The developmental needs meeting strategy: An ego state therapy for healing adults with childhood trauma and attachment wounds.* DNMS Institute, LLC.

Seijo, N. (2019a). EMDR therapy protocol for eating disorders. In M. Luber (Ed.), *Eye movement desensitization and reprocessing (EMDR) therapy scripted protocols and summary sheets: Treating eating disorders, chronic pain, and maladaptive self-care behaviors* (pp. 143–194). Springer Publishing.

Seijo, N. (2019b). The rejected self EMDR therapy protocol for body image distortion. In M. Luber, (Ed.), *Eye movement desensitization and reprocessing (EMDR) therapy scripted protocols and summary sheets: Treating eating disorders, chronic pain, and maladaptive self-care behaviors* (pp. 217–238). Springer Publishing Co.

Shapiro, F. (2018). *Eye movement desensitization and reprocessing EMDR) therapy, third edition: Basic principles, protocols, and procedures.* Guilford.

Zaccagnino, M. (2019). EMDR therapy protocol for the management of dysfunctional eating behaviors in anorexia nervosa. In M. Luber (Ed.), *Eye movement desensitization and reprocessing (EMDR) therapy scripted protocols and summary sheets: Treating eating disorders, chronic pain, and maladaptive self-care behaviors* (pp. 79–126). Springer Publishing.

SUPPLEMENTAL MATERIALS FOR CLIENTS

THE "STRENGTHENING A CONFIDENT AND JOYFUL SEXUAL SELF" SCRIPT

Preface
(You can read this slowly one or two sessions before planning to use the script. This is also in the client worksheet.)

"Confidence is knowing what is true about your body. Joy is loving what is true about your body" (Nagoski, 2016). Some things that can help body confidence:

1. Every day look at yourself in the mirror and write down everything you like.
2. For 2 minutes a day enter your calm place or think of a soothing activity, then see the door that opens to your authentic sexual self. "Shine a beacon of kindness and compassion through the door" (Nagoski, 2016).

The Script

I. Think of a time when you had a completely positive sexual encounter (with yourself or someone else). If no such encounter exists yet, you can

think of a moment in your sexual or affectional fantasy life,

a different moment when you felt particularly confident (perhaps with work, sports/athletics, movement, or a creative activity such as drawing or music),

or think of something positive you've seen or read that embodies the following skills or aspects:

You Felt

1. Grounded and present
2. Affirmed and consenting
3. Open to new and positive ways of interacting (sexually or otherwise)
4. In touch with your needs
5. Able to express your needs clearly

6. In touch with pleasant physical sensations and/or smells
7. Deserving of giving and/or receiving pleasure
8. Confident in your abilities
9. Desire to share this energy in some form (e.g., journaling, art, telling an appropriate friend or therapist, or transforming this energy into other areas)
10. And perhaps spiritually connected or in "flow"

II. **Have you identified a** *moment from your life*, either a physical moment or from your mind?

Notice the physical sensations that go along with this. _____
What image, symbol, sensation, or concept can represent this positive moment? _____
Give it a simple cue word or phrase to remember it. _____
What is a positive cognition (PC) that we can put with this image? _____ (e.g., I'm worthy of pleasure. I'm safe as I pursue pleasure. I enjoy connection. I radiate joy.)
How true is this PC feeling right now on a scale from 1 to 7 (1 is "false," 7 is "true")? _____
Hold the PC _____ with the cue word _____ (Apply BLS.)
How true is the PC now from 1 to 7? _____ BLS. (Continue to apply BLS sets until the PC gets to a 6 or 7.)
What emotion are you noticing for yourself? _____ (looking for a positive emotion.)
Where and how is that emotion in the body? _____
(Looking for a positive sensation and the location.)

III. Now let's go through each of the 10 skills I mentioned earlier. I'll have you hold the positive thought with the image and each skill. We will let each skill get strengthened, moving on to the next when you signal me. If a problem arises, let me know.

Now think of _____ image, _____ PC, notice any positive body sensation, and focus on…

1. Feeling grounded and present
2. Affirmed and consenting
3. Open to new and positive ways of sexually interacting
4. In touch with your needs
5. Able to express your needs clearly
6. In touch with pleasant physical sensations

7. Deserving of giving or receiving pleasure
8. Confident in your abilities
9. Desire to share this energy in some form (e.g., journaling, art, appropriately telling an friend or therapist, or transforming this energy into other domains)
10. Perhaps spiritually connected or in "flow"

How true is your PC now? _____ (ideally at a 7; if not at a 7, inquire about any blocking beliefs and process)

IV. **Now imagine or visualize a desired** *future* encounter, whether with yourself or someone else. Take a moment to develop the setting, determine activities, and so forth. How true is the PC _____ as you imagine this scenario? (Install to a 7 using BLS sets. Once the PC is at a 7, use slower BLS and have your client take some deeper, slower breaths, staying with the scenario for half a minute or so, breathing in the positive words and sensations.)

V. Optional: Ask client for a challenge that may arise in the desired future encounter.

When you think of this future encounter, are there any possible challenges that come to mind that may interfere with full enjoyment? _____

Notice and eliminate any negative physical disturbances, or strengthen any positive physical sensations with BLS.

Install the PC to a 7.

VI. Further insight opportunity:

When you came up with this positive moment, what good things were happening in your life at the time to help set the stage? _____

CLIENT WORKSHEET

EMDR Resource: "Strengthening a Confident and Joyful Sexual Self"
by Stephanie Baird, LMHC
(Adapted and inspired by Emily Nagoski's 2016 TED Talk "Confidence and Joy are the Keys to a Great Sex Life")

Preface: "Confidence is knowing what is true about your body. Joy is loving what is true about your body." Some things that can help body confidence: (a) Every day look at yourself in the mirror and write down everything you like. (b) For 2 minutes a day enter your calm place, see the door that opens to your authentic sexual self. Shine a beacon of kindness and compassion through the door.

I. **List of desired qualities in a positive experience (ideally sexual, but can be affectional, work-related, sensual, athletic, creative, etc.):**
   1. Present and grounded
   2. Affirmed and consenting
   3. Open to new and positive ways of sexually interacting
   4. In touch with your needs
   5. Able to express your needs clearly
   6. In touch with pleasant physical sensations and/or smells
   7. Deserving of giving and/or receiving pleasure
   8. Confident in your abilities
   9. Desire to share this energy in some form (e.g., journaling, art, telling an appropriate friend or therapist, or transforming this energy into other domains)
   10. And perhaps spiritually connected or in "flow"

II. **Identify a completely positive** *moment from your life*, either a physical moment, from your mind, or something you've seen or read?

Think of an image, symbol, sensation, or concept to represent this (write or draw in this box):

> Image or symbol can be drawn here.

Give it a simple cue word or phrase to remember it: _____
What PC can we put with this image? _____

(e.g., I'm worthy of pleasure. I'm safe as I pursue pleasure. I enjoy connection. I radiate joy.)

How true is this PC right now on a scale from 1 to 7 (one is "false," 7 is "true")? _____

Hold the cue word with the PC:

| Cue word: | + | PC: |

How true is the PC now from 1 to 7? _____.
What emotion are you noticing _____ and where/how is that emotion in the body? _____.

III. **Now think of** _____ **cue word,** _____ **PC, notice any positive body sensation, and focus on... (the 10 listed qualities).**

IV. **Now imagine a desired** *future* **encounter, whether with yourself or someone else. Take a moment to develop the setting, determine activities, and so on.** _____

How true is the PC _____ as you imagine this scenario?

I have included here a helpful article I wrote regarding pornography for my monthly newspaper column, *Sex Matters*. This can be photocopied and handed out to clients looking for more information on ethical pornography.

The Question of Pornography
By Stephanie Baird, LMHC
   Originally published March 2019 in the *Montague Reporter* newspaper monthly *Sex Matters Column*.

This month's column will briefly explore the complicated existence of pornography, a topic best suited for unbiased book-long examinations. Poll anyone on the street and you will get a wide array of emotional responses to the concept of pornography. Let's begin with a formal definition of pornography. Pornography is generally defined as showing sexually explicit content (photographs, film/videos, and/or writings in magazines and books, etc.) with the purpose of stimulating sexual excitement. Some pornography can also include a supernormal stimulus nature of more violent or extreme pornography specifically designed to quickly shock recipients into having an intense physiological and/or emotional response, in some cases numbing said viewers over time to the extreme depictions of degradation. Gloria Steinem argued in 1977 that if a ciswoman and a cisman engaging in sex were shown as having: equal power, equal pleasure, and equal choice, and the imagery is egalitarian, non-coercive, and non-degrading, this should be termed not pornography, but "erotica."

At this point most people acknowledge that porn exists and will likely continue to exist in some form. Since humans could first make marks on walls and observe ourselves and each other, we have attempted to depict our sexuality, going back to images and sculptures of genitals in the Paleolithic and Mesolithic periods such as the Venus of Willendorf.

Many folks assume that most internet activity involves searching for porn. In reality, porn represents only 4% of the top million sites, and about 13% to 25% of web searches. One in three viewers of porn are woman-identified. Research shows there has been a decrease in child sexual abuse and adult rape over the years, possibly correlated to porn availability (statistics compiled by Kate Scalisi, "Sex Tech" webinar [2018], and Dr. Rosalyn Dischiavo, "Erotophobia" webinar [2020]).

There have many sociologists, psychologists, evangelists, feminists, parents, lawyers, and justices weighing on what constitutes pornography versus something more "socially acceptable" that might land in the "erotic" category (i.e., the well-known *Fifty Shades of Gray* book series as well as "Bridgerton" and the like) versus straight-up pornography websites and magazines.

The SESTA law passed in 2018, while initially positive in the sense that it hopes to limit sex trafficking and slavery, also limits consensually working and

Chapter 5 Sexual Health EMDR Future Templates

paid sex workers and even educational sexual health internet content that can now be labeled "obscene." Ultimately, the legalities of what can be outlawed and what is acceptable have remained complicated by varying perceptions of what the "average person" considers OK or not OK. Another troubling aspect of the porn industry overall is the lack of regulations overall.

Luckily sex positive activists have defined some working elements of ethical pornography as well as the concept of porn literacy. Ethical pornography (also sometimes called "feminist" or "fair trade" pornography) includes fair payment of the filmmakers and workers, is made in a safe environment where everyone is of consenting age and is respected, shows real (not faked) sexual pleasure (especially for female bodies), is created for all viewers (including women), is 100% consensual in every way, and shows diversity across body type, age, race, sexuality, and ability.

Rebekkah Rennick in a Tapestry presentation on "Digital Sexuality and Youth" shared Responsible Sex Ed Institute's (affiliated with Planned Parenthood) porn literacy definition: "form of media that teaches individuals to think about, analyze, and evaluate the media they choose to consume and the media that is already around them, such as billboards and advertisements. Everything has a message, whether intentional or not. Knowing how, why, and for whom content was created can help youth (and adults) better understand what they see and hear and make healthy decisions."

Rennick notes that 89% of youth report the internet as their primary source of information and that "unwanted" exposures comprise 66% of youth exposure. Teaching our youth (and ourselves) how to critique the images offered is becoming more and more essential for sexual health well-being. Indeed, there are real concerns and issues with most "mainstream" porn that is made by cismen for cismen. Much of this type of porn leaves out important elements like emotional intimacy, consent, using condoms, discussing sexually transmitted infections risks, and varying body types. And it often includes degradation of women, unrealistic behaviors, poor treatment, and poor financial reimbursement of the actors.

Boston University's professor and researcher Emily F. Rothman, via the Boston Public Health Commission, created a curriculum to teach youth porn literacy called "Start Strong" and presents some of this information in her 2018 TED Talk "How Porn Changes the Way Teens Think About Sex." I highly recommending looking into this TED Talk as well as other resources on porn literacy and sex education programs like OWL (the sex education program that I co-teach through the USNF) to help yourself and those in your life gain more accurate information on sexuality in general.

The Gottman Institute, a facility famous for researching and developing science-based approaches to healing and changing problematic relationship problems, published an "open letter to porn" on their website in 2016 (https://www.gottman.com/blog/an-open-letter-on-porn/).

It's worth reading this post in its entirety as they do not outright condemn porn, noting that when both members of a couple have an interest in viewing porn together, it can actually enhance communication about each person's likes and dislikes and even increase the woman's orgasm ratio.

However, the Gottmans do acknowledge many potential detrimental impacts of porn. Viewers can report lower self-esteem, inaccurate perception of relationship and sexuality information, possible decrease in intimacy between two people in relationship (especially if one prefers engaging with porn versus a live human in the room), potential numbness to violence and degradation, and susceptibility to something called a "supernormal stimulus." Supernormal stimuli "are all around us" and include most things in advertising like "photoshopped" bodies, and even "junk food laden with unhealthy fats and sugars." The supernormal stimulus of porn can "lead to a lack of desire for sex with one's partner (which usually) is a normal sex stimulus" (Gottman). Some men who report heavy adolescent porn use and masturbation later can then suffer from "porn-induced erectile dysfunction."

The bottom line is the more we all speak to each other about consent, healthy sexuality, relationships and wellbeing, the less we will be satisfied by the more "mainstream" exploitative porn foisted on us. Hopefully we can use porn literacy strategies to find content that is appealing, inclusive, realistic, consensual, safe, and arousing. And where we help the consenting workers get paid a fair wage, through our purchases. A few places for adults to look for such ethical porn include makelovenotporn.com, Bellesa.co (porn by women), Ifeelmyself.com (focus on female pleasure). There is also a burgeoning audio porn market, possibly even more ethically minded, as there are no physical depictions. Some good places to listen include tryQuinn.com (helping people feel comfortable in their bodies), Dipseastories.com (celebrating healthy sex). Happy listening!

6

Considering Gender With All EMDR Clients

Michelle M. Marchese, LICSW

LEARNING OBJECTIVES

- The EMDR clinician will understand how gender can impact clients of all genders in regard to access to services, affect, and behavior.
- The EMDR clinician will review current language in regard to working therapeutically with transgender and gender-nonconforming communities.
- The EMDR clinician will be able to integrate gender-related concepts and language directly into Phases 1 to 6 of EMDR therapy.

INTRODUCTION

As you begin reading this chapter, you may wonder, "Why should I consider gender when using EMDR therapy?"

First, all gender identities come with stories, roles, and expectations that may or may not align with someone's personal experience and varying degrees of comfort and discomfort. Gender is such a ubiquitous force that some people are not even aware that they have internalized these stories, roles, and expectations, and/or have not had a place where they can unpack their own gender and the narratives of gender that have been thrust upon them.

Second, I once had a clinical supervisor tell me, "Your clients can only go where you can go." This does not mean that you have to question your gender or have everything figured out about your gender. But it does mean that it is important to recognize how gender operates so you can understand how it might be working—or not working—for your clients. As you go through this chapter, please keep in mind that gender is different for each person and that everything discussed here will not necessarily apply to each client of a particular gender that you encounter.

I have worked in highly gendered clinical settings: a Veterans' Administration hospital, an eating disorder clinic, a historically women's liberal arts college, and in independent practice in the vibrant and active feminist, queer, and transgender communities of Northampton, Massachusetts. This clinical background has informed much of the information in this chapter. Within these different settings, I have heard clients use gender to minimize their traumatic experiences. For example, I have heard women survivors of incest say, "I can't have PTSD, I'm not a guy who went off to war." Veteran men have said to me, "I went to war, but that's not as horrible as being a women who is raped." Or a transgender women has admitted, "My experience is not so bad because I mostly pass [read as cisgender]; it would be much worse if I were nonbinary."

Now that I have explained two reasons why you should consider gender in your EMDR practice, here are some of the ways to hold gender in mind as you work through the eight phases of EMDR therapy:

1. Point out how gender expectations and norms affect your client's behavior, emotions, and thoughts. This can be a means of externalizing common trauma reactions such as blame, shame, and guilt.
2. Explore how gender expectations train people to behave with certain tendencies, as this may help survivors understand which trauma response (fight, flight, freeze, or fawn) they experienced during a traumatic event. (Fawn is when someone tries to please the perpetrator to avoid any conflict.)
3. Watch for the impact of gender norms on the inhibition of certain emotional expressions like anger, powerlessness, and fear and explore this with your client so that they may better access those feelings.
4. Examine how your client's socialization constructs include a hierarchical, gender-based understanding of relative human "value" and "trustworthiness." This, in turn, can help a client make sense of unhelpful/harmful ways that others have reacted to their trauma. Alerting your client to this unfair gender bias may deflate the power of negative cognitions such as, "I am unworthy."
5. It is important to note that there may also be a source of conflict for individuals between their gender and other social identities like race, ethnicity, physical or mental ability, age, socio-economic class status, sexual orientation, and marital status, among others. Challenges arising from these intersections may contribute to a client's negative cognition, process looping, additional or compounded trauma, assumptions they have about EMDR therapy and who it is for, and their worthiness for engaging in this highly specific therapy with a trained mental health professional. I invite you to imagine how the intersection of gender and

other social identities may come up in trauma work with clients such as: a retired Black veteran man who now must use a wheelchair as a result of an injury during active service; a single, White woman who was homeless during a devastating hurricane; a young Indian woman, recently matched with a husband, now diagnosed with invasive breast cancer; or a Chinese nonbinary person who has been emotionally terrorized by their affluent family of origin.

This chapter is organized into three sections: EMDR therapy with women, men, and transgender/gender-nonconforming/nonbinary/gender expansive or fluid/genderqueer (referred to in the rest of the text as TGNC) people. Within those sections, I will be referring to considerations in the eight different phases of EMDR therapy. It is by no means exhaustive of the ways that gender impacts individuals, systems, or the context of traumatic experiences, or of the ways to address gender in the context of trauma treatment, specifically EMDR therapy. However, my hope is that it adds some dimension to the important work you do with each and every one of your clients.

Perhaps many of the suggestions I make here are already integrated into your EMDR practice—and I would be thrilled to know that this is case! Still, continuing to think about your current clinical interventions within the context of gender, and utilizing humility about the culture and experiences of any of your clients, will always further enhance your practice.

WHAT IS GENDER?

Theorists in many fields still debate the concept of gender identity. Aristotle planted the seeds of a biological deterministic view of gender, and more recently Judith Butler proposed that gender is merely a performance (Bodnar, 2018; Butler, 1993). We now tend to understand gender as a social construct, meaning that a gender identity is not dictated by biology but is instead prescribed by the culture someone lives in as a series of behaviors, preferences, presentation, abilities, roles, tasks, and emotional expressions.

People tend to confuse or try to connect the concepts of *sex* with *gender.* Let us look closely at this: In the United States, a parent gets an ultrasound at about 18 weeks of cells growing in a uterus. A technician squints at some pixels thought to represent external genitalia, and declares that the cells are "a boy" or "a girl." and this leads people to lay out a myriad of gender-based expectations and limits that will last a lifetime. This scenario can also happen at birth. Babies can also be born *intersex* and possess "atypical" genital characteristics or reproductive organs. Since the 1950s "gender normalizing" surgeries have been frequently performed at birth with and without parental and, of course, child consent (Creighton, 2001).

However, what does a baby's perceived genitals have to do with the kinds of clothes they may like to wear, their favorite colors, the kinds of jobs they might be drawn toward, the division of domestic and emotional labor in their homes, or their relationship with anger? When people start to tie gender to bodies, the argument falls apart. If gender is related to body parts, what does this mean for women who have had mastectomies, hysterectomies, or oophorectomies? Similarly, if we determine gender based on genetic markers, what about the thousands of people born with more or less than the prevalent 46 chromosomes? Sometimes people will argue that hormone levels explain gender norms; what implication does this have for younger and older people, or people on hormone blockers due to cancer (Burstein et al., 2019; Senefeld et al., 2020)? We all know plenty of people who, even though they feel that their gender aligns with the sex they were assigned or assumed at birth, do not conform to gender norms. Many are therapists reading this book.

It may be easier to see how gender is constructed socially when we look outside of our immediate culture and notice differences in the expectations for and attitudes about genders. In Israel, all citizens regardless of gender must register for the Israeli Army. Women were prohibited from wearing pants throughout much of European history. Many transgender people are recognized and named within their cultures such as the *hijura* of India and Pakistan, the *kathoey* of Thailand, and *muxe* of Mexico; it was the influence of British colonization that introduced judgment and discrimination of people with these genders (Chang et al., 2018). Similarly, most indigenous North American (or Turtle Island) communities recognize and accept the *Two-Spirit* gender role, in addition to the roles of women and men (Ristock, Zoccole, & Passante, 2010). You may observe that some of these examples reference the past, thus contaminating the argument. But the introduction of time only further confirms the point of gender being socially constructed, because this means that gender roles were created by the culture *of that time* and that our current culture *no longer* recognizes those distinctions.

Because gender roles, expectations, and stories are socially constructed, it becomes important to understand how each individual feels in relation to these social narratives. Even the person who seems to most strictly conform to a culture's gender norms probably has moments where something about their gender role does not feel 100% right for them.

BASIC LANGUAGE CONCEPTS

Our language is constantly evolving. For example, your great-grandparents may think of "slides" as a photographic image on a piece of glass. Your parent may think of "slides" as an individual piece of photographic film, inserted into a projector, and viewed at a much larger capacity on a blank wall. Currently, a college undergraduate student may use "slides" to denote a series of text-based images posted online via social media or used on a computer in a PowerPoint presentation. In the same way, our language regarding gender is constantly changing—and fast. In fact, some of the language I employ in this chapter may soon be out-of-date. It is important to keep this in mind and stay curious, especially when working with

Chapter 6   Considering Gender With All EMDR Clients

people whose gender is different from yours or who are at different life stages. Box 6.1 will illustrate some of the gender-related terms I will be using in this chapter and with which you may or may not be familiar. These definitions stem from literature created by TGNC individuals and communities; affirming organizations that serve them, such as the World Professional Association for Transgender Health (WPATH); my professional experience working with TGNC clients for 10 years; and my personal experience as a member of queer and feminist communities (Chang, 2017; Shlasko, 2014; WPATH, 2011). Keep in mind that terms referring to individuals should be first used by the persons themselves.

Box 6.1 Gender-Related Terminology

Assigned-Sex-at-Birth, Assigned-Male-at-Birth, Assigned-Female-at-Birth (or AMAB or AFAB): The sex marker, usually male or female, declared at someone's birth according to their perceived external genitalia. Many legal documents will refer to this marker. Some sex educators and activists also use the term "sex assumed at birth" to denote the actual complexity and variety of marker and feature combinations.

Gender Identity: The internal, felt sense of an individual's gender. You cannot tell someone's gender identity just from looking at them, even if you think you can!

Gender Presentation or Expression: The outward mannerisms, accessories, or ways of relating and communicating that people tend to describe as "masculine" or "feminine." This does not have to align with someone's internal sense of their gender.

Gender Binary: The idea that there is only the two distinct, opposite gender categories of "male" and "female."

Transgender: Someone who transitions from living their life as one gender to another. This transition may or may not incorporate physical, social, or legal changes. Many people no longer use "transsexual," so avoid this term unless the person claims this identity.

Gender Nonconforming: A term that can encompass a range of gender identities that do not fall under binary gender definitions.

Non-binary: Someone who does not identify as either or entirely "man" or "woman." A non-binary identity can fall under either the categories of "gender-nonconforming" or "transgender," or both.

Cisgender: A person whose gender identity aligns with their sex assigned at birth. Someone who is not trans.

Gender Pronouns: All personal pronouns are gender pronouns. "They/them" is a common gender/neutral pronoun for a singular person. Some people use no pronouns.

Gender Self-Reflection Exercise for Therapists

There are many ways that we have been socialized to understand gender and the gender identities of those around us. In order to be gender-affirming to all of our clients, and to avoid replicating the trauma of forced gender expectations on any individual, it is importrant to unpack our own relationship to gender. By understanding how the mechanisms of gender work within ourselves, we are more likely to see how they work for and against our clients. This type of personal reflection and deconstruction demands more than just considering these few questions, but they may provide an entry point for further exploration (see Box 6.2).

Box 6.2 Gender Self-Reflection Questions

- When you were a child, what kinds of messages did you receive about how you should dress, how you should act, or how others should treat you that were related to your assigned gender at birth?
- Who were the people who communicated these messages to you? What kinds of power did they hold over you? Were they teachers, parents, peers, celebrities?
- Did you ever receive praise for conforming to gender roles or expectations?
- What happened when you did not conform to gender expectations?
- Have there been sexual or affective expectations of you in regard to your gender?
- Are there ways that you have communicated to others when they are or are not conforming to normative gender roles? Example: Have you joked about someone's gender or gender presentation?
- How did your gender play or not play a role in your choice to become a therapist?
- How do clients of any gender react to your gender?
- How are clinicians of different genders treated in your clinical setting? Are they paid differently? Do you notice any connections between their gender and the power they hold in your setting?
- Are there assumptions you have about your clients of any genders, especially if they are coming to you for trauma treatment? Have you noticed that some genders seem to be given certain diagnoses more than others? What have or have you not noticed about the gender of clients who have been previously diagnosed with bipolar disorder, borderline personality disorder, posttraumatic stress disorder (PTSD), acute stress disorder, narcissistic personality disorder, dissociative identity disorder, among others?

(Continued)

> **Box 6.2 Gender Self-Reflection Questions *(Continued)***

- Do you notice the physical or fashion attributes of clients of particular genders more than you do of other genders? Do you expect clients to present to you a certain way according to their gender? If a client does not conform to your idea of their gender, does this make you wonder about them diagnostically?
- What theoretical models have you been trained in or have you been drawn toward? What has been their view on clients of different genders? Did any of these models particularly pathologize women or transgender people? Were they initially conceptualized by men or women or a TGNC individual? How might Francine Shapiro's gender have played a role in how she disseminated information about EMDR therapy or how the larger research community initially reacted to EMDR?

These questions were inspired by a similar exercise in the excellent book, *A Clinician's Guide to Gender-Affirming Care*, by Chang, Singh, and Dickey (2018).

EMDR THERAPY WITH WOMEN*

The psychological field has been tainted by gender values and ideas since its was birthed by a man. Sigmund Freud famously treated cisgender women who were thought to suffer from something called *hysteria*. He subsequently published a paper in 1896 called *The Etiology of Hysteria*, in which he recognized that most of his patients reported what we now call sexual assault and incest. His findings threatened the power of the cisgender men who perpetrated these crimes. In deference to that power, and to shield himself from the consequences of highlighting traumas steeped in gender bias, Freud abandoned his "seduction theory" (Masson, 1984). Instead of describing the etiology of hysteria symptoms as stemming from sexual trauma, he proposed that they were caused by graphic, upsetting "fantasies" that were a result of deficits in psychosexual development (Jahoda, 1977). What does this history have to do with EMDR therapy?

Well, many master's and doctoral level programs in psychology and social work still teach Freud's theories. Despite the fact that our field has critiqued the mechanics of Freud's original theories, this does not mean it has fully disentangled gender bias from the field of psychology. If the foundation of psychological

---

*I use the term "women" here to apply to both cisgender and transgender women. However, I have grown to prefer the term *femme* because this term can include queer or nonbinary people who do not identify as a woman or a girl but who present in a "feminine" manner and, as a result, may all experience similar effects of gender bias.

history is rife with gender bias, how might that bias have remained in some form in more modern theories, or through the work of respected teachers and experienced trainers?

Fast-forward to the present.

Women are a third less likely to report trauma than men; yet, they are two times as likely to develop PTSD and four times as likely to develop chronic PTSD than men (Kimerling et al., 2013; Tolin & Foa, 2006). (While transgender women and transgender men may have been included in those large categories of gender in the literature, TGNC individuals are not referenced in this research.) This rate discrepancy is not because of something inherent in women that makes them more susceptible to trauma or PTSD, but instead has to do with various social and cultural factors, including the fact that women are more often victims of interpersonal violence (Centers for Diease Control and Prevention [CDC], 2021). One type of interpersonal violence, sexual assault, is more likely to cause PTSD than other traumatic experiences (DiMauro & Renshaw, 2021). Our culture tends to blame victims, especially women (Kennedy & Prock, 2018). Blaming the victim works to minimize the effects and symptoms of trauma of the one who was harmed in order to preserve a sense of control in the face of upsetting events. *Rape culture* is a term used to describe the pervasive particular cultural messages, in the context of interpersonal sexual violence, that seek to normalize rape and blame women for the violence perpetrated against them (Connell & Wilson, 1974). Victim-blaming may keep them from getting help because they do not "deserve" it, which can further exacerbate symptoms.

Access Issues

At this time, the majority of EMDR therapists tend to work in outpatient settings and many of them in independent practice. This already limits access to EMDR therapy for women who are engaged in treatment in psychiatric inpatient hospitals, receiving care through the Veteran's Administration, have services monitored by departments dealing with children and families, and who use Medicaid and/or Medicare insurances. Thankfully, many members of the EMDR community are working diligently to bring the practice of EMDR therapy to all settings and all populations, but it is still a process.

Decades of economic inequality also may impede a woman's ability to pay for or take time off to attend EMDR sessions, inequalities that are even more exaggerated for women who are BIPOC (Black, Indigenous, and People of Color; Wingfield, 2020). Since insurance is frequently tied to employment in the United States, unregulated work, such as sex work, further decreases access to EMDR treatment for women who labor in those fields, compounding the increased risk of sexual violence experienced by folks working in a criminalized field.

In our culture, women still shoulder the brunt of childcare, highlighted by the recent COVID-19 pandemic (Kenny & Yang, 2021). This further constrains the time some women may have to seek out and engage in EMDR therapy, and certainly in taking advantage of EMDR therapy in an intensive format.

Interaction With Legal Systems

While interpersonal violence is unfortunately perpetrated against people of all genders, as mentioned previously, women report the highest rates of sexual and interpersonal victimization (CDC, 2021). If survivors engage in the legal system as a result of this violence, they may experience structural or individual gender bias from local police departments, school administrators, hospitals, and human resource departments. As a result, your client may not only suffer from their initial trauma, but also may suffer from trauma related to how they were treated at the police station, what was said during a medical exam at the hospital, how their college has treated similar cases in the past, or even how governmental officials, as highly-placed as the U.S. Supreme Court bench, are not fully investigated after allegations of assault have been made public.

This has two implications for EMDR treatment.

One, when creating a Trauma and Loss Inventory in Phase 1, you may need to ask your client about the initial experience of violence, as well as identify subsequent traumatic interactions with institutions that were supposed to have supported your client.

- Example: If you are treating a traditional-aged college student who has survived a rape, together you will process the rape, but you also might need to process the school administration's suggestion to not pursue legal consequences, or her lawyer's insinuation that her drinking or clothing choices were the reasons your client was assaulted.
- Two, your client may not even recognize these instances of bias and instead internalize the negative messages experienced. Incorporating interweaves in Phase 4 about gender bias may help your client externalize and restructure her beliefs and judgments about the traumatic event, and allow for the digesting of emotions these beliefs may have blocked.
- Example: If this client internalized the idea that it was her fault that she was assaulted because she had been drinking, helping her understand how gender bias contributed to that belief may aid your client in no longer continuing to blame herself. This, in turn, may allow your client to access more adaptive beliefs related to her value and/or the values of gender equality. This new understanding may permit identification of resources that she either felt she did not deserve (when she believed the assault was "her fault") or resources that can represent gender liberation. (I have found many clients gravitate to the character Olivia Benson from the TV show *Law and Order: SVU*.)

Emotional and Behavioral Considerations

People are taught what emotions are socially acceptable for them according to their gender via social and institutional interactions and media (Kennedy-Root & Denham, 2010). This can show up in treatment sessions with women in particular ways. I will highlight two examples of such emotions: anger and disgust.

Anger

In the United States, *anger* is an emotion that many people who are socialized as female are not comfortable expressing. They are told, "Anger is not productive" or "Your anger hurts other people." Showing anger contradicts the cultural expectations that women and girls should be caretakers and peacemakers. In fact, our culture has a negative and offensive term for women and girls who express anger—"bitch"—yet there is no equivalent of this term for male subjects.

Since your client may not know how to engage with her anger, she may instead over-identify with other emotions such as fear, sadness, the experience of having autonomy blocked (powerlessness), guilt, or shame. I encourage you and your client to get curious about her lack of anger, and explore how it may be impacting her other feelings.

All of this may also mean that the only "acceptable" way for her to express anger is to turn it against herself. Anticipate ways this may creep into treatment:

- Phase 1: Anger turned against the self can show up as symptoms such as self-harm, disordered eating, suicidal thoughts, stomach pains and headaches, and perfectionist behavior.
- Phase 2: You may need to offer specific psychoeducation to normalize anger and explain its function.
- Phase 3: A client might not recognize sensations of anger because she has never been allowed to have them.
- Phase 4: You may need to reorient your client toward anger. She may also require cognitive interweaves that validate her anger and/or that invite her to unpack cultural or familial messages about anger.
- Phase 5: A client may not be able to install a positive cognition because she feels guilty for the anger that emerged during Phase 4.
- Phase 6: As needed, share information about how people tend to somatically feel anger in their head, chest or hands during the body scan. This may end up bringing you back for further processing in Phase 4.

Be sure to always consider the intersection of other social identities in relation to emotions. For example, Black women are often stereotyped as "angry" (Ashley, 2014). This pejorative trope could impact your client's ability to express anger, and depending on *your* race, it may impact her ability to express it to *you*.

Disgust

I have also found the emotion *disgust* to be implicated in gender socialization. Disgust is an emotion that has a particularly strong, negative, somatic charge to it. As a result, both clients and therapists may find themselves avoiding digging into this emotion. However, disgust can be an integral part of sexual and interpersonal violence, as well as medical or any other traumas that involve the physical body. In particular, a woman may be inclined to shield you, her therapist, from her disgust or aspects of her traumatic experiences that are disgusting. While some of this may be a manifestation of the classic avoidance response to traumatic material, it also may be tied to shame from victim-blaming, as well as socialized behaviors to caretake and prioritize the comfort of others, even at your client's own expense. Consider ways to bring up and normalize disgust for your client:

- Phase 1: Assess for caretaking behaviors in your client.
- Phase 2: Talk to your client about how she might avoid or hide contact because she thinks it may upset you. Reassure your client many times that this is not necessary.
- Phase 3: While setting up a target suggest disgust as a possible emotion she may feel.
- Phase 4: Ask about emotions associated with nauseous feelings. Disgust is often characterized by an obvious, particular facial expression. If you notice even a flicker of that across your client's face, bring attention to it.

Another aspect of disgust is that, like anger, it can be easily turned toward the self. Pay attention to the language your client uses such as, "I was disgusted with myself." This could be a clue to guide her toward processing disgust during Phase 4.

In addition to emotions, gender socialization affects behaviors. One of these behaviors is caretaking, which was mentioned previously. A related behavior is the act of saying "no." The first thing that might come to your mind after reading that statement is the historical phenomenon of "no" in the context of sexual consent. This context has served to render a woman's "no" as meaningless, not to be respected, or believed. That context also highlights how women are conditioned in general to *not* say "no" to others in order to keep the peace or because her needs are valued less than the needs of others. The behavior of saying "no" has implications in the treatment of sexual trauma, but it also affects our clients' abilities to set healthy boundaries. It can also play into the tendency to be a people-pleaser. Examples of how this may appear in treatment follow:

- Phase 1: This can appear as a client who often misses sessions due to obligations in her personal and professional life. It can also mean that it is not enough simply to ask for your client's consent to treatment. You must begin from your first session to normalize her opinion and her choice to speak up if something in the treatment is not feeling helpful.
- Phase 2: Your client may jump to an imaginal resource that she has positive feelings for, but make sure that there are no other negative associations with this resource that the client is ignoring or omitting to report, as a result of being overly accommodating toward that figure.

- Phase 3: Your client may need some additional permission from you to communicate difficulty connecting with her negative cognition, feeling, or somatic sense of the target event. She also may not feel comfortable redirecting you if she realizes this is not the right target at the right time, without you first normalizing this.
- Phase 4: What is probably most obvious is that your client might struggle with the idea that she did or did not say "no" during interpersonal violence. She may also be judgmental of the fact that she "froze" during a traumatic event or that she "fawned" over a perpetrator. Interweaving explanations on how she may have been taught to not occupy physical or emotional space and to diffuse the negative feelings of others may facilitate processing in this phase.
- Phase 5: Installing a positive cognition might be challenging if other people continue to be upset with her due to her handling of, or reactions to, the incident.
- Phase 6: Tuning into the sensations she feels in her body may feel confusing because she is so used to attending to others that she has trouble with "interoception" (tuning into and recognizing her own bodily sensations).

EMDR THERAPY WITH MEN*

In general, men do not face the same issues of pay inequity, cultural pressures to be the primary caretaker of children and families, legal bias, and assumptions about their blame with which women must contend. (Although, again, age, socioeconomic class, ability and other social identities can complicate this picture.) To return to the history of psychology, half of the cases Freud published centered on male patients, and male psychoanalysts were expected to be in treatment themselves throughout their careers. So, why are men accessing therapy at lower rates, and quitting therapy at higher rates? And how might gender impact the traumatic experiences of some men and play out in EMDR sessions?

Access Issues

While cisgender men do not face the same structural issues of access that women or TGNC clients do, they do struggle to start and complete treatment (Shiner et al., 2017). Part of this is due to stigma around men needing or seeking help (Sagar-Ouriaghli et al., 2019). Furthermore, many men are not acculturated to the language around therapy and the emotional activities inherent in it. Rather, certain expectations regarding the domination of others and one's environment, toughness, physical force and violence, aggression, blaming others, being independent, and not showing emotions are messages that boys and men receive from

---

*I use the term *men* here to apply to both cisgender and transgender men. However, the term *masc* can also include queer or nonbinary people who do not identify as a man or a boy but who present in a "masculine" manner and as a result, may all experience similar effects of gender bias.

parents, media, peers, family, lovers, and people in authority like doctors or the police (Seidler et al., 2016).

While there is a spectrum of these narratives and the ways that individual men identify with them, some people refer to the constellation or phenomenon of these negative expectations as *toxic masculinity*, a term originating from men involved in the self-help movement of the 1970s. Toxic masculinity includes qualities that some cultures attribute to masculinity that are harmful to the man who exhibits them and to the people around him. The function of toxic masculinity is to keep and to consolidate power for men by devaluing qualities deemed to be "feminine," such as emotional sensitivity, tenderness, emotional connection, and warmth. However, while toxic masculinity works to hold on to certain kinds of interpersonal power, it denies the subject loving, mutual, supportive, affective experiences and relationships.

Since men may not have been socialized to seek help, they may first encounter therapy tied to their employment in some way. Some examples of this are services provided by the Department of Defense or Veterans Affairs, or through Employee Assistance Programs (EAP). These providers and programs tend to offer time-limited, brief services. Due to the nature of this, a focus on outcomes and prescribed processes are common, and, as a result, may not allow the opportunity for acculturation to therapy or titrated experimentation with, and exploration of, emotions and acts of vulnerability.

Another way that men may find themselves in therapy is through referrals from other health providers. The steps between a suggestion during a routine health exam and a connection to an individual therapist combined with the variables of stigma and lack of acculturation create layers of barriers.

Additionally, issues around a therapeutic gender "match" seem notably heightened for many men (Shiner et al., 2017). If a man is working with a female therapist he may feel the need to adhere to prescribed gender roles and expectations or may assume that she will not grasp the intricacies of his gender experiences. If he works with a male therapist, he may worry about emotionally opening up to another man who may judge him for his emotional reactions. In fact, some research shows that men are more likely to quit therapy if working with a male therapist (Shiner et al., 2017). If he works with an "out" transgender or nonbinary therapist, any of these previous issues, plus gender insecurity or fears about homosexuality (homophobia), could arise.

Emotional and Behavioral Considerations

Considering that our culture can communicate messages that masculinity requires a stoic posture, it comes as no surprise that many men may deal with some level of alexithymia, or difficulty feeling and expressing emotions (Sullivan & Brown, 2015). This may require you in Phase 1 to be more directive and specific in your questions regarding emotional experiences and symptoms, as well as in your explanations of the therapeutic process. In Phase 2 you may need to prioritize explicit psychoeducation on emotions, thoughts, and behaviors, work to restructure stigma about engaging in therapy, and identify positive resources that showcase masculinity and emotionality. In Phase 3 it may take additional time for your client to recognize an emotion during the target setup.

Whereas women tend not to be encouraged to feel or express anger, for many men the only feeling they have been socialized to own is anger (Chaplin, 2015). This is because anger can take forms that preserve the dominance and insensitivity inherent in toxic masculinity. Many men feel a range of emotions but have learned to unconsciously translate all of them into anger (Chaplin, 2015). Many men may find that *fight* is the trauma response triggered most often for them. This has implications for emotional looping and avoidance of other negative emotions in Phase 4. Interweaves that reorient, validate, and normalize other emotions, as well as ones that direct to other somatic sensations may be useful. Other men who do not engage with anger for a variety of reasons, or for whom trauma responses tend to be *flight, freeze,* or *fawn,* may experience shame or self-judgment due to not aligning with a cultural masculine ideal. All of this would need to be addressed in Phase 2 and Phase 4.

Since many men are socialized to express anger and to avoid accountability through aggression, it may be particularly challenging for them to process feelings of vulnerability, fear, weakness, fear of losing autonomy (powerlessness), and shame. Digesting these emotions may come with the secondary grief of losing the idea of the man he thought he was, that his parents wanted him to be, or who is attractive to his partner. Make sure to help your client see the benefits of a full emotional life and discuss how many people value a man who can be supportive, take responsibility, and connect on emotional levels. Resources or references to positive male role models may be helpful here. Some of the ones I use include: Coach Eric Taylor from the TV show *Friday Night Lights*, T'Challa from the *Black Panther* film, Lieutenant Commander Paul Staments from *Star Trek Discovery*, Atticus Finch from the book *To Kill a Mockingbird*, or Randall and Jack Pierson from the TV show *This Is Us*.

EMDR Future Template work might revolve around practicing emotional reactions besides anger, or learning to express anger in ways that is not harmful to your client or those around him. It also may be about cultivating compassion for himself as well as others in future relationships and situations.

Male Survivors of Interpersonal Violence

When people imagine victims of physical, sexual, or emotional abuse, the first image that comes to mind is probably not one of a man. Yet in the United States, 1 in 6 boys has experienced childhood sexual abuse and one quarter of all men will experience some kind of interpersonal violence within their lifetimes (Briere & Elliot, 2003). Rates of sexual abuse of boys by members of the clergy are in the tens of thousands (Fitzgibbons & O'Leary, 2011). Men's experiences of interpersonal violence tends to be erased due to some of those previously mentioned toxic masculinity issues. Fear of minimization, being mocked, or not being believed can silence boys and men who experience this kind of trauma.

How can your practice not collude with the erasure of these men's experiences? What language about survivors can you use on your website to be inclusive of male survivors? Do you ask about all kinds of interpersonal violence for each of your clients during the Phase 1 intake? Do you know where to find resources for referrals, additional professional supports, books and articles that you can give to these clients? Many of these men struggle with loneliness and shame due not only to the initial trauma but also to the cultural response—or lack thereof—to their experiences. As a result, group modalities may be transformative, and examples of this can include group meetings that focus on resourcing (Phase 2), sessions for men, groups focusing on the future, or group EMDR (G-TEP) that would allow clients to process in a community of other male survivors.

In addition to issues of erasure and alienation, male survivors may have fears about what their traumatic experiences mean about their gender identity or sexual orientation. This is because being a victim of interpersonal violence is the antithesis of embodying certain toxic masculine ideals. While you may truly work with clients who have survived interpersonal violence and who happen to be questioning their gender or sexual identities while being assigned/assumed male at birth, be careful not to validate incorrect causal relationships between those things for other clients.

EMDR THERAPY WITH TGNC CLIENTS

I highly recommend Dr. Sand C. Chang's chapter entitled, "EMDR Therapy as Affirmative Care for Transgender and Gender Nonconforming Clients" in Mark Nickerson's book *Cultural Competence and Healing Culturally Based Trauma with EMDR Therapy* (2017). Some of the information discussed here may overlap with some of the material found in that chapter; however, Chang's work provides a wealth of information far beyond what I can present here.

Transgender, gender-nonconforming, and nonbinary clients may seek EMDR therapy for a variety of concerns. TGNC people are at a higher risk for trauma due to discrimination in most contexts (Clements-Nolle et al., 2006; Edelman, 2011; Nadal et al., 2010). As a result, individuals may be seeking trauma processing for events related to their gender identity, such as being estranged from family members, bullying, workplace discrimination, medical trauma, religious trauma, and interpersonal violence.

However, being TGNC is in itself not traumatic, and not all TGNC people find aspects related to their gender, legal, social, or physical transition to be traumatic. Instead, TGNC people might be seeking services for the kinds of traumatic events that we work through with our cigender clients. However, as with all other genders, I encourage you to be curious about how gender may impact your TGNC client's traumatic experiences and/or their relationship to it. If you are cisgender, please approach this part of the chapter knowing that you may have TGNC people as your clients, and that TGNC people may also be your EMDR colleagues.

Access Issues

TGNC clients have faced high rates of discrimination and harm by the psychological field due to anti-trans bias and ignorance (Campbell & Arkles, 2016; Chang et al., 2018). As a result, they may avoid mental health treatment (Chang et al., 2018). Keeping this history in mind, work to create trust and believe your clients, even if they report negative experiences with one of your beloved peers. Know that you might need to help your client process interactions they have had with previous providers.

Challenges with insurance if or when someone has not legally changed their name, or insurance that is provided by a family member who does not know your client is TGNC, creates barriers to treatment. To manage some of these barriers, be thoughtful and collaborate with your client about how to bill and document services. Discuss ahead of time about how to coordinate with other providers, agencies, or family members.

Structural oppression such as homelessness, poverty, unemployment, and police brutality hinder not only the availability of services for TGNC clients, but also the opportunity to choose providers based on their gender-affirming capabilities. Some of the considerations listed under "Interaction With Legal Systems" in the section on EMDR Therapy With Women may be applicable to consider in the context of some TGNC identities. Not all TGNC people will transition physically, socially, or legally. Some of this is due to personal choice and/or the cost and challenges associated with some changes.

Understand the limits of your knowledge and seek out resources that you can share with your TGNC clients. Take care to continue to educate yourself and shift your practice to recognize TGNC identities in the first interaction someone has with you or your practice.

To that end, I encourage you to change your intake paperwork to be inclusive of all genders (See Box 6.3). This means not assuming anything related to gender with any of your clients. You may find that some of your cisgender clients question you about this, but I find explaining at the start of any intake that, "I am going to ask you questions that I ask everyone who first comes into my office. Some of them may seem obvious to you, but I just don't want to assume anything about anyone," alleviates many tensions. Many of my suggestions seem simple once you read them, but I have found that clinicians often ask me how to specifically operationalize these ideas into questions.

Box 6.3 Some Suggestions for Gender-Inclusive Intake Questions

For all clients:

What is your name?

What is your gender identity? *(With no pre-determined categories listed)*

(Continued)

Chapter 6   Considering Gender With All EMDR Clients   181

> **Box 6.3 Some Suggestions for Gender-Inclusive Intake Questions *(Continued)***
>
> What are your pronouns?
>
> What has your experience been like working with other mental health providers?
>
> For TGNC clients:
>
> Are you "out" about your gender identity to other providers I will be communicating with to coordinate care? *(Make sure to protect their privacy and honor their choices.)*
>
> Does your insurance have another name on it? *(Do NOT ask things like: What is your REAL name or the name you were given. This is considered offensive.)*
>
> How do other people in your life react to your gender identity? Who is supportive? Who isn't?

Practicing Language

I referred to gender pronouns earlier, but nouns can also be gendered. You do not have to erase all gendered nouns from your language, but it is helpful to know some gender-neutral substitutes and to practice using them when you do not specifically know someone's gender (see Box 6.4).

> **Box 6.4 Gender-Neutral Nouns**
>
> | |
> |---|
> | sister or brother … try SIBLING |
> | niece or nephew … try NIBLING |
> | girlfriend or boyfriend … try PARTNER, DATE, or SIGNIFICANT OTHER |
> | husband or wife … try any of the above or SPOUSE |
> | alumnae, alumnus … try ALUM |
> | mother or father … try PARENT |

I have found that some clinicians who are not part of the LGBTQI2 (Lesbian, Gay, Bisexual, Transgender, Queer/Questioning, Intersex, Two-Spirited) community, and even some who are, have trouble with changing names, nouns, and pronouns for their clients. That is likely because they do not often get a chance to practice. The following two short case vignettes provide you with such an opportunity (see Box 6.5).

> **Box 6.5 Case Vignettes**

1. **Practice changing this client's name, pronouns, and gendered nouns to the two suggestions that follow the formulation. Imagine that your client Jason has transitioned to Halie, a transgender woman who uses she/her pronouns.**

    Jason is a 24-year-old, White, cisgender man from Amherst, Massachusetts. He is an alumnus of a local liberal arts college and works as a mechanical engineer. He presented to treatment due to long-standing issues with acute anxiety and panic. He states that he wants to work on these symptoms so that he can more fully commit to his wife and "be a good husband."

    ...

    Halie is a 24-year-old, White, transgender woman from Amherst, Massachusetts. She is an alumna of a local liberal arts college and works as a mechanical engineer. She presented to treatment due to long-standing issues with acute anxiety and panic. She states that she wants to work on these symptoms so that she can more fully to commit to her wife and "be a good wife."

2. **Here is another example. Imagine that your client Aika has transitioned to Asao, a nonbinary person who uses they/them pronouns.**

    Aika is an 18-year-old, cisgender female, Japanese international first-year student who recently graduated from boarding school in upstate New York. She currently majors in contemporary ballet. She is estranged from her family due to parental emotional abuse and wonders what family obligations she has as an elder sister to her five brothers.

    ...

    Asao is an 18-year-old, nonbinary, Japanese international first-year student who recently graduated from boarding school in upstate, New York. They currently major in contemporary ballet. They are estranged from their family due to parental emotional abuse and wonder what family obligations they have as an elder sibling to their five brothers.

Emotional and Behavioral Considerations

TGNC people are susceptible to the cultural messages that other genders face. So while there are specific considerations for supporting TGNC clients, also know that, for example, when working with a transgender woman, issues previously discussed about women need to be held in mind: This is because transgender men are men, and transgender women are women. However, navigating gender roles and norms can be complicated when someone has been raised as one gender and is now living as another gender. They may even feel at the mercy of all gender roles and norms at different times of their lives, especially during "coming out" or transitioning periods, or if they are gender-expansive or gender-fluid. Feelings related to "passing"—meaning, whether or not someone is perceived as cisgender—may impact someone's relationship to emotions and behaviors.

Gender Dysphoria and Implications for Dissociation

Dissociation can be an adaptive strategy to cope with gender dysphoria (distress that someone feels when their gender identity does not align with the sex they were assigned at birth or with their body), navigating between places where they are "out" and "not out" about their gender identity, and environments steeped in trans bias. As trauma therapists, we are trained to screen for trauma-related dissociation because this kind of dissociation can interfere with EMDR treatment or can re-traumatize clients during processing (Schauer & Elbert, 2010). However, the most widely used dissociation measure, The Dissociative Experiences Scale II, does not distinguish among these types of dissociation and, as a result, does not account for the divergent meanings of certain questions. For example, "Some people have the experience of looking into a mirror and not recognizing themselves," is a statement that can have different meanings for people with trauma-related dissociation and people who are in various stages of physical, social, or legal transitioning. In the latter case, a positive answer may not mean that they suffer from dissociation or that their dissociation could impact trauma processing, but instead refers to the way their gender identity does not correspond to how they look right now. Note that not all TGNC individuals experience gender dysphoria.

Therefore, talk to your client about dissociation in relation to their gender dysphoria. If you assess for dissociation in Phase 1, and they give higher scores to questions on the scale, ask them more about the context of their answers. Assess to see if gender dysphoria plays a part in their answers or not.

If your client does dissociate to manage gender dysphoria, you will still want strategies to help them manage the dissociation during trauma-processing sessions. Many of you are familiar with a wide array of coping skills for dissociation. Some of these can be helpful if your client has, for example, just returned from an unsafe situation or has not been able to be "out" all day until they settle into your office or with you via telehealth. Orienting them to a safer, present moment can then be helpful. However, many times if someone is feeling a higher level of bodily discomfort due to gender dysphoria, orienting to the current distressing moment is not helpful.

I suggest talking to clients about how you both can work to decrease this kind of dissociation in sessions. It is important to note that this dissociation may be highly adaptive for your client's situations or environments, so your goal is not to necessarily eliminate the dissociation completely. Some examples of what problem-solving this dissociation with clients can look like include:

- A transgender man wears a restrictive binder to smooth out the appearance of his chest. By the time we have our session at the end of day, the binder is causing physical pain that reminds him about his discomfort with his body. This was hard to ignore. My client found himself dissociating to cope with this. As a result, we changed his appointment time to first thing in the morning when he was more physically comfortable.
- A transgender woman works alone at home as a software engineer. Her family of origin is not accepting of her gender identity. Her being "out" to me does not alleviate the stress caused by the lack of experiences feeling seen as a woman in general. This stress causes her slip into dissociation. As we explored this together, she recognized that she felt the best about herself at the gym where she could see herself running on the treadmill with her ponytail swinging behind her. As a result, she planed workouts before our therapy, and if she felt gender dysphoria coming on, she would stroke her long ponytail to reorient to the positive feelings from her gym session.
- A nonbinary client tells me that their gender dysphoria is heightened each month during their menstruation cycle. As a result, each month we spend that weekly session on supportive talk therapy rather than EMDR trauma-processing. If the client feels ready the following week, we return to EMDR therapy.

Resourcing and Imagery Considerations

Although guiding clients to imagine themselves as a child can be therapeutically powerful and an integral part of many EMDR interventions and related therapies, you must talk to your client before engaging in these activities (Chang et al., 2018). For some people, seeing themselves as a younger person presenting in a gender that they do not identify with is extremely painful. For other people, it may be clinically appropriate to invite them to imagine themselves as a child, presenting as their true gender identity. Still other clients may not imagine their child-self looking different, but may want you to use either their current name and pronouns, or to their name and pronouns assigned at birth. Discuss all of these possibilities with your client during Phase 2, if you plan on using these types of interventions. Of note, should TGNC clients decide to use different names and pronouns for a younger self, this does not imply "alters" or "multiple personalities."

Relatedly, be thoughtful about the genders of your client's resources in Phase 2. Suggest specific figures that might bring the comfort of recognizing and accepting their gender, or may even mirror their identity. When choosing resource figures culled from their life experiences, make sure those figures are not contaminated by any anti-trans bias from other interactions.

I wholeheartedly encourage you to check out one of the best resourcing interventions developed by a nonbinary therapist for TGNC clients. It is called the "Future Empowered Self" and can be found in the Sand C. Chang chapter referenced at the start of this section.

Body Attention Scan/Considerations

Now that you have read about gender dysphoria and how it relates to discomfort with one's body, carry this information over to your consideration whenever you bring attention to bodily sensations in Phase 3 or Phase 4, as well as the Body Scan in Phase 6. First, talk with your client ahead of time about the practice and the utility of bringing attention to their body during processing (Chang, 2017). During this conversation, you might explore ways to make this more comfortable. However, accept that some TGNC people may have days when this kind of attention is not an option; for others, it may never be an option (Chang, 2017).

Next, get consent for somatic work each and every session you might engage in body-based work (Chang, 2017). You may get consent from a client to focus on their body one day, but dysphoria may be higher the next day for a variety of reasons, so always check in with your clients.

Another issue with the Body Scan in Phase 6 is that there may continue to be physical discomfort for your TGNC client even if processing is complete (Chang, 2017). This may be due to possible gender dysphoria and is not necessarily related to the traumatic memory. This discomfort might also remain because it is a result of a recent gender-affirming medical procedure or a garment used to contour certain physical characteristics.

Finally, TGNC folks tend to be physically scrutinized in many situations (Chang et al., 2018). Others may attempt to figure out an individual's gender according to how their body looks, or they may be overly curious when they notice physical changes. Either way, this translates into the importance of checking in with your TGNC clients and making no assumptions about what body-based attention is best for them.

Sexual Health Considerations With TGNC Clients

When discussing sexual health with your TGNC clients, please ask about the kind of language they use. Similar to cisgender clients, your TGNC clients may use a range of words to describe their bodies and what pleasure or pain they experience in those bodies. However, words that you may be comfortable using with your cisgender clients could be invalidating, misgendering, and at worst, triggering for your TGNC clients. You will want to let your client be in control of the language used in session, as you would with all of your clients. But because you are in a position of power as a therapist, it is important to use this power to show sensitivity and anticipate challenging conversations. Do this by inquiring about language right away by using simple questions such as:

"Are there words that you would like me to use or not use when referring to your body or talking about sex?"

At the same time, as previously mentioned, many TGNC individuals have the experience of having their body scrutinized by others due to curiosity, so only explore their sexual health after they have consented to talk about this with you.

There are some particular considerations to keep in mind about your TGNC clients' sexual health if they are in the process of physically transitioning. While someone can anticipate some common changes when starting hormone replacement therapy (HRT) or after some gender-affirming surgeries, every person is different so it is important to check in with your individual client without relying on them to educate you on the basics of these experiences. To this end, it will be important to refer to the latest research on how primary and secondary sex characteristics can change when someone is new to HRT, especially since some of your clients may be surprised about these changes, too, as all medical providers do not always provide detailed information about what to expect.

Issues related to gender dysphoria, in addition to hormones or surgeries, can possibly affect your client's interest in sex, and even who they are attracted to sexually. You may find your clients talking about "a second puberty," a desire to experiment and explore different gender roles in the context of sex, or a curiosity about other sexual orientations and those orientations' cultures around sex. The latter two may also emerge if your client is newly single or opening up their relationship(s) after transitioning. In any situation, it will be important to not jump to gendered or binary conclusions about any of these changes. As we all know, change is often anxiety producing, so encourage your client to allow themselves the freedom to play and experiment!

SUMMARY

Gender impacts all people, regardless of their gender identity. Gender can be a source of pleasure or terror, with a wide range of experiences in between. Considering the effects of gender on every client, and talking with any of them about gender when appropriate, can encourage and deepen fuller EMDR processing. I encourage you to seek out consultation and explore how gender may be operating in regard to transference and countertransference, whether or not you share gender identities with your client. If gender is interfering between you and your client, perhaps seek supervision with a consultant of a gender different from your own, or one that aligns with the client you want to discuss. Gender is different for each person, so all issues and concepts will not apply to each person who identifies with a particular gender. This chapter is far from exhaustive in its exploration of gender and trauma therapy: May you continue to not only expand your knowledge and comfort on this therapeutic topic, but also to expand the rules of gender expression for liberation for all.

REFERENCES

Ashley, W. (2014). The angry black woman: The impact of pejorative stereotypes on psychotherapy with black women. *Soc Work Public Health, 29*(1), 27–34. https://doi.org/10.1080/19371918.2011.619449

Bodnar, I. (2018). Aristotle's natural philosophy. In E. N. Zalta (Ed.), *The Stanford Encyclopedia of Philosophy* (Spring Ed.), Edward N. Zalta (Ed.). https://plato.stanford.edu/archives/spr2018/entries/aristotle-natphil/

Briere, J., & Elliot, D. M. (2003). Prevalence and psychological sequels of self-reported childhood physical and sexual abuse in a general population sample of men and women. *Child Abuse & Neglect, 27*, 1205–1222. https://doi.org/10.1016/j.chiabu.2003.09.008

Burstein H. J., Lacchetti C., Anderson H., Buchholz T. A., Davidson N. E., Gelmon K. A., Giordano, S. H., Hudis, C. A., Solky, A. J., Stearns, V., Winer, E. P., & Griggs, J. J. (2019). Adjuvant endocrine therapy for women with hormone receptor-positive breast cancer: ASCO clinical practice guideline focused update. *Journal of Clinical Oncology, 37*(5), 423–438. https://doi.org/10.1200/JCO.18.01160

Butler, J. (1993). *Bodies that matter: On the discursive limits of "sex."* Routledge Classics.

Campbell, L. F., & Arkles, G. (2016). Ethical and legal concerns for mental health professionals. In A. A. Singh & L. M. Dickey (Eds.), *Affirmative counseling and psychological practice with transgender and gender nonconforming clients* (pp. 95–118). American Psychological Association.

Centers for Disease Control and Prevention. (2021). *Preventing sexual violence*. https://www.cdc.gov/violenceprevention/sexualviolence/fastfact.html

Chang, S. C. (2017). EMDR therapy as affirmative care for transgender and gender nonconforming clients. In M. Nickerson (Ed.), *Cultural competence and healing culturally based trauma with EMDR therapy* (pp. 177–194). Springer Publishing Company.

Chang, S. C., Singh, A. A., & Dickey, L M. (2018). *A clinician's guide to gender-affirming care*. Context Press.

Chaplin, T. M. (2015). Gender and emotion expression: A developmental contextual perspective. *Emotion Review: Journal of the International Society for Research on Emotion, 7*(1), 14–21. https://doi.org/10.1177/1754073914544408

Clements-Nolle, K., Marx, R., & Katz, M. (2006). Attempted suicide among transgender persons. *Journal of Homosexuality, 51*(3), 53–69.

Connell, N., & Wilson, C. (1974). *Rape: The first sourcebook for women*. New American Library.

Creighton, S. (2001). Surgery for intersex. *Journal of the Royal Society of Medicine, 94*(5), 218–220. https://doi.org/10.1177/014107680109400505

DiMauro, J., & Renshaw, K. D. (2021). Trauma-related disclosure in sexual assault survivors' intimate relationships: Associations with PTSD, shame, and partners' responses. *Journal of Interpersonal Violence, 36*(3–4), NP1986-2004NP. https://doi.org/10.1177/0886260518756117

Edelman, E. A. (2011). "This area has been declared a prostitution free zone:" Discursive formations of space, the state, and trans sex worker bodies. *Journal of Homosexuality, 58*, 848–864.

Fitzgibbons, R., & O'Leary, D. (2011). Sexual abuse of minors by Catholic clergy. *The Linacre Quarterly, 78*(3), 252–273. https://doi.org/10.1179/002436311803888276

Jahoda, M. (1977). *Freud and the dilemmas of psychology* (p. 28). Hogarth Press.

Kennedy, A. C., & Prock, K. A. (2018). "I still feel like I am not normal": A review of the role of stigma and stigmatization among female survivors of child sexual abuse, sexual assault, and intimate partner violence. *Trauma, Violence, & Abuse, 19*(5), 512–527. https://doi.org/10.1177/1524838016673601

Kennedy-Root, A., & Denham, S. A. (2010). The role of gender in the socialization of emotion: Key concepts and critical issues. In A. Kennedy Root & S. Denham (Eds.), *New directions for child and adolescent development* (pp. 1–9, 128). Jossey-Bass.

Kenny, C., & Yang, G. (2021). *The global childcare workload from school and preschool closures during the covid-19 pandemic.* The Center for Global Development. https://www.cgdev.org/sites/default/files/global-childcare-workload-from-school-closures-covid.pdf

Masson, J. (1984). *The assault on truth.* Farrar, Staus & Giroux.

Nadal, K., L., Rivera, D. P., & Corpus, M. J. H. (2010). Sexual orientation and transgender microaggressions in everyday life: Experiences of lesbians, gays, bisexuals, and transgender individuals. In D. W. Sue (Ed.), *Microagressions and marginality: Manifestation, Dynamics, and impact* (pp. 217–240). Wiley.

Ristock, J., Zoccole, A., & Passante, L. (2010). *Aboriginal Two-Spirit and LGBTQ Migration, Mobility, and Health Research Project.* https://www.rainbowhealthontario.ca/resource-library/aboriginal-two-spirit-and-lgbtq-migration-mobility-and-health-research-project/

Sagar-Ouriaghli, I., Godfrey, E., Bridge, L., Meade, L., & Brown, J. (2019). Improving mental health service utilization among men: A systematic review and synthesis of behavior change techniques within interventions targeting help-seeking. *American Journal of Men's Health, 13*(3), 1557988319857009. https://doi.org/10.1177/1557988319857009

Schauer, M., & Elbert, T. (2010). Dissociation following traumatic stress: Etiology and treatment. *Journal of Psychology, 218*(2), 109–127.

Seidler, Z. E., Dawes, A. J., Rice, S. M., Oliffe, J. L., & Dhillon, H. M. (2016). The role of masculinity in men's help-seeking for depression: A systematic review. *Clinical Psychology Review, 49*, 106–118. https://doi.org/10.1016/j.cpr.2016.09.002.

Senefeld, J. W., Lambelet, C. D., Johnson, P. W., Carter, R. E., Clayburn, A. J., & Joyner, M. J. (2020). Divergence in timing and magnitude of testosterone levels between male and female youths. *JAMA, 324*(1), 99–101. https://doi.org/10.1001/jama.2020.5655

Shiner, B., Westgate, C. L., Harik, J. M., Watts, B. V., & Schnurr, P. P. (2017). Effect of patient-therapist gender match on psychotherapy retention among United States veterans with posttraumatic stress disorder. *Administration and Policy in Mental Health, 44*(5), 642–650. https://doi.org/10.1007/s10488-016-0761-2

Sullivan, C. L., & Brown, J. S. (2015). Masculinity, alexithymia, and fear of intimacy as predictors of UK men's attitudes towards seeking professional psychological help. *British Journal of Health Psychology, 20*(1), 194–211. https://doi.org/10.1111/bjhp.12089

Tolin, D. F., & Foa, E. B. (2006). Sex differences in trauma and posttraumatic stress disorder: A quantitative review of 25 years of research. *Psychological Bulletin, 132*(6), 959–992. https://doi.org/10.1037/0033-2909.132.6.959

Wingfield, A. H. (2020). *Women are advancing in the workplace but women of color still lag behind*. Brookings Institute.

World Professional Association for Transgender Health. (2011). *Standards of care for the health of transsexual, transgender, and gender nonconforming people* (7th ed.). World Professional Association for Transgender Health. https://www.wpath.org/publications/soc

7

EMDR Therapy and Sexual/Affectional Orientation: Relationship and Pregnancy Status

Stephanie Baird, LMHC

LEARNING OBJECTIVES

- EMDR clinicians will learn the definitions of heterosexual and LGBTQ sexual and affectional/romantic orientations (including asexual and demisexual). An EMDR therapy case composite example illustrates intersections.
- EMDR clinicians will learn about different relationship statuses (monogamy, affairs, divorce, and consensual non-monogamy/polyamory). An EMDR therapy case example demonstrates how EMDR therapy can treat the impact of affairs on sexual health.
- EMDR clinicians will learn about possible infertility EMDR targets as they relate to sexual health.
- Sabrina Herman, LICSW, provides insights and an EMDR therapy case composite on working with pregnancy loss.

SEXUAL AND AFFECTIONAL/ROMANTIC ORIENTATION

Introduction

Definitions and descriptions of sexual orientation continue to evolve as we blaze onward into the 21st century. Most of us are familiar with these long-standing definitions: heterosexual (attracted to a different gender from your own), lesbian (female-identified, attracted to female-identified), gay (male-identified, attracted to male-identified), and bisexual (attracted to multiple genders).

However, sexual orientation is often about much more than sexual behavior. A former client once pointed out that when he came out as gay in his teens, he was mortified that people might imagine him engaging in sexual activity, upon hearing the label "gay." This particularly bothered him as he had no sexual experience yet, nor were his own sexual thoughts and fantasies developed. I am repeating this here as a reminder to understand that a person is much more than their sexual orientation or gender. As Walt Whitman (n.d.) famously wrote in his epic poem "Song of Myself," "I contain multitudes."

As people expand gender constructs and experiences, ideas of attraction are also expanding. We now know that orientation can include *both* sexual and affectional or romantic attractions. Someone might describe themselves as heterosexual and heteroromantic. Or they may describe themselves as bisexual (sexual attraction to more than one gender) *and* homoromantic (romantic/affectional attraction towards the same gender). Sexual and affectional orientation, like gender, can remain consistent or change over one's lifetime. It is helpful to have welcoming language in your office or on your intake forms, allowing your clients to indicate pronouns, labels, and categories, if they wish.

If you feel comfortable identifying in any of the categories described in this chapter (queer, gay, poly, bisexual, demisexual, as an asexual person ["ACE"], etc.) in your practice information, this may help certain clients who might feel invisible find their way to you, benefiting from EMDR therapy to address stigmatization, microaggressions, and/or traumas resulting from erotic marginalization (Sennott, 2020).

Microaggressions are "subtle insults that are delivered through dismissive looks gestures, and tones (verbal, nonverbal and over visual) that are often directed toward people of color" (Sue & Constantine, 2007, p. 137) and can also be experienced by other marginalized populations such as LGBTQIA+ individuals. Many of our clients from these erotically marginalized communities may report experiencing any number of microaggressions, potentially worthy of targeting with EMDR therapy. Additionally, heterosexism (cultural victimization of LGBTQIA+ individuals) and heteronormativity (privileging of heterosexual relationships) can be seen as a form of abuse that oppresses LGBTQIA+ individuals (Neisen, 1993).

If you hang rainbow flags or check off in your profile that you serve LGBTQIA+ clients, make sure you are fully comfortable treating folx from these categories (Marich, 2021). Additionally, everyone has different and unique experiences, so a lesbian client in her early twenties may not behave and/or have many similar experiences to a lesbian EMDR clinician in her late fifties. Understanding that our clients may have different definitions and experiences of sexuality and gender, even those that appear to identify the same as we do, is helpful to remember.

Denouncing Sexual Orientation Change Efforts

It is important to know that the EMDR International Association (EMDRIA) has a statement denouncing "conversion" or "reparative" therapy using EMDR therapy to "change" someone's orientation to heterosexual:

> *EMDRIA recognizes the need and responsibility to address the use of EMDR therapy approaches in any sexual orientation change efforts (SOCE) that pathologizes sexual and gender minority (LGBTQIA) persons and communities. EMDRIA does not believe that representations of sexual orientation and gender identity result from unresolved trauma. An individual's sexual orientation and gender identity are not matters of pathology. EMDRIA does not believe LGBTQIA+ individuals are in need of mental health treatment by virtue of their sexual orientation and gender identity. Therefore, the use of EMDR therapy in any SOCE program or other similar intervention is inappropriate and outside the norms and values of EMDRIA. EMDRIA prohibits the use of EMDR therapy for this purpose by its Members, Certified Therapists, Approved Consultants, Credit Providers, and Approved Training Providers. (Reprinted with permission from the EMDR International Association Professional Code of Conduct. www.emdria.org/about-emdria/emdr-international-association-policies/) (EMDRIA, n.d.)*

The American Psychological Association issued a statement in 2009 condemning any kind of sexual orientation change efforts, noting the "longstanding consensus of the behavioral and social sciences and the health and mental health professions is that homosexuality per se is a normal and positive variation of human sexual orientation" (Anton, 2010). Unfortunately, some conservative religious organizations have rebranded the word "conversion" in different ways, attempting to capture religious participants, particularly youth, who may be struggling with non-heterosexual desires and attractions. Research has shown SOCE to be particularly harmful to our vulnerable youth, leading to "depression, anxiety, drug use, homelessness, and suicide" (Human Rights Commission, n.d.).

We will certainly do harm if we "go with that" and attempt to use EMDR therapy to reduce or eliminate attractions and/or identities that have been eliminated from the *Diagnostic and Statistical Manual of Mental Disorders* (DSM 5; APA, 2013) as a disorder since the mid-1970s (Marich, 2021). Rather, we may find ourselves in the unique position to provide validation, affirmation, normalization, and psychoeducation of LGBTQIA+ identities (as well as basic information about systemic oppression) to our questioning clients. In fact, for some clients this may be the first time they have ever broached the topic of non-heterosexual attractions with anyone. We do not want to mimic or exacerbate the external oppressions, frequent traumas, and microaggressions folx with these marginalized identities already encounter regularly, by complying with requests to "get rid of" this "problem." In fact, EMDR therapy can be helpful to *survivors* of SOCE programs (SOCE remain legal in over half of our states), potentially de-programing the decreased self-image and increased shame perpetrated via SOCE.

Lastly, let us not forget that LGBTQIA+ individuals, especially those more visible in communities, tend to experience violence, microagressions and negative targeting of their identities over their lifetime versus heterosexually-identified folx. It was only about 80 years ago that Kinsey brought homosexuality out in the open with his research, only about 50 years ago that the *DSM* dropped homosexuality as a disorder (shortly after the Stonewall Riots which kicked off the modern LGBTQ movement), and only 6 years ago that gay marriage was legalized (June 26, 2015). Certain lawmakers continue to impede progress toward equality for all. The second largest mass shooting by a single individual in U.S. history occurred just 5 years ago in 2016 at the Florida gay nightclub, Pulse, killing 49 mostly Latino individuals.

John O'Brien has an informative and helpful chapter on "EMDR Therapy with Lesbian/Gay/Bisexual Clients" in Nickerson's book *Cultural Competence and Healing Culturally Based Trauma with EMDR Therapy* (Chapter 12, 2017).

Men Who Have Sex With Men/Same Gender Loving Categories

Researchers since the 1990s have also identified a group called "men who have sex with men," "males who have sex with males" or "MSM." These are (usually) cismen or cismale-identified who may answer "heterosexual" (among other identities) on questionnaires *and* engage in sexual activity with other male-identified individuals. Similarly, for females, sometimes the term "women who have sex with women" (WSW) is used in gathering data. This term was developed to solely capture the behavioral aspect of this group, originally for disease-risk based research. Cleo Manago coined the term "same gender loving" in the early 1990s, often used in communities of color as a non-Eurocentric based term (compared to the White Euro-centric "gay" and "homosexual" terms). Some of our clients may choose this language to describe themselves.

Bisexuality/Pansexual/Polysexual/Omnisexual

Bisexuality (admittedly a binary term) has frequently been misunderstood as a "transition" or "fence-sitting" phase. Many bisexual-identified folx claim this label as a lifelong identity. Kinsey and early sex researchers in the 1940s were the first to develop a sexual orientation scale (The Kinsey Scale: 0 = *completely heterosexual attraction/behavior,* 6 = *completely homosexual attraction/behavior*). They discovered in their research of thousands of anonymous Americans that noticeable percentages of Americans (up to 37% of males) reported gay or lesbian experiences (based on questions about attractions, fantasies, and actual experiences), technically placing a surprisingly large group in the "bisexual" category at that time (Kinsey et al., 1948, 1953). However, how people choose to actually identify may be very different from their behavior.

Expanding on the Kinsey Scale to understand bisexuality and human nuance more accurately, other scales were later developed. The Klein Sexual Orientation Grid, developed in 1978 (Klein, 1993), looks at past, present, and ideal sexual attraction, behaviors, fantasies, emotional/social preference, and self-identification. The Storms Sexuality Axis (1980) plots eroticism on an x/y axis, respectively. I find the "Gender Unicorn" a wonderful recent tool for looking at continuums of identity and attraction, helpful for all individuals, whether bisexual or not. See Figure 7.1.

Bisexual activists continue to fight against biphobia, and often point out that for them, they prioritize getting to know a person, not what is "between their legs." Many bisexual folx understand there are more than two genders, including those possibilities in their personal definition. Folx may call themselves pansexual/panromantic ("gender-blind" attraction to others), omnisexual (sexual or romantic attraction toward all possible genders, with some possible gender preferences), or polysexual/polyromatic (attraction toward multiple genders).

Boston-based Robyn Ochs is a bisexual activist that publishes and speaks widely. Ochs recently said, "If you are LGBTQ+, existing proudly and unapologetically in public is a form of activism. Surviving and thriving is a form of activism"

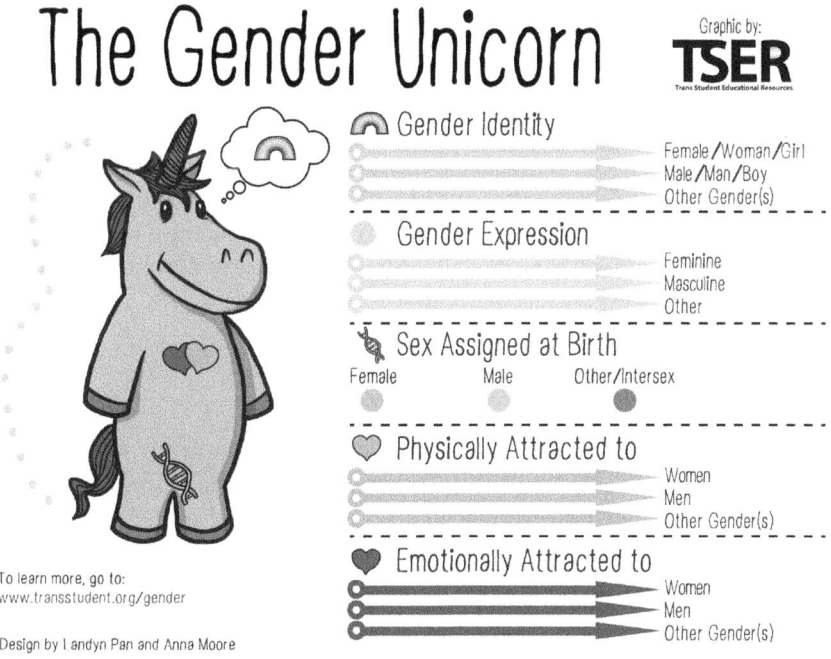

FIGURE 7.1. The gender unicorn.
Source: Courtesy of Trans Student Educational Resources (TSER). (2015). *The gender unicorn.* https://transstudent.org/gender/.

(Ochs, 2021). She and other activists have also pointed out over the years that a bi/pan/omni identity does not mean one is attracted to everyone, just like a heterosexual ciswoman attracted to cismen gets to be picky about her "type" and is not attracted to *every* cisman. Nor does a bi/pan/omni identity always guarantee a Saturday night date.

Asexual/Graysexual

Clients may also apply these descriptive terms to themselves or their partners: asexual or aromantic (no experience of sexual or romantic attraction toward anyone, and may enjoy sexual experiences on their own), or graysexual or grayromantic (rarely experience attraction toward anyone). Yes, many factors can impact sexual interest (trauma history, relationship issues, mental health issues, communication, hormones, medications, medical conditions, parenting or work fatigue, negative sexual environment or lack thereof, and/or "sexual brakes" being fully pressed, etc.), AND a growing number of individuals, regardless of any of those factors, assert this term. An ACE or graysexual identity is legitimate and real, and often still stigmatized in a culture that prizes sexual activity as part of a romantic relationship.

Asexual clients may perceive clinicians' questioning about lack of sexual interest as pathologizing. If clients (whether ACE or not) express concern about a low or decreased sexual interest, then we need to ask for their full permission and consent to inquire about the possible aforementioned mitigating factors. We can also share information about asexuality or graysexuality, particularly if those are new terms to them. I have had asexual clients over the years state "asexual" at intake and remain asexual long after our EMDR trauma targets were completed. By helping our clients discern whether they truly are experiencing a reduced sexual interest, or perhaps identify more with asexual or graysexual, we normalize and validate asexual and graysexual orientations.

Demisexual

Another orientation clinicians might encounter more frequently is demisexual and/or demi-romantic. Demisexuals/-romantics experience sexual or romantic attraction AFTER they have developed a strong emotional connection with another person. Clients may not yet know this term, so it can be helpful to introduce it and normalize their experiences, which may be the opposite of what many mainstream movies and television portray (i.e., intense erotic attraction at first sight).

EMDR master therapist Dr. Jamie Marich, who identifies as demisexual, mentioned recently (personal communication, May 24, 2021) that she, as well as many of her demisexual friends, have all received comments from therapists that their demisexual orientation must be "due to unhealed sexual trauma or religious hangups." Marich reported that one of her good friends was "scared off of EMDR *this week*" (my italics for emphasis) (personal communication, May 24, 2021) because her therapist made such a comment. As Marich further explained, "I am not letting just anyone up in my energy and my emotions, and that feels like the most organic and honest thing I can do for myself. Sometimes I get jealous of my friends who can just 'hook up,' but alas, that is not me." Again, just like with a potentially asexual client, we must perform due diligence in following our clients' lead, asking their permission for any clarification as they disclose their experiences and identities, and not interject our own theories and assumptions.

Queer

Some people, especially Millennials (in my clinical experience), reclaim and use the term "queer" to describe themselves, an umbrella term that can include living, loving, or identifying outside of binary expectations, in specific or multiple ways. A person will let you know if they use this term for themselves, so don't use this word unless they give you permission. Ideally they will feel comfortable to explain what "queer" means to them.

Preemptive Radical Inclusion

CB Beal, sex educator, uses the term *preemptive radical inclusion* (PRI; 2018) to understand that whoever walks through our office door may have experienced erotic marginalization or engaged in erotically marginalized practices (non-heterosexual, non-monogamy, kink, etc.). PRI also involves shifting away from penis-in-vagina sexual experiences, moving toward a shared language for sexual, intimate, and sensuous romantic practices, and is not orgasm focused. PRI means that "we position ourselves in the room to presuppose that everyone already, and always, is in the room…and purposely create experiences that preemptively involve them" (Beal & Alves, 2018). Rather than waiting for an individual to express their identity and need, we create experiences that *preemptively* involve them. Beal states that "PRI is a process, and justice and equity is the outcome."

Case Study 7.1: Haley, Demisexual-Identified

Haley, an early thirties White ciswoman who worked as a middle school art teacher, sought EMDR therapy to work on post-traumatic stress disorder (PTSD) symptoms related to a sexual assault in high school. Haley had been able to ignore or shrug off these symptoms (specifically nightmares, avoidance, interfering thoughts, and exaggerated startle response) for many years. We surmised that the stability of her current relationship seems to now provide a safe place for the symptoms to be recognized.

During the intake Haley openly identified as demisexual and pansexual, and in a current monogamous relationship with a transwoman (male to female). Haley was very clear that she was happy with her demisexual identity, stating that over the years she learned that her sexual interest in a person begins *after* an emotional attraction develops. She related this about her current relationship, describing how sexual interest and attraction to her partner eventually grew from a slow courtship and increasing emotional connection. She noted greatly appreciating her partner's patience. However, now that PTSD symptoms were intruding in their sexual relationship, Haley was very motivated to address the past trauma so that she and her partner might resume formerly pleasurable and desired sexual activity. I also provided information about sexual brakes and accelerators during these initial sessions, and we conceptualized that the prior trauma was fully pushing on her sexual brakes, eliminating any interest in sex.

Additionally, during medical history gathering, Haley disclosed she had recently sought medical help due to menstruation issues. An exam revealed that she possessed two uteruses. She reported feeling incredibly distressed by this information, and like a "freak." Lastly, Haley also noted growing up in Alabama in a fundamentalist Baptist household where any non-married sexually active and/or non-heterosexual identity was considered "blasphemous" and grounds for "going to hell." Although she no longer identified as Baptist, she noted some lingering internalized homophobia and entophobia.

Sorting through her background, we determined there were many EMDR targets beyond the presenting high school sexual assault. Our EMDR target timeline included:

- Several pre-teen targets of noticing same-gender attraction, yet feeling incredibly shameful.
- Occasions when she asked her pastor and parents roundabout and vague questions about sexual orientation, and being harshly rebuked and censored.
- The original reason for referral—the high school sexual assault (this occurred right after a football game where she cheerlead).
- Some early college dating experiences with cismen that involved non-consensual actions perpetrated by them.
- Shame regarding these initial sexual experiences due to her non-consent as well as the heavy "no sex" messaging in her family of origin and early religious environment.
- Two initial same-gender dating experiences in her mid-twenties where her partners moved faster sexually than she wanted.

Chapter 7 EMDR Therapy and Sexual/Affectional Orientation

- Shame around not being out as pansexual to her family of origin, and worry about eventually being outed.
- Haley's recent medical examinations where she learned of her particular anatomical configuration—both the doctor's insensitivity in relating and explaining the information, and her own medical concerns of potential fertility issues.

Thankfully, as mentioned before, Haley had a very supportive relationship, stable job, and positive community of friends and co-workers. We were able to proceed through the EMDR targets without much trouble, getting through the timeline over the course of a few months. Her negative cognitions (NCs) for the EMDR targets related to sexual identity and biological anatomy tended to be either "there is something wrong with me" or "I'm abnormal." For the sexual assaults, her NCs were "I'm not strong, I'm vulnerable, it's my fault."

Haley's positive cognitions (PCs) related to sexual identity targets and biological anatomy included "I'm worthy of being my authentic self," "I am normal," and "I'm fine as I am." PCs for her sexual assault experiences included "I'm strong/capable, I'm safe," and "it's not my fault." For emotions during Phase 3 and Phase 4 she often reported shame followed by anger and grief. Physically these emotions generally presented as tightness in her chest or throat. As the targets processed, she would report a loosening of the tightness, particularly as she found her voice during processing, often speaking aloud things she wished she had said during the various events. Once the targets were fully processed, Haley noted a return of interest in sexual activity with her partner, and an even fuller enjoyment of their sexual interactions than before.

We also completed several Future Templates which included (a) making complaints to the doctor's office of the initial handling of her anatomical difference, (b) confidently coming out to her parents as pansexual and involved with a transgender person, (c) capably handling running into the more recent assailants that continue to live in the same region, and (d) expressing some new sexual fantasies to her partner.

RELATIONSHIP STATUS

Singlehood

We encounter clients who are single, whether by choice or circumstance. Some may be proud of their singlehood. Others may express some shame or feel they are single due to some sense of unworthiness. It can be beneficial to spend some time unraveling their attitudes on relationship and singlehood, as there may (or may not) be EMDR targets accessible through any negative beliefs they may hold.

Heteronormativity and Romonormativity

In mainstream media, *heteronormativity* contributes to the privileging of representations portraying a cisman and ciswoman as the ideal sexual/romantic couple. In her article "Rom-com Without Romonormativity, Gays Without Homonormativity: Examining the People Like Us Web Series" (Ng, 2020), Eve Ng (Associate Professor of Media, Women's, Gender, and Sexuality Studies at Ohio University) coined the term *romonormative* to describe privileging "monogamous romantic relationships," a phenomenon that also often involves "downplaying same-sex eroticism." Finally, a word for all the Disney-forced monogamous romance plots (not to mention the all-too-common heteronormativity of mainstream media)!

Monogamy

Many of our Westernized clients will experience monogamy (one person committed sexually and/or romantically to one other person) as their relationship status at some point in their lives. Many clients might identify as serial monogamists (having one monogamous relationship after the other) or fervently desiring a committed long-term or life-long monogamous relationship. However, a surprising number of clients may report experiences and preferences that do not meet that definition, despite the heavy societal coercion toward relationships and monogamy.

The United States has a powerful $60 billion a year wedding industry, further enforcing the monogamous relationship as the highest pinnacle of romantic (or interpersonal) achievement. Many fortunes ride on the fairytale notion of two people falling in love, committing, then getting married. However, the marriage rate in the United States is 6.5 per 1000 people, dropping considerably since the 1990s. Zimmer (2013) explains that only 17% of human cultures across the world are strictly lifetime monogamous—many cultures embrace some flexibility regarding sexual and emotional relationships such as serial monogamy, polygamy, secret dual monogamous relationships, and so on. And in the United States, reports from the Pew Research Center reveal that only "half of Americans ages 18 and older were married in 2017... down 8 percentage points since 1990" (Geiger & Livingston, 2019). And while marriage rates are declining (potentially due to folks waiting till later ages, more economic independence for ciswomen, and/or lack of access and high expense for some), cohabitation rates have steadily increased. Divorce rates have dropped overall 18% between 2008 and 2016, according to a recent study on divorce by sociologist Philip N. Cohen (2019), yet are on the rise among baby boomers and older (Geiger & Livingston, 2019).

Consensual Non-Monogamy / Polyamory

Monogamy, marriage, and divorce are not the only options for sexual and/or romantic relationships. While monogamy has been the Western puritanical default assumption of what humans should aspire to, more and more folx, especially

Millennials, are also exploring and claiming non-monogamous orientations, defining and ascribing to "consensual non-monogamy" (CNM) or "polyamory"—being intimate with more than one person at a time. Polyamory tends to be defined as ongoing emotional and/or sexual relationships with more than one partner. CNM is often defined more broadly and can include things like one-night-stands. Any kind of CNM involves the knowledge and consent of all partners involved (Tallon-Hicks, 2016). Fluid-bonded is another term clients may use to describe their relationships. Individuals in the defined group may be intimate without barriers such as condoms or dental dams, with other individuals in that bonded group.

A favorite illustrated book *How to Have Feminist Sex* (Perry, 2019) has a wonderful section on the history of non-monogamy. She essentially notes that many other cultures and similar species (chimps and bonobos) do not have an overriding monogamous expectation. She mentions several human peoples from non-Western cultures that have these ideas: Any child in that group could potentially have any number of fathers (Naskapi tribe, Canada), and therefore all children are loved and cared for, and every woman is possibly a little bit pregnant by more than one man (some Amazon tribes). Some tribes have a built-in agreement in romantic relationships about not getting too jealous of other lovers (the Canela in Brazil) and making sure no one is neglected (the Siriono in Bolivia). There are folks on many fronts (academic, artistic, civilian, you name it) challenging the Western monogamy paradigm.

Many CNM clients are well-informed and utilize the ethical ideals of honesty, communication, and transparency as detailed in these books: *The Ethical Slut* (Easton & Hardy, 2009), and *Opening Up* (Taormino, 2008), among others. Other clients may be new to CNM and in exploration mode, having had learning experiences worthy of EMDR therapy. According to various research investigations ranging from 2,000 to 8,000 participants, anywhere from 4% to 20% identified some type of non-monogamous practice. Folks who practice CNM or polyamory might mention being part of a polycule (the group of folks romantically or sexually connected to each other in this way) or having a metamour (a person who is in an intimate relationship with one of their intimate partners).

Compersion

Folks in poly relationships might report feeling "compersion," the opposite of jealousy. Compersion means feeling happy and delighted that an intimate partner had a wonderful sexual experience with another person. Compersion can also exist alongside jealousy (Tallon-Hicks, 2016). Joli Hamilton, sex educator/activist, has a TEDx Talk on "Compersion—The Opposite of Jealousy" (TEDx Talks, 2020). However, some of our openly CNM clients, just like our monogamous clients, may struggle with jealousy at times, adding unwanted jealousy to their list of EMDR targets. We can also ask our clients about any positive and negative experiences with CNM. This can help ascertain possible EMDR resourcing (i.e., the RDI) and/or EMDR targets.

New Relationship Energy

Both monogamous and CNM clients might mention and/or experience new relationship energy (NRE). This often occurs at the beginning of a new relationship, when giddiness, excitement, and endorphins for the new partner are high. CNM clients may notice that NRE with a new partner may cross over into current long-term relationships, infusing the more established relationships with zest as well. Conversely, unskillfully navigated NRE (i.e., spending all one's free time with the new partner) can sometimes result in long-term partners feeling neglected and jealous. Experienced polyamorists anticipate, accept, and plan for NRE. Community wisdom advises folks to put off making major decisions during NRE, and to make extra effort to do special things for the current partner(s) (Sheff, 2019).

Infidelity

Infidelity can occur in both monogamous and CNM relationships. Sixteen percent of married folks report cheating at some point in their marriage (general social survey, 2010–2016). If two people have committed exclusively to each other, then the experience and discovery of a sexual, romantic, or emotional affair, whether via the internet or in person, can be gut-wrenching for all involved. Conversely, infidelity can occur in open relationships when one person violates the terms of the consensual non-monogamy (e.g., seeing a new sexual/romantic interest yet not informing their partners; not using a condom when the agreement included universal condom use; spending the night at a partner's house when that was not an agreed option). It is important for clients in relationships to check in regularly with each other about what constitutes cheating for them, especially with the opportunities and possibilities made available by technology of emotional to cyber affairs.

Jealousy, break-ups, divorces, and infidelity, whether from short-term, long-term, monogamous, married, or CNM relationships can provide a wealth of EMDR targets.

Case Study 7.2: Kai, Infidelity and Low Sexual Interest

Kai is a late-forties, heterosexual, Southeast Asian cisman, working as an anesthesiologist. He is married and in a consensual non-monogamy (open) marriage. He sought EMDR therapy after discovering his wife's (similar age, working professional, White) affair with a much younger man. Although they had a CNM relationship, Emily had chosen to keep this new partner, a younger cisman, from him.

After Kai learned of the affair, some time prior to entering therapy, he spent many hours pressing Emily for details (which she gave) and listening to her apologies and renewed professions of loyalty, love, and commitment to him as her primary and fully informed partner. Kai searched the internet and found images of the man. Armed with details of their affair, plus a visual of the person, Kai conjured unshakable mental images of the sexual details of the affair. Kai noted previously enjoying compersion for Emily and her other lovers (and enjoying her compersion for him). His goal for treatment was to find a way to forgive her, be comfortable and trust her again, and stay married (they had children together and Emily stated over and over that she wanted to stay married to him and was willing to do anything).

We were able to develop a timeline of the events now corroborated as cheating moments (i.e., when Kai was away at a conference or working late) and populate them with the mental images he formed. Other targets also included the events surrounding the disclosure and early conversations about the affair. Kai's NCs over the course of many targets included: "I'm abandoned, unimportant, not worthy, a loser, tricked/betrayed, second rate," and so on. His PCs included: "I'm important, I have power, choices, I'm desired, able to trust and move on." He reported emotions of betrayal, anger, disgust, grief, and sadness, and experienced the associated disturbance as tightness in his chest.

Once we worked through most of these EMDR targets, Kai spoke of wanting to be able enjoy some affection from his wife. We were able to develop and install EMDR Future Templates of effectively "enjoying being touched by her." This was his explicit goal, as he adamantly wanted to remain married, despite having trouble regaining full respect for her. These EMDR Future Templates helped him to begin enjoying touch with Emily again.

As we wrapped up individual EMDR therapy, Kai and Emily entered couples therapy. Kai acknowledged that their marriage health was not yet fully restored. He felt optimistic about their marriage moving forward, resolving the lingering notes of betrayal and recently identified off-balance dynamics of their relationship (Emily felt he made more of the decisions and rules, contributing to some of her unhappiness).

FERTILITY, PREGNANCY LOSS, SEXUAL HEALTH, AND EMDR THERAPY

Clients may seek EMDR therapy due to disturbing events related to childbirth and fertility. Some clients who want to have children may have gone through years of fertility treatment, arriving at your office discouraged, in despair, and perhaps holding medical trauma related to some of the fertility procedures, miscarriages, or stillborn births.

Other clients may report harrowing childbirth experiences that continue to haunt them physically and/or emotionally, impacting their desire to engage in penis-vagina intercourse, or in any sexual activity, for that matter. It can be a good idea to gently inquire about any difficulties with getting pregnant, the pregnancy, and/or birth in your search for potential EMDR targets.

Infertility

For reproductive-aged individuals in the United States, about 9% of people with testes, and about 11% of people with ovaries, have experienced *fertility* problems. In one third of infertile couples, the difficulty is with the testes and/or related organs. In one third of infertile couples, the difficulty is with the ovaries and related organs. In the remaining third, the difficulty cannot be identified, or is with both people (Chandra et al., 2013). Overall, people are more and more delaying giving birth to their first child. A recent *Forbes* article noted that the worldwide average age of an individual giving their first birth has moved back to 31; in the United States the age has moved from 21 to 26 (Stahl, 2020).

Infertility, Sexual Health, and EMDR Therapy

Marina Lombardo and Regina Morrow developed the Infertility Protocol with EMDR published in *Eye Movement Desensitization and Reprocessing (EMDR) Scripted Protocols: Special Populations* (2009) to assist with infertility-related trauma. In the interest of space and time, I will include the pieces most relevant to sexual health in this section. For the full protocol chapter, please go to the Supplementary Files page offered as a companion to this book at https://connect.springerpub.com/content/book/978-0-8261-86768.

Excerpts From the Infertility Protocol With EMDR

General Fertility Questions
"When your issues with fertility began, what was happening in your life?"
"Do you have a current diagnosis for a fertility issue?"
"Are you currently in the midst of a treatment cycle and taking any hormones or fertility drugs? If so, which ones? Any reactions to this medication?" "History of any past treatments or procedures and the results of these efforts, including fertility medications and physical and emotional reactions?"
"How do you feel about the medical care you are receiving now" (i.e., supported or unhappy)?

Chapter 7 EMDR Therapy and Sexual/Affectional Orientation

Assessment and Improvement of Partner Relationship System Concerning Infertility
"Assess the quality of romantic relationship and explore ways to bring balance and increased communication into the relationship if necessary…based on client or couple's needs, particular strategies can be incorporated" such as improved "decision-making and boundary setting, particularly with friends and family" (Lombardo & Morrow, 2009). Approaching the issue in this way normalizes a wide variety of responses and allows you to assess specific concerns and needs.

"Do you feel pressured, supported by, or do you feel like you are disappointing your partner?"
"Have you discussed the boundaries of your fertility treatment? How much will you spend? How long will you continue?"
"How do you make these decisions? Does one person have more power in decision-making? Any conflict in this regard?"
"Has infertility treatment become the center of your world as a couple, or do you regularly engage in other activities as well?"

Assessment and Improvement of Sexual Health, Body Image, and Infertility
"Assess the client's relationship with their body and construct an action plan that can allow for support and healing including cognitive strategies. Clients who struggle with infertility often feel betrayed by their bodies and this can manifest in poor self-care" (Lombardo & Morrow, 2009). We can take this opportunity to help transform the client's relationship with their body into something more nurturing and to see their body as an ally on this journey (Lombardo & Morrow, 2009).

"How has infertility impacted your sex life?"
"Has sexual intimacy become exclusively linked with procreation and fertility treatment?"
"How has your body image or relationship with your body been affected?"
"What emotion(s) and beliefs arise when you think about your body?"
"Do you believe that your body is doing the best it can or do you feel betrayed or let down by your body because you are struggling in this way?"
"When you think about the organs in your reproductive system, what is the picture or mental image that comes up for you?"
"How have you been treating your body as a result?"

Assessment of Possible Negative Cognitions
"Infertility clients often carry within them a strong sense of blame and misplaced personal responsibility. The two primary negative cognitions that appear most often are: 'There's something wrong with me,' and 'I must have done something wrong.' It can be helpful to ask clients if what they believe about themselves is a

result of infertility struggles. If there is more than one belief, responsibility is usually primary, followed by safety, then control" (Lombardo & Morrow, 2009).

"Please tell me what you are believing about yourself as a result of this struggle you are having concerning getting pregnant and issues of infertility?"
"If there were a particular incident that represents that struggle, what would it be?"

Check for triggers for each belief that you have talked about. For fertility clients, this often appears in the form of ongoing treatment, dealing with friends and extended family, relationship with spouse, including intimacy and body image issues. Many fertility clients may have divorced any desire for body pleasure from their fertility journey, and may eventually identify EMDR targets related to cutting off sexual interest and pleasure.

Preparation and Resources
"If the client is in need of fertility resources for education, patient advocacy, or social support, there are various professional organizations available. These include the American Society for Reproductive Medicine (www.asrm.org), and Resolve (www.resolve.org), both of which provide support and information through public education and advocacy. Clients are also encouraged to make their own well-being a priority and discover choices and set boundaries that reflect this awareness. The clients are educated that the skills that they gain from navigating this issue will serve them in meeting all of life's challenges more successfully" (Lombardo & Morrow, 2009).

Reassessment and EMDR Future Templates
"Reassessment helps to evaluate treatment effects and monitor how these changes are occurring in the client's world. Future templates can facilitate this by allowing the client to try on and project a desired emotional or behavioral response in a certain situation. Specifically, future templates may be used to strengthen relationships or set boundaries with family members, communicate with healthcare providers, or improve self-image or lifestyle choices. Future templates need to be consistent with the client's goals and consider where they are on their fertility journey" (Lombardo & Morrow, 2009).

"Future templates, however, are *not* used to project specific outcomes in terms of treatment. In fact, with infertility clients, it is often important to separate the desire to conceive from the way that infertility challenged that choice. As grief resolves, and a client is able to regain a healthy self-image, they can often make the distinction between parenthood and pregnancy … consider the choice to live child-free" (Lombardo & Morrow, 2009), and perhaps re-engage with sexual behavior for non-reproductive reasons.

Grief
Many clients identify infertility as a "life crisis." It is helpful to educate them about the "grief inherent in the diagnosis, as well as the cycle of ongoing grief (hope to disappointment) that (can) occur every month they are unsuccessful in becoming pregnant (or) if there is a procedural failure" (Lombardo & Morrow, 2009). This possible ongoing grief can certainly keep the client's sexual brakes fully slammed on, impacting on any interest in sex for pleasure or connection's sake.

The Whole Person Fertility Program Fill-in-the-Blank Questionnaire
The 13-question questionnaire (Paulsen-Payne, 1997; adaptation by Marina Lombardo), included in the Infertility Protocol, can help the client crystallize information, negative cognitions, possible EMDR targets, possible EMDR resource installation, and/or EMDR future templates related to their own history and fertility. I have included a few sample questions here.

1. The biggest message I learned from my family is _____.
2. In my family, we kept _____ a secret.
3. I learned from an early age that women _____.
4. I learned from an early age that men _____.
5. I think I have trouble conceiving or holding onto a pregnancy because _____ happened in my family.

Fertility Questionnaire: Deciding When Enough Is Enough
This 12-question quiz, also included in the Infertility Protocol, can help your client determine when it is time to "take a break or put an end to treatment and consider alternatives" (Lombardo & Morrow, 2009). Here are a few sample questions:

1. Do you often find yourself mentally and emotionally tired?
2. Are you losing hope about the outcome of your medical treatment? Do you assume failure to guard against disappointment?
3. Does it seem as if your whole world is about infertility and that little else matters?
4. Do you find yourself irritable and resentful on the days when you have a doctor's appointment? Are you resisting following medical instructions?

Pregnancy Loss, Sexual Health, and EMDR Therapy

Miscarriages and pregnancy loss affect many people. "About ten to twenty percent of known pregnancies result in miscarriage" (Mayo Clinic Staff, n.d.). About one in 100 pregnancies are stillborn (babies lost at 20 weeks of pregnancy or later; MacDorman et al., 2015). Any or all of these losses can result in ongoing grief and PTSD symptoms for the people involved. EMDR therapy can assist in targeting and working through the emotional aftershocks. Sabrina Herman is an

EMDR clinician who specializing in working with pregnancy loss and infertility concerns. Her observations and reflections follow in this next section.

EMDR Therapy Reflections and Case Example of Working With Pregnancy Loss, by Sabrina Herman, LICSW

Terminology

I encourage all of us to use inclusive gender language when referring to perinatal, postpartum, and parenting support. Please recognize, and not erase, trans-bodies, non-binary, gender fluid, genderqueer and Two-spirit folx in the world of reproductive health and sexual health. Out of deep respect for my clients and all people pursuing pregnancy, and/or who have become pregnant by a planned or unplanned pregnancy, in-vitro fertilization (IVF), intrauterine insemination (I.U.I.), or natural, via donor or not, please use the terms "pregnant person" and "parent," as opposed to only assigning "women" or "mother" to pregnancy. "Spouse" and "partner" can be included in this inclusive terminology, in addition to "husband" and "wife" if stated by the client. It can also be more inclusive to use the terms "nursing," "chest-feeding," "feeding," or "lactating" versus "breast-feeding."

My own primary practice includes clients identified as non-binary and transmen who have given birth, are pursuing pregnancy, or whose partners are pursuing pregnancy. With that said, I would like to see more research on stillbirth, loss, postpartum mood disorders, and trauma, for a range of gender identities and expression.

It can be important to refer to someone as "parent" (if the client is comfortable with this) regardless of whether their child is alive or deceased.

Intake Information Gathering

During intake I strongly encourage providers to gather information about any deceased babies and miscarriages, alongside birth order and client's reproductive history. A person who has experienced loss often does not feel safe to acknowledge the deceased baby/fetus for societal taboos, or for the clinician's (dis)comfort. Holding space to recognize the existence of the lost pregnancy is a critical part of healing.

When gathering intake information, ask clients about their physical and emotional experience of prior pregnancies, any abortions (including why or why not they chose abortion), and sexual assault trauma. Clients' perceptions of these events play a key role in how they heal or highlight particular areas of their experience that may sabotage healing. We must hold our own inherent biases at bay when inquiring about a client's pregnancy experience. It is also important to recognize that clients can experience postpartum trauma and postpartum mood disorders many years beyond the first year after pregnancy/birth.

In addition, I inquire about clients' cultural or religious perspectives on death and parenting, respecting clients' viewpoints and beliefs of life and death. People of Color (in particular, Black ciswomen and/or female-identified in the United States) have suffered from generations of oppression that directly impacts their pregnancies and birthing process. Inherent biases in reproductive health and the devastating impact of racism on fetal and maternal/parental health are disproportionate and must be addressed as a serious heath crisis in our work. Acknowledgment and recognition (not erasure) are keys to facilitating healing.

It is particularly challenging for clients to heal and regain trust in their body if there has been an added layer of past childhood molestation or prior birth trauma either via C-birth or vaginal birth. If body image issues, body dysphoria, or present or past eating disorders are a part of the client's past, then those issues will also need to be addressed before their overall health can be regained.

Pregnancy loss and grief demand astute attention to the unique reconfiguration and challenge to a person's physiological, spiritual, emotional, socio-economic, and familial system. Ideally, we attend to ancestral trauma components, as well as cultural influences that may play a role in our clients' healing and regaining comfort in their body and mind.

Clinical Observations and Insights
The clinical observations I share here are based on years of working directly with parents who have struggled with fertility, are on the fertility journey, experienced birth trauma, postpartum depression, and/or have had a loss during pregnancy (miscarriage, stillbirth, or loss of an infant in postpartum periods). My own personal and professional interests were birthed from my process, using EMDR to heal from my birth trauma and regain health and a positive relationship with my own body after an emergency C-birth and resulting trauma. I believe we providers cannot sincerely do the work unless we have delved deep into our own wounds and trauma.

Anecdotal client themes that have been pervasive throughout my clinical work include: loss of trust in one's body, shame, blaming one's own body or (perceived lack of) ability to do the right thing to "save" or "protect" one's baby or fetus from harm, and "failure" to become a mother/parent/father. Understanding and processing the extended family's loss history can also be integral to healing (e.g., client's mother's stillbirths, grandparents' experience).

Sexual Intimacy and Pregnancy Loss, Fertility Concerns, and So On
Sexual intimacy and pleasure can be a part of the fertility journey. However, it is not necessarily a part of all individuals' paths. I encourage clinicians to keep this in mind as we respectfully work with clients, following clients' leads regarding their presenting concerns, as well as allow for a space for sexual health to enter the room if the client desires. Making room and giving permission for eventual

sexual pleasure conversations can be accomplished by asking about positive sexual experiences during the intake, in questionnaires (Chapter 3 has an extensive questionnaire about sexual health), or displaying books and posters affirming sexual pleasure. Additionally, sexual intimacy can become a means to reproduction, regaining trust in one's body, as well as claiming one's motherhood/fatherhood/parenthood/personhood. Other sexuality themes clients may articulate include sex *only* for reproduction's sake and goal, or sex as the means to create a corrective experience to have a living child.

EMDR Targets and Pregnancy Loss
I have had to be flexible with the prioritizing of various EMDR target memories. Sometimes a client presents in my office with acute stages of trauma and grief from a pregnancy loss. The pain and distress may be so intolerable and overpowering that stabilization and containment are the only focus of the treatment. Clearing the most recent devastating trauma might take precedence. Holding space to witness grief can profoundly impact healing. Conversely, a client who has experienced early childhood molestation, loss of a loved one, or prior loss by stillbirth can benefit tremendously from working on chronological trauma/loss target memories, eventually regaining a sense of trust for their body and body integrity.

Case Study 7.3: A., Impact of Pregnancy Loss on Sexual Health, Treated With EMDR Therapy

In this writing, I focus on one case example, primarily on the deep and profound impact that stillbirth has on this person's sense of connection to body integrity, body dysmorphia, and sexual health.

The client (referred to as A.) is a White cisgender heterosexual woman in her mid thirties, familiar with psychotherapy prior to seeking EMDR. She identifies herself as a "mother" and includes prior miscarriages in her history of pregnancies and motherhood. She has given birth to three children, two of which are living, one who is not living. However, her deceased baby continues to be a "blessed memory" and a "spirit guide" as well as a "resource" for her in her clinical work, via EMDR.

A. was referred to me after the stillbirth of her second child. For the first session, her husband was present but decided to discontinue work together as they both felt it was most important for her to do individual trauma work. I will address partner dynamics later in this writing as couples' work is often imperative in stillbirth/miscarriage work.

Finding ways to ritualize the reality of loss, and naming and offering permission to speak aloud about death, can be healing parts of a pregnant person's journey. Naming the need to continue to remember and honor the baby is often a common theme. The anniversary of the birth and death of her stillborn baby, and the subsequent birth of her living third child, occurred over the course of a year and a half of weekly psychotherapy sessions with myself. Once these markers passed, she was able to tolerate examining how the loss of her baby, loss of her mother, birth trauma, and past childhood molestation and sexual assault impacted her own sexual health.

EMDR therapy initially focused on processing A.'s early childhood loss of her mother and molestation. Later, while addressing her and her spouse's desire to have a fourth child, she noted disconnection to sexual intimacy and her body. A profound statement was made as she reflected on her mistrust for her body, her dissociation during sexual activity, and her primary focus on "reproduction." As I gently inquired, showing respectful curiosity about her expressed thoughts, she professed, "my body is a crime scene." I paused and acknowledged that statement, reflecting on it with her with respect and compassionate curiosity.

She described intimacy with her spouse as "my goal is procreation and just to get it over with." She expressed a repeated sense of dissociation from her body and a shame around enjoyment of sexual intimacy after the loss of her baby. "My dissociation keeps me defending myself from deeper enjoyment as a way simply to deal with my grief." On hearing this, I invited A. to explore these fixed, NCs through a session of EMDR.

For this particular EMDR therapy session, her target memory was an ultrasound where they (she and her spouse) discovered that her baby no longer had a heartbeat. This was near the end of an otherwise healthy pregnancy. Her Subjective Units of Distress (SUD) for this memory was an 8 out of 10. Her installed resource was the "spirit" of her deceased mother, whom she described as being "a feminist" who would remind her "you deserve pleasure." Her negative cognition was the statement: "My body is the scene of a crime." Her positive cognition was "my body is capable." The Validity of Cognition (VOC) was 4 (out of 7) at the start. She reported "sadness" for her emotion and "tightness" in her neck and heart region for body sensations.

Themes that arose during Phase 4 EMDR processing were: "Does my husband believe I betrayed him? He put trust in my body to protect our baby and now I betrayed him." She continued to ask "How could this happen?" She expressed anger at herself. Self-blame shifted to trying to find meaning and to a "higher power." Thoughts of her body being the place of loss/death shifted to deeper existential religious questions about death. "Do we need to blame anyone or anything?" Her neurological pathways had her travel back to a time of being wounded by an ex-boyfriend who reportedly was sexually manipulative and exploitive. Her processing went to the break-up with him and a past belief of "everything happens for a reason"(referring to the break-up). A. recalled a time when she wanted a tattoo after the break-up that said "EHFAR." She began to smile and said: "shit happens" (stating that she was imagining a tattoo "SH"). After more bilateral stimulation (BLS) she took a deep breath on her own. I inquired "What came up?" She stated with enthusiasm, "Wow, the place I wanted that tattoo after I broke up with him is now the place I have a tattoo for N." (her deceased baby)! She proudly showed me the tattoo.

A.'s cognition shifted to "my body has wisdom." Her tight heart region shifted to feelings of love and softening. She then was able to notice a shift in belief as she accessed the "soul" of her deceased baby stating that "N.'s soul perhaps has a higher meaning and that her soul doesn't want us to be in pain."

Through tears and expressions of profound grief, she was able to bring curiosity and inquiry to her installed resource (her mother). The questions shifted from "Who is to blame?" to "How can I change my belief so I don't keep punishing my body?" Her thoughts progressed to "I don't' need to punish myself and sexuality. My body does have wisdom! I carried three perfect babies, two miscarriages, one death but they all were perfect!"

With some silence and holding sacred space for her to process, she spoke out loud, "I wouldn't blame my body if it was a car accident that killed my baby. I need to trust my body more." Which led her positive cognition to shift to "My body is functioning perfectly, really!"

Once her SUD decreased steadily, arriving at 1, we checked in with her VOC: "My body is capable of doing great things, is not a failure, this happened to my body. It is a miracle that my body still works." Her SUD eventually went down to 0; the VOC rose to a 7. She noted feeling lighter in her body and more expansive. In a follow-up session, A. expressed relief and that she had an open honest conversation with her husband about their sex life. She reported that he shared "deeper love and respect" for her and that he loves that "I carried our babies."

This case illustrates the intricate weaving of sexuality, body integrity, trust, and cognitive confusion of death after birth, and the pain and somatic manifestations of grief, blame, shame, and societal demands of "the good mother." Experiencing one's body as the place of loss/trauma is profoundly difficult. Another client once shared that pregnancy loss was like living in the "house of abuse and I can't escape healing." It reinforces the deep somatic wounds that occur in one's womb as life and death coexist as one.

Conclusion

I would be remiss if I only focused on the pregnant client and did not mention the work that needs to be done with any potential or available partners. While it is obvious the pregnant person is typically the "identified client," their partners can also experience postpartum depression, postpartum anxiety, and postpartum trauma and loss. The partner's lens can be vastly different (from emotionally removed to visceral) and can directly affect how they support the client's grief. The partner may also experience fear of death of their spouse/partner. The partner's healing affects the client's and the couple's continued sexual health and intimacy. The family system (including existing immediate or extended family members, plus other supports) may also feel the wounds of grief and loss. Couples (and/or family) therapy, as well as individual therapy for the partner, can all be crucial parts of the healing process.

In conclusion, it is a privilege and an honor to hold space for the vast intricacies of body, mind, spirit, partnership, grief, loss, and sexuality as part of adulthood. Finally, I would like to thank the spirits of those precious souls lost who have guided my/our work. The work demands us all to speak the truth about loss. Grief is a deep expression of life, love, and can transform into gratitude while healing our deepest wounds.

SUMMARY

Sexual and affectional attraction and orientation can be important parts of our clients' relational identities and can remain stable, or change, throughout their lifetimes. Sexual and affectional orientations encompass a wide range of healthy and normal human experience including attraction to other genders, similar genders, many or all genders, or little to no attraction. A very short list of the enumerable descriptors clients might utilize include: heterosexual, gay, lesbian, same gender loving, bisexual, pansexual, omnisexual, demisexual, graysexual, asexual, and/or queer. It is helpful to know and remember that homosexuality was removed from the *DSM* nearly 50 years ago (1973), based on the consensus that "homosexuality (et al.) is a normal and positive variation of human experience."

Both EMDRIA and the APA have formal statements denouncing any kind of Sexual Orientation Change Efforts (SOCE). Unfortunately SOCE is legally allowed in some states, despite research showing the harm it can cause people subjected to it (especially youth). We must never use EMDR therapy as a SOCE, and in fact, our clients who have SOCE may need EMDR therapy to process and ameliorate the trauma from any harmful and deleterious SOCE experience.

Bisexuality, pansexuality, and/or omnisexuality are often misunderstood as transitional or fence-sitting identities, when in actuality a surprisingly large number of individuals have had experiences and attractions to similar and different genders. Clients may also identify as asexual (very little or no sexual interest) and/or demisexual (sexual attraction grows once an emotional connection is established). Both of these are valid and do not need to be seen as a result of trauma or pathologized as a hyposexual disorder. Preemptive Radical Inclusion (PRI) presupposes that any or all of our clients may possess marginalized (erotically or otherwise) experiences and/or identities. We must perform due diligence in understanding each unique client, their experiences, and attractions.

Our clients may be single (by choice or default), committed to one person, married, or in a consensual non-monogamy (CNM) relationship. Our society puts incredible pressure on people to comply with heteronormativity and romonormativity. Compersion can occur in CNM and is when one partner derives happiness from their partner's enjoyment of another romantic or sexual relationship. Jealousy can occur in any type of relationship. Infidelity can create trauma responses, potentially treated by EMDR therapy.

Issues can arise with fertility, pregnancy, and childbirth. The "Infertility Protocol with EMDR" has a wealth of information and suggestions on helping someone process infertility. Pregnancy loss can be devastating and traumatic. Sabrina Herman, LICSW, shares insights and observations on using EMDR therapy to work with pregnancy loss and sexual health concerns.

REFERENCES

American Psychiatric Association. (2013). *Diagnostic and statistical manual of mental disorders* (5th ed.). Author.

Anton, B. S. (2010). Proceedings of the American Psychological Association for the legislative year 2009: Minutes of the annual meeting of the Council of Representatives and minutes of the meetings of the Board of Directors. *American Psychologist, 65*, 385–475. https://doi.org/10.1037/a0019553

Beal, C. B., & Alves, C. L. (2018, March). *OWL facilitator training for young adult, adult, and older adult levels*. New England Region UUA.

EMDR International Association. (n.d.) *EMDR International Association policies.* https://www.emdria.org/about-emdria/emdr-international-association-policies/

Chandra, A., Copen, C. E., & Stephen, E. H. (2013). Infertility and impaired fecundity in the United States, 1982–2010: Data from the national survey of family growth. *National Health Statistics Reports, 67*, 1–19. https://www.cdc.gov/nchs/data/nhsr/nhsr067.pdf

Cohen, P. N. (2019, January 1). The coming divorce decline. *Socius: Sociological Research for a Dynamic World, 5*. https://doi.org/10.1177/2378023119873497

Easton, D., & Hardy, J. (2009). *The ethical slut: A practical guide to polyamory, open relationships, and other adventures*. Celestial Arts.

Geiger, A. W., & Livingston, G. (2019, February 13). *8 facts about love and marriage in America*. Pew Research Center. https://www.pewresearch.org/fact-tank/2019/02/13/8-facts-about-love-and-marriage/

Human Rights Commission. (n.d.). *The lies and dangers of efforts to change sexual orientation or gender identity*. Human Rights Commission. Retrieved September 17, 2021, from https://www.hrc.org/resources/the-lies-and-dangers-of-reparative-therapy

Kinsey, A., Charles, P., Wardell, B., & Martin, C. E. (1948). *Sexual behavior in the human male*. Philadelphia, PN: W.B. Saunders.
Kinsey, A. C., Pomeroy, W., Baxter, M., Clyde E., & Gebhard, Paul H. (1953). *Sexual behavior in the human female*. Philadelphia, PN: W.B. Saunders.
Klein, F. (1993). *The bisexual option*. Taylor and Francis.
Lombardo, M., & Morrow, R. (2009). Infertility protocol with EMDR. In M. Luber (Ed.), *Eye movement desensitization and reprocessing (EMDR) scripted protocols: Special populations*. Springer Publications, 168–198.
MacDorman, M. F., & Gregory, E. C. (2015). Fetal and perinatal mortality: United States, 2013. *National vital statistics reports: From the Centers for Disease Control and Prevention, National Center for Health Statistics, National Vital Statistics System, 64*(8), 1–24.
Marich, J. (2021, June 13). *EMDR therapy and LGBTQ+ experiences* [Webinar]. The Institute for Creative Mindfulness. https://icm.thinkific.com/courses/emdr-therapy-lgbtq-experiences-webinar-replay
Mayo Clinic Staff. (n.d.). *Miscarriage*. Retrieved September 17, 2021, from https://www.mayoclinic.org/diseases-conditions/pregnancy-loss-miscarriage/symptoms-causes/syc-20354298
Neisen, J. H. (1993). Healing from cultural victimization: Recovery from shame due to heterosexism. *Journal of Gay and Lesbian Mental Health, 2*(1), 49–63. https://doi.org/10.1300/J236v02n01_04
Ng, E. (2020). Rom-com without romonormativity, gays without homonormativity: Examining the 'People Like Us' web series. *New Review of Film and Television Studies, 18*(1), 83–100. https://doi.org/10.1080/17400309.2019.1664057
Ochs, R. (2021). *Surviving and thriving is a form of activism*. https://robynochs.com/2021/05/04/surviving-and-thriving-is-a-form-of-activism/
Paulsen-Payne, N. (1997). *The whole person fertility program: A revolutionary mind-body process to help you conceive*. Three Rivers Press.
Perry, F. (2019). *How to have feminist sex: A fairly graphic guide*. Penguin Random House.
Sennot, S. (2020, May). *Sex therapy with erotically marginalized clients: Nine principles of clinical support*. [Workshop]. Smith College School for Social Work.
Sheff, E. (2019, October). New relationship energy: What it is & how to deal with it. *Psychology Today*. https://www.psychologytoday.com/us/blog/the-polyamorists-next-door/201910/new-relationship-energy-what-it-is-how-deal-it
Stahl, A. (2020, May). New study: Millennial women are delaying having children due to their careers. *Forbes*. https://www.forbes.com/sites/ashleystahl/2020/05/01/new-study-millennial-women-are-delaying-having-children-due-to-their-careers/?sh=18f10a0d276a
Sue, D. W., & Constantine, M. G. (2007). Racial microaggressions as instigators of difficult dialogues on race: Implications for student affairs educators and students. *College Student Affairs Journal, 26*(2), 136–143.
Tallon-Hicks, Y. (2010, June). *Polyamory for professionals*. [Workshop]. Northampton, MA.
Taormino, T. (2008). *Opening up: A guide to creating and sustaining open relationships*. Cleis Press.
TEDx Talks. (2020, January). *Compersion – the opposite of jealousy / Hamilton, Joli* [Video]. YouTube. https://www.youtube.com/watch?v=bIojP4MnTwg&t=11s
Trans Student Educational Resources. (2015). *The gender unicorn*. www.transstudent.org/gender

Whitman, W. (n.d.). *Song of myself, 51*. https://poets.org/poem/song-myself-51
Zimmer, C. (2013, August 2). Monogamy and human evolution. *New York Times*.

ADDITIONAL RESOURCE

TristanTaormino.com

8

Other Marginalized Populations, Sexual Health, and EMDR Therapy

Stephanie Baird, LMHC

LEARNING OBJECTIVES

- EMDR clinicians will learn basic sexual health concerns of physically marginalized populations, illustrated with an EMDR case study.
- EMDR clinicians will learn about basic sexual health concerns and the sexual rights of intellectually marginalized (those with intellectual disorders) and neurodiverse populations.
- EMDR clinicians will learn about *erotically* marginalized populations (e.g., kink/bondage, discipline or domination, sadism, and masochism, fetish) and EMDR therapy, illustrated with EMDR case studies.
- EMDR clinicians will learn about fetish versus paraphilias and EMDR therapy.
- EMDR clinicians will explore issues facing sex workers. EMDR therapy case studies are included.
- EMDR clinicians will learn about sex offenders in general. One EMDR therapy case study is shared.

INTRODUCTION

"Marginalized communities are those excluded from mainstream social, economic, educational, and/or cultural life. Examples of marginalized populations include, but are not limited to, groups excluded due to race, gender identity, sexual orientation, age, physical ability, language, and/or immigration status. Marginalization occurs due to unequal power relationships between social groups" (Sevelius et al., 2020).

This chapter looks at a few specific marginalized communities. It would take several more volumes of this book to perform adequate justice with all the types of marginalized groups and individuals in this country (and abroad). Mark Nickerson (2017) does an excellent job of encouraging cultural humility and expanding cultural competence for EMDR clinicians with many different groups, including refugees, immigrants, folks with addictions, and folks from the uniformed services, among other groups. I wholeheartedly encourage you to study the excellent chapters in his book to increase your awareness of different groups, some of which you may or may not consider yourself a part.

Marginalized groups are also addressed throughout this book and in other specific chapters. Chapter 6 entirely explores marginalization based on gender. Chapter 7 provides information on people with LGBTQ sexual and affectional orientations, groups that continue to be marginalized despite many advances like equal marriage and anti-discrimination laws.

The communities explored in this chapter are marginalized due to external characteristics (like a prosthetic leg), internal characteristics (such as an intellectual disability), and/or some are erotically marginalized due to sexual behaviors. The last groups investigated are those that are legally or criminally marginalized.

Constantinides et al. (2019) have written the highly informative and valuable book *Sex Therapy With Erotically Marginalized Clients: Nine Principles of Clinical Support* detailing principles to consider when working with people from marginalized groups. Briefly, the nine principles are:

1. Maintain transparency and name systemic/individual oppressions.
2. Challenge binary thinking and its constrictions.
3. Support willingness to experience the anxiety of uncertainty.
4. Practice a relational and dialogic approach (not "expert").
5. Emphasize the client's own words, knowledge, and narratives.
6. Locate oneself and respond to client's meta-communication (non-verbal cues).
7. Support participation of family and network.
8. Practice active allyship.
9. Build a community of colleagues.

PHYSICALLY MARGINALIZED POPULATIONS

According to the Centers for Disease Control and Prevention (CDC; Okoro et al., 2018), nearly one in four U.S. adults report a disability. Categories of disabilities in this ongoing survey of more than 400,000 adults each year include hearing, vision, cognition, mobility, self-care, and independent living. More specifically, individuals may have central nervous system damage (e.g., cerebral palsy), musculoskeletal conditions (e.g., scoliosis), congenital malformations (e.g., diabetes, asthma, cystic fibrosis, cancer), or accident-related injuries (Bruess & Schroeder, 2018). Many of these clients will make their way to our offices. Some of their disabilities may be visible (such as using a wheelchair or walker) while other disabilities may be invisible to some degree (such as hearing difficulties, chronic illness, or now, "long-haul COVID"). Some of these clients have been living with their disability for their lifetime (e.g., type 1 diabetes, life-long hearing impairment). Still other clients may have a newly acquired disability due to a recent disease, injury, or an aging complication (e.g., cardiovascular disease, hypertension, stroke, arthritis, and/or osteoporosis).

Many illnesses and diseases can impact sexual functioning. A cancer diagnosis and treatment can reduce desire and interest in sex. A majority of clients with chronic fatigue syndrome or fibromyalgia report difficulties with having an orgasm, vaginal irritation, and decreased interest in sex (Buehler, 2021). Diabetes can result in erectile dysfunction, low sexual interest, and delayed ejaculation. Vaginal dryness, uncomfortable intercourse, and decreased blood flow to the clitoris and vulva can also occur more frequently (Buehler, 2021). With my apologies, the types of disabilities that can occur to all of us are too numerous to mention and do justice here. Please continue to seek current information from trusted sources on sexuality and disability.

Some clients recognize and name "ableism": discrimination and social prejudice against people with disabilities and/or people who are perceived to be disabled (Wikipedia). Some clients are new to this term and could greatly benefit from learning about this type of prejudice. EMDR therapy can help target the few or many instances of discrimination and prejudice they may have encountered. Avoid using the term "differently abled"; this term is dismissive of people with disabilities. The *Social Model of Disability* views disability not as the impairment itself; rather, it is the result of a particular impairment's interactions with social and environmental barriers. Solutions to disablism (prejudice and discrimination against people with disabilities) include everyday equality strategies like making all buildings wheelchair accessible.

There are many myths and prejudices in play with how society tends to view people with disabilities. The most recent *Our Whole Lives (OWL)* curriculum (Davis, 2019) lists these common but incorrect stereotypes: people living with disabilities and chronic conditions are not sexual (false), not desirable (false), and cannot have "real" sex (also false—sex includes many, many kinds of erotic and sensual activities), and lastly, that people living with disabilities and chronic illness are not sexually adventurous or are perverted (false). Every human being has the capacity to be sexual and enjoy sexuality, in whatever consenting form that takes. Every human body can experience some form of pleasure. People with disabilities, depending on the changes in how their body parts and organs work, may need to get creative about exploring their bodies or learning to orgasm. They may need partners and/or devices (e.g., vibrators) to help them figure out paths to pleasure if they have no sensations in genitals. They may experience "emotional orgasms" (more full body relaxation) versus traditional orgasms (Joannides, 2017). Encouraging exploration, knowledge acquisition, communication, and empowerment (as we do with temporarily able-bodied people) all remain great strategies for safe and pleasurable sexual health.

> **Case Study 8.1: Terry Has Cerebral Palsy and Wants a Sexual Relationship**

Terry, a 25-year-old graduate student, identifies as a White bisexual cis-woman. She was born 8 weeks prematurely with cerebral palsy, limiting her mobility and her use of her right hand and leg. She has a visible impairment with her gait and hand mobility. Her very supportive parents "mainstreamed" her in public school as her intellectual abilities matched and often exceeded those of the "mainstream" students.

Terry's reason for seeking therapy was that she "struggled to be vulnerable," yet was "tired of being alone" and urgently "wanted to be in a romantic and sexual relationship, yesterday." She reported a lack of experience with dating and intimacy, somewhat due to her academic focus for many years, but also due to fears that no one would want to date her. Additionally, she had experienced one unrequited love with a college peer, Alex. Although they had enjoyed emotional closeness, the peer sent mixed messages about engaging romantically. Ultimately nothing romantic or sexual transpired. At this point Terry confessed she did not feel like a worthy sexual being.

During the intake Terry shared many negative incidents related to her cerebral palsy, despite the good intentions of her parents and much of the community she grew up in. She reported bullying incidents in elementary school. One incident involved a peer calling her a "cripple"—the first time she heard that word. Another incident involved a teacher humiliating her by calling out her inability to tie her shoes. Fortunately she had told her parents about this when she got home. Her parents complained to the school resulting in the teacher being disciplined and Terry switched to a different class. She also reported two incidents at dances of not feeling desired in high school (compared to the "able-bodied" peers around her), and then several events related to the unrequited love with Alex. As Terry was open to the idea of EMDR therapy, we solidified the timeline, installed several resources (including an Resource Developement and Installation (RDI) that featured supportive friends, family, a beloved pet cat, Stephen Hawking, Franklin Delano Roosevelt, and Frida Kahlo).

As we processed through the timeline, her negative cognitions (NCs) tended to be "I'm not worth anything, something is very wrong with me." Her positive cognitions (PCs) tended to be "I'm worthy, fine as I am, and deserve love and respect." Additional targets arose concerning coming out to herself and others as bisexual. One target included a college acquaintance snickering and implying that Terry did not get to be a sexual being due to her cerebral palsy. Her NC for this target was "I'm worthless, nothing, a broken, sexless human." Her PC was "I am worth a lot, I'm amazing as I am, I get to be sexual like everyone else." At last Terry was beginning to see herself as a sexual being.

Once we processed these targets we then created and installed several Future Templates oriented toward building confidence around dating and sexual intimacy (including a template about feeling sexy and desirable). During this time Terry asked out a fellow graduate student, Mary, who said yes. They began dating and Terry noted that as they increased their physical and sexual intimacy, she was able to keep her PC in mind of "I am worth a lot, I'm amazing as I am, I get to give and receive sexual pleasure like everyone else," quelling her fears of being undesirable. Months passed and their relationship solidified into a healthy, sexually vibrant bond. Terry discharged, feeling confident and joyful in her sexual, romantic, and relationship skills.

NEURODIVERSE POPULATIONS

Neurodiverse generally refers to people with ADHD diagnoses, dyslexia (trouble with number and letter decoding), dyspraxia (having difficulties in planning and executing fine and gross motor operations), Tourette syndrome, and/or on the autism spectrum. Just as temporarily abled individuals are considered and assumed to be sexual beings from the day they are born until they die, so, too, does this apply to individuals with any type of disability or neurodiversity (Bruess, 2018). Individuals with neurodiversity deserve and need sexuality education and counseling like the rest of our planetary companions. It is important to recognize these clients as individuals with sexual needs, verbalizing and inquiring about any sexual goals or lack of information. One excellent sex education resource that serves many populations well is the *Drawn to Sex* (Moen & Nolan, 2018, 2020) book series (also useful for individuals with intellectual disabilities). The best gift we can give anyone, especially those frequently dismissed as non-sexual, is accurate, affirming, and empowering sex education.

Neurodiverse individuals may report self-esteem issues and lack of worthiness for romantic and sexual relationships. EMDR therapy (along with accurate sexual health information), addressing any doubts, prior negative incidents, and their ideal Future Template for romance and sexuality can be a godsend in boosting confidence and social ability.

INTELLECTUALLY MARGINALIZED POPULATIONS

(Written by Melanie Peele, MA, MEd, LPC, and Stephanie Baird, LMHC)

Clients with intellectual disabilities (IDs) are a vital population to engage in trauma treatments, including EMDR. IDs refer to "limits to a person's ability to learn at an expected evel and function in daily life" (CDC, n.d.). Some causes of IDs include Down's syndrome, fetal alcohol syndrome, head injury or stroke, and/or birth defects (CDC, n.d.). Levels of ID can vary greatly, and individuals with IDs can have a more difficult time letting others know their wants and needs (CDC, n.d.).

Individuals with ID are more likely to experience traumatic events (Kildahl et al., 2020; Mevissen et al., 2016). Unpublished U.S. Department of Justice data show adults with intellectual disability are **seven times** more likely to be sexually assaulted than those without disabilities (Shapiro, 2018). Compounding their increased risk, individuals with ID are also less likely to receive appropriate sexual health education (Roden et al., 2020). Individuals with IDs are also more prone to develop PTSD after a traumatic experience (Kildahl et al., 2020; Mevissen et al., 2016). Given this greater vulnerability, increasing the focus on trauma resolution rather than simply behavior modification (Barol & Seubert, 2010) could greatly benefit individuals with IDs and improve their quality of life.

Sexual Health Rights

The Better Health Channel (n.d.) website on Cognitive Disability and Sexuality details sexual health rights for people with IDs. They state that people with IDs have the right to receive accurate and understandable sex education that affirms their right to have satisfying and pleasurable sexual lives. Sex education should be tailored to the individual, and "cover age-appropriate sexual issues that may be associated with their particular disability."

Better Health Channel also spells out that some people with IDs need assistance and support from family members and caregivers to explore sexuality and relationships. Support can include finding ways for them to have privacy, learning about private versus public behavior, utilizing appropriate contraception, learning how to give informed consents, and remaining free from sexual exploitation. Comprehensive, cognitively and developmentally appropriate, and recurring sex education can help people with IDs learn what is acceptable and unacceptable behavior from others and learn ways to resist, protest, and report inappropriate transgressions against them.

EMDR Therapy With Clients With Intellectual Disabilities

On the whole, the literature about the use of EMDR to treat those with mild to moderate IDs is supportive, showing consistent symptom reduction and acceptance by clients (Barrowcliff & Evans, 2015; Jowett et al., 2016; Keesler, 2020; Mevissen & de Jongh, 2010; Mevissen et al., 2012; Rodenburg et al., 2009; Smith et al., 2021). A small randomized controlled trial found EMDR effective and well-received by clients (Karatzias et al., 2019). Mevissen et al. (2012) also provide four case studies describing the successful use of EMDR with clients with severe IDs.

A few important considerations for the use of EMDR with clients with IDs must be addressed. First, the definition of "trauma" for this population must be expanded by clinicians to better include the totality of their life experiences (Seubert, 2005), including systems-related violations as well as interpersonal ones. Second, clinicians must guard against misjudging PTSD symptoms as ID symptoms (Mevissen et al., 2016). Third, clients' possible limited expressive and receptive verbal capacity (Mevissen et al., 2016) may prove to be a barrier in the early phases of EMDR, necessitating the involvement of caregivers. Fourth, the lack of appropriately adapted assessment and evaluation tools to measure the effectiveness of treatment (Mevissen & de Jongh, 2010) must be adapted for by clinicians. Many case study articles describe how clinicians have been creative in their assessment of symptom disturbance and improvement (Barrowcliff & Evans, 2015; Mevissen et al., 2011, 2012; Seubert, 2005). Finally, due to the increased vulnerability to exploitation of individuals with IDs, specialized ethical considerations in treatment and research (Gilderthorp, 2015) must be employed.

While clients may find EMDR different or more technical than other types of treatment to which they have been exposed (Unwin et al., 2019), EMDR also offers unique benefits for use with clients with IDs. EMDR does not require a high level of verbal expression, and can even be conducted with minimally verbal clients (Mevissen et al., 2016). Unlike other modalities, EMDR does not require homework outside of session (Mevissen et al., 2016). In addition, the use of visual and artistic modalities, such as picture cards and drawing, provide increased options for expressive communication (Dilly, 2014). Finally, given the cognitive and emotional differences among clients with IDs, clinicians may benefit from checking in more frequently on Subjective Units of Disturbance (SUD), more frequent redirection to positive resources, and greater verbal engagement by the therapist (Barol & Seubert, 2010).

Yaskin and Seubert (2017) have a chapter in Mark Nickerson's book *Cultural Competence and Healing Culturally Based Trauma with EMDR Therapy* (2017). In this chapter Yaskin and Seubert (2017) encourage EMDR therapists to "replace culturally (enforced) negative stereotypes (of people with ID as a "burden") with a compassionate and humane understanding of people with ID as *individuals*." They provide EMDR therapy case studies addressing stigma, shame, and grief related to being excluded, as well as dissociation and attachment. Their case examples also describe modifications they made in communicating the protocol to clients, such as using hand gestures for the SUD scale and or drawing out feelings on paper.

EMDR THERAPY WITH EROTICALLY MARGINALIZED POPULATIONS

Introduction

As you bring more sexual health concepts into your EMDR practice, it is helpful to be aware of erotically marginalized populations' behaviors, needs, and identities. While there are many books and articles that explore the world of kink in depth (see References and Additional Resources), this section provides some basic information around terminology.

Kink is an umbrella term that covers any sexual, sensual, or erotic behavior not considered *vanilla*. Kink does not necessarily have to involve genital contact. Vanilla generally refers to non-kink/bondage identities and interactions (sexual activities like mutual masturbation, oral sex, and penis–vagina intercourse).

The word *polysemicity* is helpful to keep in mind as you read through this section (and book). Polysemicity essentially means that another person's experiences may not mimic or duplicate your own experience, even if you both perform the exact same behavior (Klein, 2010). "Don't yuck my yum" (every person is entitled to their own preferences and interests regarding consenting adult sexual activities) is a useful catch phrase I learned at my Sexual Attitude Reassessment Class and can help our clients embrace and affirm their sexual desires and interests.

When people hear the terms kink and BDSM they may assume that only a small portion of the population practices these behaviors. A recent study (Joyal & Carpentier, 2017) found that actually about half of around one thousand Canadian subjects have a desire for one or more kinky acts (e.g., voyeurism, fetishism, masochism), with about a 40% of that sample having had engaged in such an act. There were no gender differences in this sample

Trauma Reenactment Versus Trauma Play

Some professionals assume kink/BDSM behavior is pathological and/or trauma reenactment. BDSM activities were removed as disorders from the *Diagnostic and Statistical Manual of Mental Disorders* (5th ed.; *DSM-5*) in 2013.

"*Trauma reenactment* is when people recycle the events and relationships from childhood, repeating old wounds by placing themselves at emotional risk or in physical danger in a compulsory mimicry of the past" (CRSH, n.d.). An example is someone who was emotionally and verbally abused by a parent, suffering successive abusive relationships as an adult. *Trauma play* involves "learning how to play with their childhood traumas without putting themselves in danger or stunting emotional growth" (CRSH, n.d.). For example, someone who had their knuckles hit by a ruler-wielding teacher may now, as an adult, notice, experience, and purposely enhance sexual arousal in a sexual role-play where their partner pretends to be their teacher.

Clients who engage in kink/BDSM do not have higher rates of trauma than the general population, and very often insightfully understand and communicate their trauma-free interest in kink/BDSM. For BDSM, the practitioners purposely play with the particular act to enhance a sexual experience. Jack Morin's book *The Erotic Mind* (1996) explores and examines how childhood experiences and relationships shape adult preferences and fantasies (for all individuals, whether vanilla or kinky). He encourages people to explore favorite and peak sexual experiences and fantasies to help discern *core erotic templates* (CETs). CETs are our arousal imprints, and can "transform old wounds and conflicts into excitation." His approach is sex-affirming and erotic-positive, seeing our CETs not as problems, but solutions. It is helpful to keep all of this in mind when clients disclose interests and activities that diverge from mainstream heteronormative, vanilla, and erotophobic culture.

Kink/BDSM Definitions

Bondage can involve using physical restraints such as cuffs, rope, fabric, zip ties, and so on, to prevent or limit movements of a consenting person as well as psychological or verbal restraint (Moore et al., 2014). The purpose of bondage can include immobilizing the person, making the person "accessible" for others, and/or displaying the person. Any of these may be "intended to cause humiliation" (if desired by all consenting participants).

Discipline involves providing specific rules and/or punishments to a consenting person in order to exert agreed upon control over them (Moore et al., 2014). Punishment can involve physical (e.g., spanking or whipping) and/or emotional (e.g., verbal or nonverbal humiliation) actions.

Domination involves someone (consensually) assuming total power in a "scene, situation, or relationship." The names of dominants are typically spelled with a capital letter (Moore et al., 2014).

Submission involves an individual agreeing to be controlled or dominated by another individual. This power/control/authority could be granted for single scene, or for an ongoing relationship. The names or designations of submissives are usually referred to with a lowercase letter (Moore et al., 2014). For example, mike granted Timothy total domination.

Sadism involves the experience of sexual pleasure and/or excitation by the consensual giving of emotional and/or physical pain or force in a scene, whether single or ongoing (Moore et al., 2014).

Masochism involves the experience of sexual pleasure and/or excitation by the consensual receiving of emotional and/or physical pain or force in a scene, and so forth (Moore et al., 2014).

Consent in Kink/BDSM

Another important concept in the BDSM or Kink world is *consent*. "Consent is critical to the BDSM community as it separates kink from pathological or abusive behaviors" (Taylor & Ussher, 2001). Consent is an agreement to engage in BDSM activity and has two major schools of thought within the community. The first consent guidelines are "safe, safe, and consensual" (SSC). Some, however, prefer to define their consent as "risk-aware consensual kink" (RACK) to allow for going beyond the possibly limiting SSC if engaging in *edgeplay*, which is meant to challenge the conventional parameters of SSC.

Anyone engaging in these practices needs to be intimately familiar with consent, able to communicate their boundaries and limits, and be willing to dialogue with their partners about "responsibilities, expectations, and potential risks." Safe words or phrases need to be established and respected, often during the negotiation that precedes a scene (a period of play). "After a scene, it is encouraged and standard for the people in the scene to engage in aftercare which is also discussed during the negotiation period and may include eating to restore blood sugar, cuddling, being wrapped in a blanket, or spending a brief time alone" (Moore et al., 2014). Purposeful and conscious BDSM behavior that involves any pain, between consenting adults, is meant to be performed with "caring intent" (Kort, 2018).

It is also important to note that many folks engage in kink or BDSM type behaviors (like spanking, blindfolding their partner, or role playing), yet do not consider themselves part of the BDSM community or define themselves in that way. However, the same concepts of consent still apply to their interactions and behaviors with others.

Additionally, sexual sadism and masochism are only considered *DSM-5* diagnosable conditions if the person practices these behaviors with nonconsenting individuals or if the client reports duress regarding their participation in these behaviors. Certainly, if someone discloses disturbance around wanting, performing, and/or receiving these behaviors, exploring the origins of any BDSM-related erotic templates and behaviors can be helpful, particularly if they also report a trauma history.

If clients are practicing their kink safely, sanely, and consensually, with the experience of pleasure and satisfaction, then the work may be around helping them reduce any unwanted shame and/or stigma regarding these desires and behaviors. This may involve identifying and processing past EMDR targets related to kink/BDSM desires or scenes where they felt shame. For example, a client may report being shamed by asking a partner to tie them up and blindfold them. Once those EMDR targets no longer cause disturbance, processing EMDR Future Templates of self-identified enthusiastic and desired participation in SSC scenes and activities may help the client move beyond any reported unwanted shame into joyful, confident, and empowered initiation and participation.

Lastly, I have had clients who requested EMDR therapy because a partner went beyond the agreed limits and boundaries of their negotiation, or a partner began enacting behaviors such as spanking, restraint, or even strangling, with no discussion, warning, or consent.

Case Study 8.2: Leslie, Sadism Gone Too Far

Leslie, a late twenties pansexual, demisexual gender non-conforming individual (Asian-identified) experienced an unwanted strangling attempt during sexual activity with their partner Josh. They were both in their early twenties. They had enjoyed mutually consenting sexual activity in their 5-month sexual relationship and added in bondage, dominance, and sadism activities such as being tied up and spanking. Josh had assumed the dominant role, with initial appropriate negotiation of consent and safe words, and Leslie noted enjoying this dynamic until one scene when Josh put his hands around their neck, while they were restrained, and began choking them. Leslie immediately verbalized their safe word, yet Josh did not stop. It escalated to Leslie fighting back then suddenly blacking out.

Leslie left Josh's apartment that night, attempting to break up with him, but Josh began harassing them (texting Leslie videos and photos he had taken of them without their knowledge), culminating 3 weeks later in a sexual assault. Because of their initial agreed upon BDSM activities, Leslie felt ashamed and embarrassed to disclose the choking, harassment, and final sexual assault. Leslie eventually sought EMDR therapy, noticing "kink-aware" on the EMDR therapy profile. Once Leslie felt at ease with the EMDR therapist, Leslie was able to disclose these incidents. After some resourcing, an EMDR timeline was formed, and the EMDR targets of the choking incident, harassment, and assault were processed over several sessions. Leslie's NCs were "I have lost total control, my consent is gone." The PCs were "I am truly consenting because I have fully negotiated my limits, and I can trust again."

Leslie then decided to press charges upon completing EMDR therapy, feeling more empowered. Leslie also reported meeting a new partner, Mary, for BDSM activities, who was well vetted by other BDSM community members. After some time getting to know her, Leslie was then able to continue exploring submission and masochism giving full consent and enjoying ongoing safe, sane, and consensual communication and activities.

> **Case Study 8.3: Derek, Boundary Crossed Submissive**

Derek is a "mostly heterosexual-identified" professional cisman in his early thirties. Over the course of a few months, Derek had become one of Nia's three submissives. Derek gradually watched Nia, a dominant, methodically cross some of the boundaries and agreements with the other two submissives. Nia also began pushing some of his boundaries (i.e., leaving him tied up for longer periods of time than agreed, requiring many days and weeks of grunge chore work with no reciprocal sexual contact). Nia rationalized this behavior by saying she was engaging in "edgeplay," working to ensure the submissives were getting "what they truly needed."

Derek eventually left the relationship, entering EMDR therapy due to PTSD symptoms of nightmares and interfering thoughts, mostly related to behaviors he witnessed her enact toward the other two submissives. He had tried to convince them to leave Nia's dominance, but both refused for a variety of reasons. This contributed to negative cognitions of "I am helpless, my consent is gone. I have no control of any kind."

The EMDR timeline included earlier targets in grade school and with his family of origin where he reported difficulty speaking up for himself and others, eventually concluding with the Nia-related targets. Other NCs included "I have no voice, I'm not worthy of speaking up." He emerged from EMDR therapy with a clearer sense of his boundaries in daily life as well as in kink/BDSM scenes. His positive cognitions included "I have choices, I am capable, I can speak up for myself and others, I choose when I consent to give." We also successfully completed EMDR Future Templates on seeing Nia at an upcoming kink/BDSM play event. Derek was able to install his PC of "I can speak up for myself and others" to a 7 regarding this chance of running into her.

Fetishes and Paraphilias

Fetishes involve relying on "props, body parts, scenes, or scenarios in order to get off sexually" (Joannides, 2017). This can occur in real life or fantasy. If this is done alone, or with a willing and consenting adult partner, then there is no reason to pathologize a particular fetish, especially if the person with the fetish can enjoy other types of sexual activity. Problems can arise if the formerly willing partner no longer wants to engage with the fetish, begins to feel like the person is only interested in the fetish not them, or the person with the fetish can only experience sexual arousal and/or orgasm with the fetish present.

If the fetish becomes indispensable for sexual arousal/orgasm, then the individual may be meeting criteria for a paraphilia. Again, if the adults involved are happy with their paraphilia, treatment is likely unnecessary. However, if a client seeks therapy stating they feel alone and disconnected from the relationship, relying on their paraphilia to supply non-demanding acceptance, then the work may be in helping the client gain social skills and confidence to combat fear of closeness and reduce loneliness (Joannides, 2017). Any reports of anxiety, trauma, or distress around relationships with other humans may be good EMDR therapy targets to ultimately reduce fear of getting close to others. Additional treatment can involve helping the client understand their CETs, finding ways to create new or additional CETs and sexually arousing scenarios (independent from the fetish), and/or approximating the fetish to more generic/universal sexual behaviors.

The *DSM-5* (2013) distinguishes between paraphilias and paraphiliac disorder. Paraphiliac disorder is when the paraphilia causes distress, interferes with the person's daily functioning, and/or harms (or potentially harms) self and/or other individuals. If your client reports a harmful or imminently harmful situation, you may need to take steps to prevent such harm through mandated reporting to local, state, or criminal agencies. Make sure you have gathered adequate information for your next step. Seek consultation with a specialist if you are in any doubt about what to do.

SEX WORK

This section is included to help correct misinformation and terminology. Activists (sex activists, academics, etc.) no longer use the word *prostitute* to describe someone who receives money (or other valued items) for sex. Instead, the term "sex work" is now the umbrella term for any consenting adult engaging in the exchange of sexuality-related activities for money (making or appearing in pornography, stripping, providing sex for money, phone or web cam sex work, etc.). Certain activities are arbitrarily legal or illegal in different states and countries.

Sex trafficking (enslaving a person for sexual purposes) is a different issue altogether and is considered a huge human rights issue with estimates between 12 and 27 million victims enslaved or forced into some kind of sexual activity a year. It is the second largest criminal industry in the world, at $32 billion a year. Sex trafficking, as it is defined under federal law, requires "force, fraud, and coercion"; sex work does not (Grant, 2018). The passing of FOSTA-SESTA in this country in 2018, making it illegal to assist, facilitate, or support human trafficking, has created many difficulties for sex workers and inconsistencies in how sex work is legally considered.

Rather than resulting in high numbers of sex traffickers being indicted and charged, critics note that the law simply seems to allow more legal targeting of sex workers (Chloe, 2018). Activists talk about how "these bills not only do nothing to actually reduce sex trafficking, but they also create dangerous conditions for both sex trafficking victims and consenting sex workers" (Chloe, 2018). This is because the ability to use the internet to advertise or screen sex work clients has been greatly hindered (as all parties, including the internet platform such as

Craiglist, could be charged with sex trafficking), resulting in increased difficulty in screening clients (Chloe, 2018). Additionally, many sex workers who were able to operate independently due to internet screening and unrestricted access to harm-reduction information now use pimping services or solicit outdoors, much more dangerous scenarios. In fact, Chloe (2018) cites recent research that shows that when Craigslist introduced the Erotic Services section, violence against women had actually dropped by 17.4%.

It is important to remain nonjudgmental and open if a client discloses a background of sex work, whether providing or receiving. *If* the client reports distress around sex work, *then* it can be helpful to obtain your client's consent and permission to inquire about the circumstances surrounding the distress, whether any coercion was involved, if your client of age at the time, if there were any substances forced upon them, and how they perceive the events now. People may choose to go into sex work for a variety of reasons, including positive reasons such as higher wages than other available jobs, and having their sexuality and defined boundaries work for them. Therefore, it is crucial that we do not impose our own values or beliefs. Feminist sex-positive activists has long regarded sex work similarly to The Netherlands (where it is legal and regulated). Put parameters in place that protect the sex workers and make it safe for them to report any abusive behavior, versus forcing them into the shadows for fear of being criminally charged themselves (and potentially suffering more abuse at the hands of law enforcement; Chloe, 2018).

In the case of a sex trafficking victim, there will most likely be traumatic memories and events associated with their enslavement, particularly as many victims are trafficked by foster homes, their caregivers and family members, or intimate partners (Chloe, 2018). Some of their trauma may be more related to a sense of betrayal from the groomer who enticed them into this path (similar to survivors of childhood incest, who sometimes report that the betrayal by the trusted person was worse than the actual acts). Not many folks (usually children or teenagers) simply "stumble" into trafficking. There is usually a process of getting to know the child, grooming, and attaining their trust, before moving into enslavement.

Many sex workers maintain intimate relationships with partners and have families, experiencing both positive and negative elements in their intimate relationships, similar to non sex workers.

Case Study 8.4: Liliana, Stripping to Pay for College

One EMDR and sex work case example is Liliana, a Latinx ciswoman college student who sought EMDR therapy for middle school and high school sexual assaults. At intake Liliana described a fairly typical college existence:

juggling classes, friends, and a supportive boyfriend. After a few sessions Liliana disclosed that she earns her college tuition by stripping at a couple of strip clubs in the state. She noted making more than enough cash each weekend to pay for her private college tuition. She reported feeling empowered by using her sexuality in a way that was also furthering her education. She stated her boyfriend did not mind her stripper work, although he did not attend any of her shows.

Consistent with her referral and intake information, Liliana prioritized working on the pre-teen and teen sexual assaults she had experienced by older neighborhood kids and one older cousin who sometimes babysat her. She noted these memories were bothering her more and more, often interfering with her sexual interest in her boyfriend. Once we worked through these targets, she then determined that a couple of prior situations at work also bothered her. One occurred a year earlier and involved another staff member who became obsessed with her, eventually stalking her via text messaging and arranging to work the same shifts she did. Liliana had explicitly informed this person she was not interested in dating or a relationship. Eventually Liliana informed the management, who responded by scheduling the stalker on opposite days.

Liliana's EMDR targets for this situation included (a) telling the person to leave her alone (yet the person stayed in her physical space) and (b) seeing the harassing text messages on her phone. Liliana no longer worked at that particular club, nor had any recent contact with the stalker, at the time of processing these targets with EMDR therapy. She had found work at a different striper club managed by women, which felt safer to her. Once these targets were resolved, Liliana was able to process EMDR Future Templates on the possibility of running into the stalker again. Her positive cognition of "I have boundaries, choices and, can act" remained completely true throughout the future template. She also noted interest in sexual activity with her boyfriend returning. She continued to do stripper work as that was the highest paying hourly rate available to help her pay for college.

Case Study 8.5: George, Sex Cam Work Preferred Over in Real Life (IRL)

Fred, a Black gay cisman working as an accountant, sought EMDR therapy for domestic violence (DV) targets that occurred in a prior relationship in his early twenties. He also had witnessed DV between his caregivers growing up. He was eventually interested in dating again, but felt quite nervous, as he did not want to fall into that same rabbit hole. After a few sessions he disclosed enjoying sex cam work (performing and verbalizing sexual activities over live video with paying customers). This felt very safe, as the other person was not in the same room and therefore could not physically hurt him. He was also released of any possible emotional connection, as these customers were and remained strangers, further reducing any risk of abuse.

Once we worked through the EMDR DV-related targets, Fred pondered what it might be like to date again. After completing much boundary work and several EMDR Future Templates of meeting new people and asserting boundaries (based on the PCs of "I am strong, capable, and worthy of care and respect"), Fred eased into in-person dating. His sex cam work slowly ebbed away as time with a new loving and respectful partner steadily increased.

SEX OFFENDERS

My First Post-Graduate Work—Assessing Sex Offenders

My first post-graduate work in 1999 was assessing male-identified sex offenders for psychopathy at the maximum security Bridgewater Treatment Center for Sexually Dangerous Persons (in Bridgewater, Massachusetts), as well as providing group treatment for female-identified sex offenders at MCI-Framingham (both facilities are prisons). I was not yet EMDR trained, so I utilized the assessment resources and relapse prevention/cognitive behavior models available to me by the Justice Resource Institute, the organization responsible for providing treatment.

Most of the group therapy with the female-identified sex offenders (often convicted as accessories to a partner's crimes) involved treating the very high rates of sexual abuse they themselves had experienced as children, as well as victimization in adulthood by other adults (usually their co-perpetrators who orchestrated the grooming and sexual abuse of their child victims). Looking back, I certainly wish I had been EMDR trained at that time. EMDR therapy likely could have helped them process their own trauma history more effectively and efficiently. This healing, along with potentially more stable and symptom-free mental health, may have then increased their capacity to address their own criminal sexual offending behavior more authentically and insightfully.

As for working with the inmates at Bridgewater, a great many of their substantial files also noted a history of their own experiences of sexual or physical abuse during childhood, and/or high Adverse Childhood Experiences Scale (ACES) scores. Obviously, the great majority of survivors of childhood sexual trauma grow up to become productive members of society, many even going into

Chapter 8 Other Marginalized Populations, Sexual Health, and EMDR

the helping professions (versus harming others). However, this group of incarcerated individuals were caught and convicted of heinous sex offenses.

At the time there was a huge divide in how the correction officers versus the treatment providers (psychiatrists, psychometrists like myself, psychotherapists, and clergy) viewed these inmates. The corrections officers would have happily executed the offenders, as severe as that sounds. The treatment providers believed in the goal of sentencing. We believed in treating and reforming these individuals as best as possible as most of the convicted offenders experienced incredible victimization during their own childhoods.

As an aside, while much of the population at Bridgewater met the criteria for antisocial personality disorder (APD), about 20% of this particular inmate population at Bridgewater were rated as having *severe* APD (aka "psychopaths") via the Hare Psychopathy Checklist. Hence, their treatment typically involved behavior reform, close supervision, and relapse prevention.

Definitions and Statistics

Adult rapists tend to reoffend across several violent crime categories, not just sexual assault, and assault out of "anger, hostility, and vindictiveness." They may have more social competence than child molesters, on average, but also have poor self-regulation, offense-supportive attitudes, negative peer influences, and intimacy issues (Simons, 2015). Acquaintance rapists are less violent than stranger rapists, using an opportunity to transgress a boundary (Simons, 2015). It is well known that many offenders are motivated by a desire to gain power and control over their victim. Many of the sex offenders of adults at Bridgewater had been charged against one more than victim.

According to the Race Against Abuse of Children Everywhere website (https://www.raace.org/statistics-information) the average serial child molester may have "400 victims" across their lifetime. Certainly at Bridgewater many of the inmates who committed child sexual abuse were charged with crimes against several known victims. It was impossible to know how many other victims were out there, unnamed.

The *DSM-5* (2013) makes a distinction between pedophilic and non-pedophilic child sexual abusers. For a diagnosis of pedophilia, and individual has recurrent, intense and sexually arousing fantasies, urges, or behaviors directed toward a prepubescent child (generally 13 years of age or younger) over a period of at least 6 months. The individual will have acted or be distressed by these urges; and must be at least 16 years old and at least 5 years older than the child victim.

Child sexual abusers can also be categorized into extrafamiliar (outside of the family, having trouble maintaining adult relationships) or intrafamiliar (incest offenders, inside the family). Intrafamiliars have few victims (generally only those children that are easily accessible) and lower recidivism (Simons, 2015).

The treatment providers felt wholeheartedly that any sex offender capable of experiencing remorse and insight deserved to be treated for their own trauma histories, and deserved a chance to live as a healthy, functioning adult (including learning how to and having healthy sexual relationships with consenting adult partners, upon release from prison).

EMDR Therapy With Sex Offenders

There is some research in recent years that EMDR therapy with sex offenders can provide many positive treatment results (such as decreased recidivism), particularly as most sex offenders have higher levels of ACES than the general population (Ricci & Clayton, 2016). If you are interested in working with this client population, I highly recommend consulting the article "EMDR with Sex Offenders: Using Offense Drivers to Guide Conceptualization and Treatment," available in the *Journal of EMDR Practice and Research*, Volume 10, Number 2 (Ricci & Clayton, 2016). This article provides a summary of the EMDR therapy and sex offender research to that date, as well as a description of the authors' "offense drivers" model. They posit that "sexual offenses are propelled by offense drivers which may be implicitly held beliefs, vulnerability factors, maladaptive coping strategies, or any combination thereof that contribute to crossing the line between legal and illegal sexual behavior" (Ricci & Clayton, 2016).

Another article (Wright & Warner, 2020) described a case study of using EMDR therapy to treat an "adult male who had sexually offended against prepubescent children." The EMDR therapy was used to treat his own childhood sexual abuse, and took place over about a year (33 sessions). At the 3-year follow-up he reported a "reduction in the strength and frequency of sexual arousal to children," although not the direct target (Wright & Warner, 2020).

Another case study used EMDR therapy to treat the cognitive distortions of a male sex offender who did not think his offending behavior was wrong (Ten Hoor, 2013). Although he had been sexually abused as a child, he initially did not perceive those experiences as negative, therefore justifying his adult abuse. Nine sessions of EMDR therapy resulted in eliminating these cognitive distortions, increasing openness and authenticity around continued group therapy treatment.

Encountering Clients With a Background of Sexual Offending

Some of us will encounter clients in our offices that reveal a sex offense of some kind. Most offenses will likely have been committed in late childhood or young adulthood (this has been my experience with client disclosures). We can still provide relief for their own trauma history in the form of EMDR therapy, working our way to their targets of offending behavior.

Chapter 8 Other Marginalized Populations, Sexual Health, and EMDR

If a client discloses to you, possibly for their first time, desire or interest in engaging in sexually offending behavior (i.e. sexual assault or molestation, frottage, voyeurism, etc.), or discloses distant, prior offending (and if no one is in immediate or recent danger), take care not to scare them off with immediate discussions of turning themselves into the police. We may be presented with a first chance opportunity to help these clients begin to rework their neural networks, client willing, away from any potentially harmful, offending, and nonconsensual behaviors and dysfunctional "erotic templates" towards healthier, adaptive, and adult/consent-oriented behaviors.

If you chose to continue to work with this client, the process will likely begin with helping them identify and process their own childhood traumas—sexual or otherwise—with the goal of breaking through any denial. Once they have worked through their own trauma, as well as any disclosed past (or possible future) offending behaviors, referrals to sex offender treatment programs may then be the best course of action.

Unanticipated clients in this category may be very challenging for the general EMDR clinician. If you feel in over your head immediately seek specialized consultation or coordinate a more appropriate referral for the client. Hopefully more EMDR therapy studies and guidelines regarding this population will emerge, and any individual experiencing nonconsensual urges will have direct and speedy access to proficient treatment. This section is but a cursory introductory look into working with this small population, as we will most likely all encounter at least one client who will disclose some type of prior offending behavior.

Case Study 8.6: Joe, Soldier With Juvenile Conviction of Sex Offense

Joe, a 28-year-old heterosexual White cisman, sought therapy for a recent diminished interest in sex and arousal (trouble having and maintaining erections) with his wife (Clarissa), with whom he had a 6-year-old son named Leo. Joe was stationed at a local military base. During the intake he was very forthcoming about a juvenile sex offense conviction. He disclosed that at age 14 he had molested a much younger female cousin. This incident was essentially immediately discovered, and he was arraigned, tried, and convicted as a minor with indecent sexual assault, serving probation and receiving counseling for the remainder of his youth. During that period of counseling it was learned that he had been abused around the age of six. This abuse was treated with talk therapy.

Upon further compassionate inquiry, it was determined that all of the sexual events of Joe's youth continued to hold disturbance, and some shame, for him. We made a timeline and after much EMDR resourcing, including using the Developmental Needs Meeting Strategy (DNMS) Healing Circle to help him develop Adult Nurturing, Protecting, and Spiritual Core selves, processed these events (the sexual victimization he received, then perpetrated) with EMDR therapy. His NC for the abuse he experienced was "I'm vulnerable and powerless." His PC became "I am safe and have choices." His NC for the abuse he perpetrated was "I'm rotten, disgusting, and can't be trusted." His PC evolved into "I acknowledge and accept my crime, and am now living my life safely, healthfully, and respectful of others." We often called upon his adult Nurturing and Protector selves during EMDR processing, and as we progressed through the targets, his Spiritual core self became more active, as well.

During this work we made the connection that Joe had been abused around the age of six, his own victim was age six when he abused her, and now he himself had a child around the age of six. He reported no sexual attraction to males, and that during the first 2 years of his marriage, he very much experienced sexual attraction to his wife. He had also been in other adult relationships prior to this marriage where he reported healthy consenting mutual sexual interest. Once his child was born, however, he noted a gradual decline in sexual interest. We surmised that the addition of the child in his life had slowly started pressing on his sexual brakes, for many of the same reasons this happens to non-offending folks: lack of time and energy for consistent sensual connection with his wife.

Additionally, whereas Joe's sexual interest within his marriage had diminished slowly for a few years, his own child approaching the age of six (linking up of all these age sixes) had put a screeching halt to his emergency sexual brake. We then used EMDR therapy (bringing in his Healing Circle often) to target and process two separate fears: (a) his fears that he would molest Leo, (b) worries that others might molest Leo. Throughout our treatment he mentioned that he spoke openly to his wife about his EMDR therapy, having her full support. He was encouraged to engage in Sensate Focus with Clarissa and learn relaxation and mindfulness skills to stay in the moment. He was also given permission to explore his new erotic templates emerging post EMDR therapy. While he maintained no sexual interest in youths, he did notice a wish to be submissive to his wife. As she was open to this, they began to explore dominance and submission dynamics together.

After about a year of therapy, Joe discharged, feeling more in charge of his adult sexuality (and factors conducive for erections), more free from his past, hopeful about Leo's chances to experience a much better (and appropriately boundaried) life, and some burgeoning excitement for his own developing adult-oriented erotic templates.

SUMMARY

Our clients come from different walks of life, many of them belonging in some way to *marginalized* groups.

Clients may disclose engaging in marginalized erotic practices such as kink and or BDSM. Healthy kink/BDSM practice is "safe, sane, and consensual" or "risk aware consensual kink." For most participants (who have the same percentage of trauma history as the general population), kink/BDSM is NOT trauma reenactment. Some clients may report experiencing negative kink/BDSM experiences. EMDR therapy can help process those experiences allowing clients to successfully re-engage with desired activities.

Fetishes involve relying on "props, body parts, scenes, or scenarios in order to get off sexually" (Joannides, 2017). If all adult parties consent, and potentially enjoy the fetish, then there is no treatable concern. If an individual can only operate sexually via the fetish, then this may qualify as a paraphilia. Again, it is only a concern if it begins to negatively impact the person's daily functioning, livelihood, relationships, and so on. A paraphilia rising to the level of a paraphiliac disorder involves considerable daily distress, impacts daily functioning, and/or harms (or potentially harms) self or others.

Sex work and sex workers have been criminally marginalized in our country through many laws, including the 2018 FOSTA-SESTA bills, making it more difficult for sex workers to remain autonomous and safely screen clients. While this bill is targeted toward sex trafficking, a global problem, it has not been shown to increase true sex trafficking arrests. Victims of sex trafficking will benefit from EMDR therapy to treat any traumatic symptoms as a result of their experience. Independent sex workers maintain relationships, marriages, and family life just like any other individual. They may seek EMDR therapy for disturbing events not at all related to their sex work. We must remain nonjudgmental and follow their lead should they chose to disclose their sex work.

Treating sex offenders is very complicated. The sex offenders that are actually convicted also themselves generally had experienced being sexually abused as children. They usually receive some kind of trauma and relapse prevention treatment in prison. Clients may reveal a history of sex offending. How we respond to this disclosure can greatly impact whether the client continues to seek services. Try to remain nonjudgmental, particularly if the crime was convicted and adjudicated a long time ago. Offer EMDR therapy for any abuse they themselves experienced as this can help redirect their Core Erotic Templates, if any remain related to the abuse. If there is imminent harm or danger, you may need to involve local or state agencies or authorities. When in any kind of doubt, seek consultation from someone who regularly treats sex offenders.

REFERENCES

American Psychiatric Association. (2013). *Diagnostic and statistical manual of mental disorders* (5th ed.). American Psychiatric Publishing.

Barol, B. I., & Seubert, A. (2010). Stepping stones: EMDR treatment of individuals with intellectual and developmental disabilities and challenging behavior. *Journal of EMDR Practice and Research, 4*(4), 156–169. https://doi.org/10.1891/1933-3196.4.4.156

Barrowcliff, A. L., & Evans, G. A. L. (2015). EMDR treatment for PTSD and intellectual disability: A case study. *Advances in Mental Health and Intellectual Disabilities, 9*(2), 90–98. https://doi.org/10.1108/AMHID-09-2014-0034; https://www.cdc.gov/ncbddd/childdevelopment/facts-about-intellectual-disability.html

Better Health Channel. (n.d.). *Cognitive disability and sexuality.* Retrieved September 17, 2021, from https://www.betterhealth.vic.gov.au/health/ConditionsAndTreatments/intellectual-disability-and-sexuality

Bruess, C. E., & Schroeder, E. (2018). *Sexuality education: Theory and practice* (7th ed.). ETR.

Beuhler, S. (2021). *What every mental health professional needs to know about sex, 3rd edition.* Springer Publishing.

Centers for Disease Control and Prevention. (n.d.). Facts about intellectual disability in children. https://www.cdc.gov/ncbddd/childdevelopment/facts-about-intellectual-disability.html

Center for Relationship and Sexual Health. (n.d.). *Shades of play: Trauma enactment versus trauma play.* Author.

Chloe. (2018, July 19). *Offline shadows: How sex workers become marginalized victims of morality-based legislation.* Astrostraddle. https://www.autostraddle.com/offline-shadows-how-sex-workers-become-marginalized-victims-of-morality-based-legislation-426191/

Constantinides, D. M., Sennott, S. L., & Chandler, D. (2019). *Sex therapy with erotically marginalized clients: Nine principles of clinical support.* Routledge.

Davis, M. (2019). *Our whole lives: Sexuality education for older adults.* UUA and UCC.

Dilly, R. (2014). Eye movement desensitisation and reprocessing in the treatment of trauma with mild intellectual disabilities: A case study. *Advances in Mental Health and Intellectual Disabilities, 8*(1), 63–71. https://doi.org/10.1108/AMHID-06-2013-0036

Gilderthorp, R. C. (2015). Is EMDR an effective treatment for people diagnosed with both intellectual disability and post-traumatic stress disorder? *Journal of Intellectual Disabilities, 19*(1), 58–68. https://doi.org/10.1177/1744629514560638

Grant, M. (2018, January 30). In 'anti-trafficking' New Orleans strip club raids, police make no trafficking arrest. *The Appeal.* https://theappeal.org/in-anti-trafficking-new-orleans-strip-club-raids-police-make-no-trafficking-arrests-a51f374b4e9/

Joannides, P. (2017). *Guide to getting it on: Unzipped. V.9.0.* Goofy Foot Press.

Jowett, S., Karatzias, T., Brown, M., Grieve, A., Paterson, D., & Walley, R. (2016). Eye movement desensitization and reprocessing (EMDR) for DSM–5 posttraumatic stress disorder (PTSD) in adults with intellectual disabilities: A case study review. *Psychological Trauma: Theory, Research, Practice, and Policy, 8*(6), 709–719. http://dx.doi.org/10.1037/tra0000101

Joyal, C. C., & Carpentier, J. (2017). The prevalence of paraphilic interests and behaviors in the general population: A provincial survey. *The Journal of Sex Research, 54*(2), 161–171. https://doi.org/10.1080/00224499.2016.1139034

Karatzias, T., Brown, M., Taggart, L., Truesdale, M., Sirisena, C., Walley, R., Mason-Roberts, S., Bradley, A., & Paterson, D. (2019). A mixed methods, randomized controlled feasibility trial of eye movement desensitization and reprocessing (EMDR) plus standard care (SC) versus SC alone for DSM-5 posttraumatic stress disorder (PTSD) in adults with intellectual disabilities. *Journal of Applied Research in Intellectual Disabilities, 32*(4), 806–818. https://doi.org/10.1111/jar.12570

Keesler, J. M. (2020). Trauma-Specific treatment for individuals with intellectual and developmental disabilities: A review of the literature from 2008 to 2018. *Journal of Policy and Practice in Intellectual Disabilities, 17*(4), 332–345. https://doi.org/10.1111/jppi.12347

Kildahl, A. N., Oddli, H. W., & Helverschou, S. B. (2020). Potentially traumatic experiences and behavioural symptoms in adults with autism and intellectual disability referred for psychiatric assessment. *Research in Developmental Disabilities, 107*, 107388. https://doi.org/10.1016/j.ridd.2020.103788

Klein, M. (2010, April). *When sex gets complicated: Pornography, kink, cybersex, and other clinical challenges* [workshop]. AASECT, Florence, MA.

Kort, J. (2018). *The trauma survivor and sexual health: How therapists can help*. Presentation. The Brattleboro Retreat.

Mevissen, L., & de Jongh, A. (2010). PTSD and its treatment in people with intellectual disabilities: A review of the literature. *Clinical Psychology Review, 30*, 308–316. https://doi.org/10.1016/j.cpr.2009.12.005

Mevissen, L., Didden, R., & de Jongh, A. (2016). Assessment and treatment of PTSD in people with intellectual disabilities. In C. Martin, V. Preedy, & V. Patel (Eds.), *Comprehensive guide to post-traumatic stress disorder* (pp. 1–15). Springer. https://doi.org/10.1007/978-3-319-086132_952

Mevissen, L., Lievegoed, R., & de Jongh, A. (2011). EMDR treatment in people with mild ID and PTSD: 4 cases. *Psychiatric Quarterly, 82*, 43–57. https://doi.org/10.1007/s11126-010-9147-x

Mevissen, L., Lievegoed, R., Seubert, A., & de Jongh, A. (2012). Treatment of PTSD in people with severe intellectual disabilities: A case series. *Developmental Neurorehabilitation, 15*(3), 223–232. https://doi.org/10.3109/17518423.2011.654283

Moen, E., & Nolan, M. (2018). *Drawn to sex, volume 1: The basics*. Erika Moen Comics and Illustration, LLC.

Moen, E., & Nolan, M. (2020). *Drawn to sex, volume 2: Our bodies and health*. Erika Moen Comics and Illustration, LLC.

Moore, L., Pincus, T., & Rodemaker, D. (2014). *What professionals need to know about BDSM*. Printed by the authors.

Morin, J. (1996). *The erotic mind: Unlocking the inner sources of passion and fulfillment*. Harper Perennial.

Nickerson, M. (2017). *Cultural competence and healing culturally based trauma with EMDR therapy*. Springer Publishing.

Okoro, C. A., Hollis, N. D., Cyrus, A. C., & Griffin-Blake S. (2018). Prevalance of disabilities and health care access by disability status and type among adults – United States, 2016. *Morbidity and Mortality Weekly Report, 67*, 882–887. http://doi.org/10.15585/mmwr.mm6732a3

Ricci, R. & Clayton, C. (2016). EMDR with sex offenders: Using offense drivers to guide conceptualization and treatment. *Journal of EMDR Practice and Research, 10*(2), 104–118. http://doi.org/10.1891/1933-3196.10.2.104.

Roden, R. C., Schmidt, E. K., & Holland-Hall, C. (2020). Sexual health education for adolescents and young adults with intellectual and developmental disabilities: Recommendations for accessible sexual and reproductive health information. *The Lancet Child and Adolescent Health*, *4*(9), 699–708. https://doi.org/10.1016/S2352-4642(20)30098-5

Rodenburg, R., Benjamin, A., de Roos, C., Meijer, A. M., & Jan Stams, G. (2009). Efficacy of EMDR in children: A meta-analysis. *Clinical Psychology Review, 29*(7), 599–606. https://doi.org/10.1016/j.cpr.2009.06.008

Seubert, A. (2005). EMDR with clients with mental disability. In R. Shapiro (Ed.), *Emdr Solutions: Pathways to healing* (pp. 293–311). W. W. Norton & Company.

Sevelius, J. M., Gutierrez-Mock, L., Zamudio-Haas, S., McCree, B. Ngo, A., Jackson, A., Clynes, C., Venegas, L., Salinas, A., Herrera, C., Stein, E., Operario, D., & Gamarel, K. (2020). Research with marginalized communities: Challenges to continuity during the covid-19 pandemic. *AIDS Behavior, 24*, 2009–2012. https://doi.org/10.1007/s10461-020-02920-3

Shapiro, J. (2018, January 8). The sexual assault epidemic no one talks about. *NPR*. https://www.npr.org/2018/01/08/570224090/the-sexual-assault-epidemic-no-one-talks-about

Simons, D. (2015). *Adult sex offender typologies*. SOMAPI Research Brief. https://smart.ojp.gov/sites/g/files/xyckuh231/files/media/document/adultsexoffendertypologies.pdf

Smith, A. N., Laugharne, R., Oak, K., & Shankar, R. (2021). Eye movement desensitisation and reprocessing therapy for people with intellectual disability in the treatment of emotional trauma and post traumatic stress disorder: A scoping review. *Journal of Mental Health Research in Intellectual Disabilities*. https://doi.org/10.1080/19315864.2021.1929596

Taylor, G. W., & Ussher, J. M. (2001). Making sense of S&M: A discourse analytic account. *Sexualities, 4*(3), 293–314. https://doi.org/10.1177/136460014003002

Ten Hoor, N. M. (2013). Treating cognitive distortions with EMDR: A case study of a sex offender. *Interpersonal Journal of Forensic Mental Health, 12*, 139–148. https://doi.org/10.1080/14999013.2013.791350

Unwin, G., Willcott, S., Hendrickson, S., & Kroese, B. S. (2019). Eye movement desensitization and reprocessing for adults with intellectual disabilities: Process issues from an acceptability study. *Journal of Applied Research in Intellectual Disabilities, 32*(3), 635–647. https://doi.org/10.1111/jar.12557

Wright, L. C. & Warner, A. (2020). EMDR treatment of childhood sexual abuse for a child molester: Self-reported changes in sexual arousal. *Journal of EMDR Practice and Research, 14*(2), 90–103. https://doi.org/10.1891/EMDR-D-19-00060

Yaskin, J. & Seubert, A. (2017). Left out and behind: EMDR and the cultural constriction of intellectual disability. In M. Nickerson (Ed.). *Cultural competence and healing culturally based trauma with EMDR therapy*. Springer Publishing.

ADDITIONAL RESOURCES

BDSM/Kink Beginner's Manuals

Bannon, R. (1993). *Learning the ropes: A basic guide to safe and fun S/M lovemaking.* Daedalus Publishing Company.

Califia, P. (2001). *Sensuous magic: A guide to S/M for adventurous couples* (2nd ed.). Cleis Press.

Easton, D., & Hardy, J. W. (2001). *The new bottoming book.* Greenery Press.

Easton, D., & Hardy, J. W. (2003). *The new topping book.* Greenery Press.

Green, L. (1998). *The sexually dominant woman: A workbook for nervous beginners* (2nd ed.). Greenery Press.

Henkin, W. A., & Holiday, S. (2003). *Consensual sadomasochism: How to talk about it & how to do it safely* (2nd ed.). Daedalus Publishing Company.

Jacques, T., Dale, D., Hamilton, M., & Sniffer. (1993). *On the safe edge: A manual for SM play.* Whole SM Publishing Corporation.

Ortman, D. M., & Sprott, R. A. (2013). *Sexual outsiders: Understanding BDSM sexualities and communities.* Rowman & Littlefield Publishers.

Rinella, J. (2004). *The complete slave: Creating and living an erotic dominant/submissive lifestyle* (2nd ed.). Daedalus Publishing Company.

Taormino, T. (2012). *The ultimate guide to kink.* Cleis Press.

Taormino, T. (2013). *50 shades of kink: An introduction to BDSM.* Cleis Press.

Varrin, C. (2004). *Female dominance: Rituals and practice.* Citadel Publishing.

Warren, J. (2000). *The loving dominant* (2nd ed.). Greenery Press.

Sex and Disability

Kaufman, M., Silverberg, C., & Odette, F. (2007). *The ultimate guide to sex and disability.* Cleis Press.

Kroll, K., & Klein, E. L. (2001). *Enabling romance: A guide to love, sex, and relationships for people with disabilities (and the people who care about them).* United Spinal Association.

9

Aging Sexual Health and EMDR Therapy

Ashley L. Mader, PhD, LICSW

LEARNING OBJECTIVES

- EMDR clinicials will be able to describe the current aging population and research on aging and sexuality.
- EMDR clinicians will be able to list the common concerns and changes that affect the sexuality of aging women.
- EMDR clinicians will be able to list the common concerns and changes that affect the sexuality of aging men.
- EMDR clinicians will be able to list the common concerns and changes that affect the sexuality and well-being of LGBTQ individuals.
- EMDR clinicians will be able to describe the social influences on sexuality and aging (loss of a partner, ageism, myths, etc.)
- EMDR clinicians will be able to describe what healthcare professionals know about sexuality and aging and how they can better serve and communicate with the aging population about sexuality.

GENDER LANGUAGE

In this chapter the term *man* refers to individuals with a penis, testes, prostate, and so on, and/or socialized into a masculine gender (generally speaking, *cis-men*). The term *woman* refers to individuals with a vulva, labia, clitoris, vagina, ovaries, and uterus, and/or socialized into a feminine gender (generally speaking, *ciswomen*). This particularly pertains to how researchers have categorized individuals in the studies mentioned, as well as some of the self-identified gender of individuals featured in case studies. Transgendered individuals and their aging are also addressed.

INTRODUCTION

As of 2018 there were 52 million adults that were 65 years and older. In 2020, the expected number of Baby Boomers will be upward of 73 million people. Baby Boomers are individuals born between 1946 and 1964 after World War II (United States Census Bureau, 2019).

The Silent Generation are those adults born between 1928 and 1945 during the Great Depression and during World War II. There are an estimated 23 million people in this generation (Howe, 2014). In 2020, there were 20% of Americans over the age of 65. That last time there was this high of a percentage of people past the age of 65 was during the Black Death, around 1350. This may come as a surprise given the death toll of the plague, however it did not affect older adults as much (Minois, 1989).

A BRIEF HISTORY OF AGING

With modern medicine people can now live well past 65 years of age, however this was not always the case. Between the years 1650 and 1850, older adults accounted for about 2% of the population. Because of this, older adults were highly regarded and deemed very wise. If one lived to an old age, one was most likely of a higher socio-economic status. There were very few poor older adults, and if there were poor older adults they were thought to be a tax burden to society and looked down upon (Fleming et al., 2003).

The shift in how older adults were viewed was around the time of the American Revolution. Before the Revolution, powdered wigs were worn to give the impression of being aged and wise. Many older adults did not save for retirement thus becoming a burden to their family. Aging became more of a disease rather than looked at in fascination (Fleming et al., 2003). In some cultures aging is still revered, such as in Greek, Native American, Korean, and Chinese cultures (Huffpost, 2017).

OLDER ADULT SEXUALITY EXPERIENCES

The Baby Boomers tend to have more liberal attitudes toward sexuality and be more satisfied with their sex lives than the Silent Generation. This may be due to

Boomers growing up during the sexual revolution. Each subsequent generation seems to have more openness about sex (Beckman et al., 2008).

Many assume that advanced age negatively affects sexual quality of life. Although there is a change in the frequency of sex, the number of partners, and older adults' perceived control over sexual aspects of their lives, many older adults report a higher level of sexual quality of life than younger adults. In older adults, the quality of sex appears much more important than quantity of sex. Older men tend to have a higher level of sexual quality of life than women (Forbes et al., 2017). Women are often widowed and live 6 to 8 years longer than men, which may account for the lower level of sexual quality of life (Murphy et al., 2018).

Sexual frequency among older adults can decrease. This is mostly due to lack of a partner. However, even among partnered women, the frequency of sex is less than that of men. Other contributing factors to the decrease in sexual activity are health related such as heart conditions, physical limitations, and sexual dysfunctions. Lifestyle and health factors have a major impact on the sexual functioning of older adults. High cholesterol, diabetes, hypertension, and other heart conditions may cause sexual dysfunction. Medications that are used to treat these conditions may also cause sexual dysfunction. It is very important that helping professionals rule out medical problems when a person comes to them with a sexual dysfunction. Sometimes a sexual dysfunction, such as erectile dysfunction or pain during intercourse, is a sign that there is an underlying medical condition (Lindau et al., 2007).

Sexually Transmitted Infections

Sexually transmitted infections (STIs) are on the rise in the senior population. Half of the people currently living with HIV/AIDS are over 50 years old. STIs such as chlamydia, gonorrhea, syphilis, HPV, and herpes are also being diagnosed at a higher rate than they were previously. There are several reasons for this uptick in STI rates among older adults. There are more divorces in middle age, thus people may enter the dating world online and potentially have more partners than before. Older adults often do not think they are at risk for STIs. When they were young adults, there was not as much focus on STIs and HIV/AIDS did not exist before the 1980s. The major prevention concern was an accidental pregnancy, not STIs. Given that older adults do not have to worry about pregnancy, they may not use protection.

Older adults today are also generally more sexually active than they were as adults in the 1990s. With the invention of Viagra and other erectile enhancement drugs, older adults are able to continue engaging in sexual activity. Lastly, medical professionals often misdiagnose STIs in older adults as "afflictions of old age." They may not ask if the patient is sexually active, therefore disregarding the possibility of an STI (Benjamin Rose Institute on Aging, 2019).

Older adults may be very distressed by an STI diagnosis. EMDR therapy can help reduce or eliminate any distress or shame.

CHANGES IN AGING WOMEN'S SEXUAL HEALTH

Menopause

What is menopause? Menopause is simply when the menstrual cycle ends. The average age of menopause is 52 years old. Some may experience it years earlier or later. Other than the cessation of the menstrual cycle individuals may experience hot flashes and vaginal changes during menopause. Though hot flashes may be uncomfortable, they generally do not impact sexuality. A hot flash can be defined as a sudden wave of heat that may cause severe sweating.

Some people experience vaginal changes such as dryness or the thinning of the walls of the vagina or vaginal atrophy. Vaginal dryness can range from minimal discomfort to severe discomfort. This can have an impact on the experience of sexuality. Individuals may experience pain during penetration and therefore more planning may be needed before engaging in sexual activity. Hydrating and over-the-counter water-based lubricants have proved helpful for vaginal dryness. Douches, perfumed sprays or toilet paper, and antihistamines may irritate the vulva and vagina more (Doress-Worters & Siegal, 1994).

Like other parts of the body, the vagina may become weaker if not engaged. There is the idea of "if you don't use it you lose it" (Burry, 2018). Though the vaginal canal is not exactly a muscle, it is made up of elastic tissue that is connected to the pelvic floor, which is a muscle. According to the Memorial Sloan Kettering Cancer Center, it may be helpful to strengthen the pelvic floor with pelvic floor exercises, such as Kegels (2018). Moreover, more penetrative sexual activity may result in less vaginal atrophy (Burry, 2018).

According to the North American Menopause Society (NAMS), women may experience orgasm changes as they age. Orgasms may become shorter in duration and the clitoris may become less sensitive (2020). Sexual desire increases and decreases over time. Many women say the reason they are not engaging in partnered sexual activity is because of the lack of a partner, not necessarily the lack of desire (Mader, 2014). Although some women report a lack of sexual desire as they get older, some aging women experience an increase in desire. Pregnancy fears have finally terminated, physically and mentally freeing for some, thus increasing sexual interest and activity (Rogers, 2019).

Hormone Replacement Therapy

Some women may opt for hormone replacement therapy (HRT). HRT is a medication that replaces the estrogen that the body loses during menopause. It can make menopause more comfortable, decrease hot flashes, and help vaginal discomfort. Some studies also show that it can prevent bone loss and fractures in post-menopausal individuals (Mayo Clinic, 2020).

Not everyone is a good candidate for HRT. Certain medical histories, such as heart disease, hypertension, liver disease, certain cancers, and blood clots may not be suited for HRT (Mayo Clinic, 2020). There has been research on HRT and how it can increase the risk of both breast and endometrial cancer. Some people who experience only vaginal discomfort may opt for estrogen cream and avoid pills. There can be drawbacks or side effects to taking HRT such as a recurrence of vaginal bleeding. Others have reported side effects, such as nausea, weight gain, bloating, and depression. It is important to weigh both the risks and benefits of HRT (Doress-Worters & Siegal, 1994).

Avoid completely medicalizing menopause. Certainly, there are times that medical treatment is needed, but menopause is also a natural occurring process that people have experienced for millennia. Having open and candid conversations about the menopause process with both peers and helping professionals should not be underestimated (Doress-Worters & Siegal, 1994).

If individuals report distress around menopausal symptoms, unpleasant sexual experiences due to aging-related changes, or other loss or change in sexual functioning, EMDR therapy may help reduce or eliminate this emotional distress.

Something to Consider: Cultural Differences

Not every culture treats menopause or experiences menopause the same. Mayan women are excited for menopause, eat a diet high in carbohydrates, with very little consumption of meat or dairy, and report no hot flashes. Greek women have a diet similar to the women in the United States, have more anxiety about menopause, and also experience hot flashes. Japanese women report taking more herbal supplements and having fewer hot flashes. Cultures that have more ageism and medicalization around menopause may make the experience worse for women (Doress-Worters & Siegal, 1994).

Black women often experience heavier bleeding, which is often overlooked by healthcare providers or not treated appropriately. Black women also have a higher rate of hysterectomies than White women. It is not known whether those are absolutely necessary. They also experience a higher rate of symptoms with uterine leiomyomas or fibroid tumors than White women (85% vs. 63%, respectively; Weiss et al., 2009). Before 1996 women of color were underrepresented in menopause research. The Study of Women's Health Across the Nation started surveying women's experiences of menopause and have found that both Black and Hispanic women experience menopause 2 years earlier than White women (Velez, 2020).

Hysterectomies and Oophorectomies

A hysterectomy is the removal of the uterus and an oophorectomy is the removal of the ovaries. As people age through menopause, their risk for uterine and ovarian cancers increases; therefore, Pap smears and pelvic exams remain extremely important. Hysterectomies and oophorectomies are often performed when the person has cancer or another life-threatening illness. Conversely, some of the gynecological issues that plagued female-bodied individuals pre-menopause may be alleviated after menopause (Doress-Worters & Siegal, 1994). However, many of these procedures are performed electively, rather than for life-threatening conditions. It is estimated that one in five hysterectomies are unnecessary (Whiteman, 2015).

It is a common belief that after menopause and the childbearing years female-bodied people do not need their reproductive organs. However, the uterus and ovaries have a purpose after menopause. Ovaries can continue to function long after the uterus is removed through a hysterectomy (Doress-Worters & Siegal, 1994). Both a hysterectomy and oophorectomy can cause a drop in hormones, which is often related to loss of sexual desire and vaginal dryness (Whiteman, 2015).

Even if the ovaries are left in place and the uterus is removed, an entire system is disturbed, which includes the vagina, ovaries, clitoris, cervix, blood and nerve supplies. The uterus is cut out, leaving the connective tissues and nerves to heal and scar. Though some health professionals report that these procedures do not affect sexual functioning, many patients report decreases in sexual desire, less powerful orgasms, vaginal pain, and dryness (Doress-Worters & Siegal, 1994).

If there are problems with lubrication, estrogen creams can be inserted in the vagina to help increase comfortable and pleasurable vaginal–penis intercourse. However, Medicare does not pay for these medications. There have been some recent improvements in Medicare's covering of medications related to menopause. Medicare Part D now covers drugs that treat severe dyspareunia.

Case Study 9.1: Katie Grieves Her Hysterectomy

Katie is a 67-year-old woman who had a hysterectomy 15 years ago. It was a surgery she was told that she needed and that nothing would change about her sex life, except eliminating the possibility of pregnancy. When asked about how it affected her, she reported that it not only affected her orgasms, but also how she felt about being a woman. As an educator herself, she researched sex after a hysterectomy and learned how sexual satisfaction was measured most often by the frequency of sex, rather than someone's actual sexual response. While she remained functionally able to engage in sex, the quality of her experience dramatically diminished. "I said back then that the woman that I was died on the operating table. I had to evolve into a different person in many ways after that" (Mader, 2014, p. 83).

EMDR therapy could potentially help Katie grieve through these orgasmic and gender identity changes. In this case, the earliest instances of orgasm change could be targeted and processed. The death of "the woman that I was" might potentially be another EMDR target.

Case Study 9.2: A Partner's Perspective on Hysterectomy

Frank is a 65-year-old man whose wife had uterine cancer. They had a very active sex life up until her cancer treatment necessitated a hysterectomy. In their sexual routine she would have an orgasm, and then he would have one. Once she had the hysterectomy, her lubrication decreased, which was discussed before the surgery. However, she would have severe pain right before her orgasm. He did not want to see her in pain, so he pretended to have an orgasm or avoided sex altogether (Mader, 2014).

EMDR therapy could target Frank's distress regarding his wife's pain. She may also benefit from EMDR therapy, particularly pain protocols. They may both benefit from EMDR Future Templates oriented toward finding new ways to be intimate, or enhancing their advocacy skills with medical professionals as they search for ways to reduce or eliminate her pain.

Yes, some hysterectomies and oophorectomies can be life-saving and beneficial, however it is extremely imperative that people weigh both the pros and cons of these surgeries, and do their own research for their own bodies.

Body Image

Changes in hormones and metabolism may affect aging bodies. The physical signs of aging that any gender may experience include weight gain, graying hair, loss of skin elasticity, loss of hearing and/or sight, and physical limitations. Any or all of these can have an effect on one's body image. A negative body image is also correlated with lower sexual desire (Quinn-Nilas et al., 2016). In an extremely youth-focused culture it is hard to find aging bodies to compare oneself. Body image issues can also include physical limitations, making certain activities more difficult than they once were. Many find it helpful to talk through the process (Hofmeier et al., 2017).

EMDR therapy can help reduce or eliminate individuals' distress and/or focus on negative body image. An EMDR timeline can be developed based on specific dislikes. A positive cognition to work toward can include "I'm fine as I am," "My aging body is normal and beautiful/handsome," "I'm still worth something."

CHANGES IN OLDER MEN'S SEXUALITY

Erections

Erections start changing around the age of 40. This does not mean erectile dysfunction (ED), but erections may change in firmness or frequency. Given there is not much information communicated about the changes that happen as one ages, men often become anxious thinking it is the beginning of ED, when it is a normal sign of aging. Because of this anxiety some men end up with ED due to anxiety, rather than actual physical causes (Rienzo, 1985).

What actually constitutes ED? ED is essentially the inability to hold an erection long enough for satisfying sexual activity (Urology Care Foundation, 2018). ED becomes more prevalent as one ages. About 40% of men experience some kind of ED in their 40s, and by the age of 70, 70% of men are affected (Lakin & Wood, 2018). There are some factors that put older men at risk for ED, such as diabetes, high cholesterol, hypertension, low testosterone, obesity, and certain medications (Danoff, 2015).

Case Study 9.3: Hugh's Nervous Penis

Hugh, a 70-year-old healthy man, came to treatment for his erectile dysfunction (ED). He was extremely healthy with no underlying health conditions or medications that would contribute to his ED. The only health condition of historical significance was Peyronie's disease from 10 years ago, which had caused tremendous pain when having intercourse, but was treated in its early stages. Hugh at times used erectile enhancement drugs, but they did not always work. After taking a detailed sexual history and through numerous sex therapy sessions, it was revealed that Hugh had anxiety around lasting long enough to please his partner, and worried that he may never have sex again, which he linked to the prior Peyronie's disease. The more Hugh worked on reducing his anxiety the more he was able to have successful intercourse both with and without the help of erectile enhancement drugs.

EMDR therapy could target Hugh's prior Peyronie's disease experiences, his anxiety around "lasting long enough," and his worry that he may "never have sex again." Positive cognitions to work toward can include "I'm fine as I am," "I am lovable no matter how I perform," and "I am capable and can handle what comes my way."

Treatment for Erectile Dysfunction

ED can be very troublesome to men. As stated, some ED is psychological and psychotherapy may be able to help. For biological ED there are numerous medications; Viagra, Levitra, Cialis, Staxyn, and Stendra are the most common of PDE-5 inhibitors. They all work in similar ways; they relax the muscles in the penis and when the penis becomes aroused the arteries in the penis become wider, allowing the penis to fill with blood and the veins to expand. The blood is trapped for a period of time, thus leading to an erection. It should be noted that if a person without ED uses these drugs for sexual performance, the drugs do not behave in the same way (Danoff, 2015).

Other more invasive treatments of ED are surgical implants with a vacuum device (Danoff, 2015). With the invention of PDE-5 inhibitors this is not as common. Injectables are also used for ED treatment. The more recent treatment is when prostaglandin-E1 or PGE-1 is directly injected into the shaft of the penis. Injectables are used when other medications have been tried but failed. The idea of inserting something into the penis is generally not a pleasant thought for many. Dr. Danoff speaks of a newer drug called Muse that is inserted at the tip of the penis through a urethral suppository. It is extremely important to talk to one's doctor to decide what treatment is right for them (2015).

Are Erections a Privilege?

Many Americans over the age of 65 use Medicare as their healthcare benefits. Viagra, Cialis, and other drugs for ED are not paid for under Medicare. A non-generic version of Viagra may cost approximately $60 per pill and a generic version may be about $35 a pill. Nevertheless, many sexual enhancement drugs are still not covered by Medicare Part D, and many individuals cannot afford to pay out of pocket for these types of treatments, leaving them impotent, sad, frustrated, and in pain (Andrews, 2019).

Changes in Sexual Desire

Changes in sexual desire are common among aging men. Many older men report they do not crave sex as much as they did when they were younger. As with most people, many problems with sexual desire have psychological underpinnings. However, lower testosterone may cause low sexual desire. If the change in sexual desire is rapid, it is important to consult with one's physician to see what could be the potential cause. It may be related to medication or another underlying health condition (Nippoldt, 2020).

Ejaculation Changes

Ejaculation may also change with aging. Delayed (slow), or retrograde ejaculation may happen. Retrograde ejaculation is when ejaculate reverses back into the bladder rather than coming through the penis. There is no cause for concern; the semen will make its way out during urination (Danoff, 2015). Diabetes, spinal cord injury, multiple sclerosis, and certain medications are all related to retarded ejaculation. Medications such as anti-depressants are especially linked to this condition (Villines, 2017).

> **Case Study 9.4: No Ejaculation**

Will (age 68) and Barbara (age 66) had been dating for 6 months. Will had been diagnosed with Parkinson's disease 2 years ago and was able to control some of the physical decline by diet, exercise, and physical therapy. When they started engaging in sexual intercourse Will was unable to ejaculate. He could maintain an erection, but had no ejaculation. Barbara was saddened by this because she wanted her partner to enjoy sex as much as she did. Sexual intercourse eventually became emotionally painful for Barbara because of Will not being able to ejaculate. They decided to consult a sex therapist. When the sex therapist was taking a history she found out that Will was taking Citalopram, an anti-depressant. Will said that he did not need to take it anymore and that he was on a really low dose. After consulting with his primary care physician, Will stopped taking the medication and his ejaculation returned. Both he and Barbara were much happier in their sexual relationship with each other.

Benign Prostate Hypertrophy

Benign prostate hypertrophy (BPH), or "enlarged prostate" as it is commonly known, affects about half of men over 50. It is not life-threatening, but may be very uncomfortable. Signs of BPH are decreased urine flow, difficulty fully eliminating the bladder, and weak urine flow. The prostate surrounds the neck of the bladder and may become larger with aging. This in turn can cause a change in urine flow. If the BPH is severe enough, a prostatectomy (full or partial removal of the prostate gland) may be recommended. It should be noted that, although this may sound scary, when done for a benign disease, it is not related to erectile dysfunction. Medication is a non-invasive way to treat BPH. Older medications such as Proscar may lower the patient's sexual desire. New medications such as Avodart have minimal side effects. It is vitally important for an individual to talk to their primary care doctor and/or urologist about potential medication and side effects (Danoff, 2015).

Body Image

It is often thought that only women struggle with body image as they age. Men, and other genders, may also struggle with their aging bodies and appearance. Some men report the loss of their hair and physical capabilities may be troublesome to them. As one gets older, body image does not only concern how the body looks, but also the physical functioning of the body. Losses such as hearing, sight, and movement may make one feel like one's body is betraying them. This is true for any body. Certain previous enjoyable hobbies may be more difficult. Arthritis in one's hands may prevent a person from sewing, knitting, or playing the piano. Losses of sight and hearing may cause people not to feel as independent. Common activities such as driving may now be less available. This can be an adjustment for the older adult (Jankowski et al., 2014).

> **Case Study 9.5: Jack and His Aging Body**

Jack is a 65-year-old man who has struggled with some erectile dysfunction due to medication issues. When asked about how he felt about his body and how it relates to his aging, he spoke about what it is like to look in the mirror and see his reflection. He sees his thinning hair and weight gain, and these changes diminish how he feels about himself. He views himself differently now and knows that he has changed, which also negatively impacts how he feels about himself sexually (Mader, 2014).

EMDR therapy can target these various negative self-perceptions, working toward the positive cognitions of "I am fine as I am," "I'm worthy and deserve sexual pleasure like any other body."

LGBTQ AGING

Along with what has been mentioned previously about the changes that happen when one ages, LGBTQ elders face different challenges as they age. About 5% of the 65 and older people reside in nursing homes. By 2030 the last of the Baby Boomers will have reached 65 years old and this population will make up one fifth of the total population. It is estimated that there are 1.5 million LGBTQ adults over the age of 65 in the United States. Many of them will rely on assisted living and nursing homes to take care of them in their old age. LGBTQ older adults are more likely to be single and childless as they age compared to their heterosexual peers. Some LGBTQ older adults have come out of straight marriages and then come out as LGBTQ, which may have caused a strain on their family relationships, leaving them more isolated (Rhode, 2018).

The experience varies among older adults. Lesbians and people of color are more likely to struggle economically than White gay men. Older bisexual individuals may experience more social isolation and depression.

Only 50% of LGBTQ older adults who reside in nursing homes or assisted living feel comfortable being out about their sexual orientation. There have been cases of mistreatment in long-term care facilities by homophobic staff. Same-sex partners have been separated in the living situations as well (Rhode, 2018).

There is a light at the end of the tunnel. In certain cities LGBTQ assisted living, long term care facilities, and retirement communities are being created.

Legislation, such as the SB 219—A Bill of Rights for LGBTQ elders was passed in 2017 in California. Though change is being made, there is still much room for improvement (Rhode, 2018).

Transgender Aging

Some transgendered older folks have an increasing likelihood of going back into the closet and not having their health needs met, such as continuing on their hormone treatments for gender affirmation (Rhode, 2018). However, some individuals choose to come out later in life rather than when they were younger. Transgender individuals face a much bigger stigma in the past than they do now, although Transphobia still exists. Many individuals chose to stay in the closet, but with more mainstream acceptance and representation, such as Caitlyn Jenner, some folks decide it is time to come out. In mid life, individuals may be more aware of the time they have left, want to live their lives as authentically as possible, and decide to transition (Fabbre, 2014).

There is a widely held fear among aging transgendered individuals that if they become dependent or have to reside in a nursing home that their genders will not be affirmed, or they will not receive proper care. Furthermore, there is a concern of violence and sexual abuse in nursing homes. Not affording proper care can leave some more vulnerable to violence and abuse in nursing homes. Not all nursing homes and facilities are educated or competent in transgender care and issues. They may be concerned that for the first time in a while, they will be outed. They may have lived in their gender for decades and may have never come out to certain people. Unfortunately, this leaves many transgender individuals vulnerable to depression and suicide. Some create "end of life plans" in case they reach the point where they can no longer take care of themselves (Witten, 2013).

> ### Case Study 9.6: The Impact of April's Transition
>
> Patrick (age 63) and Johanna (age 57) originally sought couples therapy to work through some infidelity issues. Patrick had always had a desire for BDSM (bondage, dominance, dado-masochism) and would pay Dominatrixes to engage in the behavior. Johanna was trying to accept this as she wanted their marriage to work. In one session, Patrick shared he really enjoyed wearing women's clothes and he became alive when he wore them. He always thought it was a kink behavior, but realized it has been something more. Soon, Patrick came out as a transwoman and changed her name to April. April very much wanted to stay married to Johanna, but Johanna was not attracted to women and they ended up divorcing.

April had difficulty coming out to her family. Her daughter, a teenager, was not comfortable with this and insisted that April present as male when she would visit her. April, not wanting to lose connection with her daughter, obliged, but it was painful to do so. April lost complete contact with her adult son. Though April is much happier and has created a wonderful LGBTQ community, she still struggles with the loss of some family contact and having to present as male at times.

April certainly can benefit from EMDR therapy, targeting these very sad instances of abandonment and invalidation by her family members. An EMDR Future Template might help strengthen her ability to explain and assert a refusal to appear male to her daughter. April could work toward these positive cognitions: "I'm fine as I am," "I can be myself and be loved," and "I do the best I can." Her family members, if open to EMDR therapy, could also greatly benefit from exploring and reducing their potential anger, sadness, and disappointment at losing a "man" as their father. EMDR therapy might even help April's daughter come to terms with, accept, and affirm April's transition. Their positive cognitions might include "I can handle my parent's transition" and "I accept myself and others."

Case Study 9.7: Staying in the Closet

Robert is a 70-year-old man. He has been married to his wife for 45 years. He is very active in his church as well as his senior center. He volunteered to be a part of a dissertation research study focusing on the experiences of older adults' sexuality as they age. He found the research both interesting and important. Throughout the interview, the researcher felt like Robert was holding something back. It was not until the end of the interview when the researcher asked, "Do you know anyone who is lesbian or gay who may want to participate in the research study?" Robert let out a giant sigh and said that he had same-gender sexual relations throughout his marriage. He admitted he knew it was wrong to cheat, but he got much more emotional and sexual satisfaction from men than he ever did from his wife. He admitted to the researcher he had never told anyone else about this and the researcher was the first person he told. He had no intentions of ever getting out of his marriage. (Mader, 2014, p. 95)

If Robert did choose to explore his same-gender history, EMDR therapy could help him identify and reduce any distress about potentially identifying as gay and leaving his marriage so that he may eventually more authentically pursue emotional and sexual satisfaction. His negative cognitions might be "I don't have a choice, I'm trapped." His positive cognitions could potentially be "I have choices, I can handle big changes, I deserve to openly pursue what I want."

SOCIAL INFLUENCE ON SEXUALITY AND AGING

Ageism

Ageism is discrimination based on one's age. It usually pertains to older adults rather than younger folks. Unlike other prejudices, racists are not going to wake up and find themselves with a different skin color. Someone who is anti-Semitic is not going to wake up and find themselves Jewish. However, if we are lucky, we will all one day grow old. "About the most unproductive prejudice is one directed against a group you're going to join" (Dailey, 1981, p. 312).

It is not just younger people who hold ageist attitudes. Older adults also can have internalized ageism, which can be particularly harmful, especially in terms of sexuality. These views are usually developed when one is young, then carried to old age. Take something as simple as going to the grocery store and looking at the magazines in the check-out line. What do you see? Usually, it is a younger person gracing the cover. The ads in the magazine promote how one can look younger. Even when shopping for a birthday card one will find negative stereotypes, albeit humorous, depicting aging. Seeing these images on a regular basis may be detrimental in how an older adult feels about themselves. Dr. Dennis Dailey (1981) refers to this phenomenon as the "laughter curtain." The laughter curtain basically is how people manage their feelings with uncomfortable life topics. This is just as detrimental to older adults as is silence. Having a helping professional or a family member laugh at the sexuality of an older adult causes shame. This in turn may become a self-fulfilling prophecy for many older adults. If people believe that older adults are asexual, older adults may very well shut down this part of their lives.

Internalized stereotypes and/or internalized ageism begins at a very young age and continues across the life span. Negative depictions of aging in the media, and different stories heard when one is young, affect how people feel about aging and older adults. It is easy for children to feel removed from the experiences of older adults because they are not yet in that stage of life. Given that our society is very youth focused, in some ways young adults benefit from this ageism, which exacerbates the stereotype (Levy, 2009).

Stereotypes on sexuality and aging are profound. Older women in the media are depicted as the sweet grandmotherly types or very unkempt, eccentric women. If they are depicted as sexual, "the cougar" stereotype is often presented. Older men in the media who have interest in sex are thought of as sex obsessed, hence the "dirty old man" stereotype, or they are the grouchy curmudgeons yelling at children to "get off their lawn" (Walz, 2002).

As of 2020 there has been a refreshing turnaround on how older adult sexuality is depicted in mainstream media. TV shows such as "Grace and Frankie" and movies like "Book Club" show older women and men enjoying sex well into their later years. Even with these advances there is a need for improvement so that the negative stereotypes are no longer perpetuated.

Stereotypes can also negatively impact older adults' health. Older adults may not seek the medical treatment they need because of the idea that "it's just old age." By accepting these stereotypes, older folks may not take care of themselves in the ways that are needed (Levy, 2009). This is especially true when it comes to sexuality. Often older adults do not talk to their healthcare providers about sexuality due to embarrassment or the notion that this is "just a normal" aging process. Conversely, healthcare professionals do not address sexuality with their older patients because of this ageism and general embarrassment (Gore-Gorszewska, 2020).

> **Case Study 9.8: Cathy, Minimized Vaginal Dryness**

Cathy, a 68-year-old woman on dialysis, went to her primary care doctor for a check up. She brought up a sexual concern of vaginal dryness, which is a common experience with dialysis. The doctor became very uneasy and replied, "That's what gynecologists are for." Cathy's concern was never addressed. Due to her doctor's discomfort, she never brought it up to her gynecologist, either. This example makes it clear how lack of communication hinders older adults from the treatment that they need (Mader, 2014, p.110).

If Cathy learned about and entered into EMDR therapy, this conversation with her primary care physician could be targeted as a disturbing event. An EMDR Future Template could help her find her voice and practice speaking up to medical professionals about her needs. Her positive cognitions could be "I deserve to be listened to" and "My needs are important."

LOSS OF A PARTNER

Many older adults experience loss of a partner. The World Health Organization (WHO) has found that women tend to outlive men, thus are more likely to be widowed, living 6 to 8 years longer than men (WHO, n.d.). This leaves many individuals alone for the first time in a long while and without a sexual partner. Many older adults would like to find some sort of companionship, and others are happy with friends and family (Mader, 2014). Finding a companion may prove to be difficult for some. Being out of the dating world for a long time, as well as internalized stereotypes, may prevent older adults from finding the companionship that they so desire. One of the main reasons older adults report not being sexual is because they do not have a partner (Parker-Pope, 2019).

Family Influence

Even when older adults choose to date and enter a new relationship, it is not always smooth sailing. Family and especially adult children can be very critical about their aging parents being in a new relationship. This may be due to a plethora of reasons, such as the adult child's own ageism, their grief around the loss of the other parent, and/or fear of financial loss or loss of inheritance (Hughes & Fredenburg, 2020).

It is difficult for children of any age to think of their parents as sexual beings. Sexuality is not often a conversation topic in families, so it can be a big surprise to adult children when their parents want to engage in new relationships. This may be even a bigger problem if an aging parent in a nursing home begins a relationship. As difficult as it may be, adult children should not infantilize their aging parents and need to realize that people are sexual from the day they are born to the day they die. Although it may be hard to conceptualize depending on one's age, it is important to think about how one would want to be treated in a similar situation. These aging parents had a life before their children and they can continue having one after their children are grown (Love & Harmony, 2010).

Older adults' sexuality is often infantilized, especially in nursing homes. Once they are in a nursing home, they often do not have automatic rights to sexual expression. Their rights are left up to their families and the staff. Often the families have to give permission for their loved one to engage in sexual behavior. In turn, the older resident may feel shameful about their very natural sexual behavior. In some cases, nursing home staff are more accepting of intimacy between two residents if those residents are married to each other. However, that same privilege is not always allowed to single older adults. Autonomy of older adults is often promoted and advertised by nursing homes, however sexuality is often not included in that autonomy (Doll, 2013).

Sexual contact in nursing homes can be sometimes considered an ethical dilemma. In 2014, Henry Rayons (age 78), a state legislator from Iowa, was arrested for a third-degree felony sexual abuse after engaging in sexual acts with his wife in a nursing home who was diagnosed with Alzheimer's disease. This was after the nursing home staff stated that Mrs. Rayons was not able to consent to sex. Consent and dementia can be difficult to figure out. Some researchers believe that consent may happen through facial expressions and body language. Intimacy is often very beneficial to dementia patients. While the family may be upset by sexual activities of their relative with dementia, many nursing homes are also caught in an ethical quandary. Most nursing homes do not have a sexual health policy that addresses these issues. Moreover, most nursing staff historically have not considered older adults as sexual. Fortunately, more people are researching consent and dementia, and more nursing homes are getting trained on how to manage the sexual rights of their patients. (Belluck, 2015).

The Hebrew Home Nursing Home located in Bronx, New York, created a sexual rights policy for their residents in 1995. Families are informed of this policy at the beginning. Staff are trained to look for cues of consent as well as knocking before entering a resident's room. They are also trained to ask residents certain questions regarding sex and consent (Belluck, 2015).

> **Case Study 9.9: Ethel and George's Relationship in a Nursing Home**

Ethel is a widowed, 94-year-old woman residing in a nursing home. She has lived there for the past 4 years. In the past few months she has sparked a relationship with George, a 96-year-old widower. The nursing home staff sees how happy the relationship makes them and allows them privacy to engage in intimacy. George's daughter came to visit and became irate that her father was in a relationship. She forbade her father to see Ethel and had the nursing home staff move George to another part of the nursing home. Soon after the move George died. Ethel wanted to go to the funeral, but the family had the police there to escort Ethel away from the funeral and forbade her to be there. Ethel became extremely depressed.

Ethel may also be experiencing some traumatic responses to how George's family handled their relationship, as well as grief and/or self-blame over his death. EMDR therapy could help reduce and eliminate any distress she continues to experience from their cruel treatment. Her negative cognitions might include "George's death is my fault, I don't deserve happiness, I'm all alone." Her positive cognitions could be "I did the best I could, I deserve happiness and love (like anyone else), and I have some positive connections."

HEALTHCARE PROVIDERS AND AGING SEXUAL HEALTH

Older adults account for a substantial number of patients that seek care from different healthcare providers such as primary care doctors, physical therapists, and social workers. Although there is a significant number of older adults receiving care, healthcare professionals do not usually have formal training in gerontology, and there is even less training on gerontology and sexuality. In one study it was found that psychology students had a better understanding of older adult sexuality than medical students did. It was also found that the more exposure and interest in the aging population a person had, the more open minded that person would be regarding older adult sexuality (Snyder & Zweig, 2010).

Even if a helping professional has knowledge about older adult sexuality, it does not necessarily mean that they have positive attitudes about it. It was found that the older the helping professional was, their attitude was less permissive (Langer-Most & Langer, 2010). This may be due to internalized ageism discussed previously in the chapter.

In a web-based survey of 3,000 self-identified women, 40% said that they did not seek help for sexual functioning. Fifty-four percent did seek help; however, they did not rank their experience with the helping professional high. Communication may be difficult for older adults, especially those socialized as women, in regard to sexuality. Older women may be conflict avoidant and want to remain neutral in their relationships, so sexual concerns may not be communicated. This lack of communication may impede the relationship between the helping professional and the older adult, thus older adults may not receive the help they need (Laumann et al., 2005).

If older adults do communicate with their healthcare provider about sexuality, it is most often their primary care doctor. This may be because they do not realize there are specialists available to help them. Even still, older adults are often reluctant to bring up sexuality with their helping professionals because they perceive that the professional has a negative attitude about sex. Furthermore, many older adults have adopted the "that ship has sailed" mentality and do not bring up concerns (Gott & Hinchliff, 2003).

Mental health professionals do not fare much better in the comfort of addressing sexuality and aging. Sexual histories are often taken with new patients coming into a mental health setting. Mental health professionals often omit taking a sexual history with their older clients because they deem it inappropriate. In one study, psychiatrists were given two different scenarios about sexuality: one with a middle-aged adult and another with an older adult and were asked what they would do. Most of them chose to refer the middle-aged adult to a sexual health professional and the older adult to community-based care. (Bouman & Arcelus, 2001).

Older adults who prioritize their sexuality are more likely to shop around for a helping professional that is comfortable with the topic. Moreover, some doctors have aged along with their patients and there may be a comfort already established, thus they may bring up the topic of sexuality more. Comfort and a good bed-side manner are both imperative with communicating with older adults about sexuality and aging (Mader, 2014).

The good news is sexuality and gerontology knowledge can be taught and helping professionals can become more comfortable with the topic. Students who study more sexuality topics are more comfortable and are more likely to bring up the topic with their clients. Not communicating about sexuality may lead to misdiagnosis, such as mistaking HIV/AIDS for a disease of older age. This is extremely detrimental for older adults. In line with the vision for and purpose of this book, all helping professionals benefit from sexuality education (Verrastro et al., 2020).

EMDR THERAPY AND AGING SEXUALITY

As illustrated throughout this chapter, just like with younger populations, EMDR therapy may be an excellent treatment modality to assist in identifying, targeting, and processing the many emotional and mental disturbances that may accompany aging and changing relationships. Hopefully all individuals get to experience aging, and hopefully everyone can turn to a trained EMDR clinician when the time comes to help us make peace with body changes and body image, differently functioning (or surgically removed) reproductive/generative organs, changing erectile organs, loss of partners, and any poor responses from family and/or healthcare professionals.

Case Study 9.10: Irene's Marriage "Slump"

This final EMDR therapy case study is contributed by Sandra Stephenson Murphy, LICSW (EMDR Certified Clinician), to further illustrate how EMDR may be of use and benefit for our aging adults.

Irene sought treatment to have support during the transition for her upcoming retirement. She is a 63-year-old White ciswoman who has been a school guidance counselor for 36 years. Irene is worried that so much of her identity and social life has been through her career and reports that her current marriage of 23 years has been in a "slump." Irene describes her husband as a recovering alcoholic who is about 2.5 years sober, who is kind and caring, and "would do anything for me." Yet Irene also describes her husband as "boring and sedentary," and has already been retired for 10 years. Irene also describes a lack of intimacy, both emotionally and sexually (no sex for the past 2-plus years). Her husband shows sexual interest periodically, yet Irene describes herself as feeling irritable by his overtures due to her perception of a lack of emotional connection. "I'm just not into the sex because of that."

Through extensive Phase 1/History Taking, three targets were identified:

1. Earliest/Touchstone Memory: Irene's mother told Irene as she began puberty (age 10 or 11), that if she ever had sex and became pregnant before marriage she would "kill herself." Her mother was a devout Catholic and Irene is a practicing Catholic. An early link between sex, sexual urges, and causing pain to her mother was established. To this day Irene reported hearing those words in her head at the stirring of any sexual interest.
2. During her first marriage, Irene's previous husband had an affair with her close friend. Even after the affair was discovered, and they both wanted to "save" their marriage by going to couples counseling, the husband continued the affair. They eventually divorced and Irene describes the entire experience as devastating. She felt suicidal and ashamed at the time. She currently worries about running into her husband and her ex-friend who is now his wife, in the community or at social events.

3. Irene wants sexual intimacy with her husband yet struggles with the lack of trust. Three years ago when her husband was drinking Irene threatened to end the marriage if he continued to drink. He supposedly stopped drinking and began participating in Alcoholics Anonymous. A friend then told Irene that she saw her husband buying alcohol at a package store. Irene said she "flipped out" and described this as a betrayal similar to her first husband's affair. Since that time he has stopped drinking, yet Irene has also stopped having sex.

All three targets were successfully processed to a 0 SUD (Subjective Units of Distress). The first target, not surprisingly as it occurred at a pivotal developmental moment, with an attachment figure, took six sessions. The second target took four sessions and the third target took three sessions.

Three EMDR Future Templates were identified and processed:

1. Envision having a healthy relationship with sex free from guilt and shame. Her positive cognition (PC) is "I deserve a fulfilling and pleasurable sexual life."
2. Imagine running into her ex-husband and his partner, feeling strong and confident, and seeing them as smaller. Her PC is "I am worthy, capable, and can handle it."
3. Sexual intimacy with her husband that feels "safe and sexy" for her. Her PC is "I can safely trust and enjoy sex again."

Irene reported the return of quality and frequency of sexual intimacy with her husband, noting that their communication has improved greatly, resulting in greater emotional intimacy, safety, and trust as well. She reported enjoying the sexual intimacy, and mentioned that for the first time she experienced sex and orgasms without any resulting pain, "Catholic" guilt, shame, or hearing her mother's voice in her head. Irene also stated that her husband was now interested in EMDR therapy to look at his previous drinking as a possible escape or avoidance of intimacy.

SUMMARY

This chapter shared information about the current aging population and their sexual behaviors. Female-, male-, and transgender-specific aging, and what each group may generally encounter as they age, was explored in detail. Social influences such as ageism, family, grief, myths, and stereotypes about aging and sexuality were addressed. The aging needs and barriers of LGBTQ folks were considered. Finally, the importance of communicating sexual health topics, questions, and concerns with helping professionals was emphasized, so that all older adults can continue to have enriching lives.

REFERENCES

Andrews, M. (2019, February 19). The high cost of sex: Insurers don't often pay for drugs to treat problems. *Kaiser Health News.* https://khn.org/news/the-high-cost-of-sex-insurers-often-dont-pay-for-drugs-to-treat-problems/

Beckman, N., Waern, M., Gustafson, D., & Skoog, I. (2008). Secular trends in self reported sexual activity and satisfaction in Swedish 70 year olds: Cross sectional survey of four populations, 1971–2001. *British Medical Journal, 337*(a279), 1–7. https://doi.org/10.1136/bmja279

Belluck, P. (2015, April 15). Sex, dementia, and a husband on trial at age 78. *New York Times.* https://www.nytimes.com/2015/04/14/health/sex-dementia-and-a-husband-henry-rayhons-on-trial-at-age-78.html?auth=login-google

Benjamin Rose Institute on Aging. (2019, June 12). *Sexually transmitted diseases in older adults.* https://www.benrose.org/-/resource-library/health-and-wellness-services/sexually-transmitted-diseases-in-older-adults

Bouman, W. P., & Arcelus, J. (2001). Are psychiatrist guilty of 'ageism' when it comes to taking a sexual history? *International Journal of Geriatric Psychiatry, 16*(1), 27–31. https://doi.org/10.1002/1099-1166(200101)16:1<27::AID-GPS267>3.3.CO;2-J

Burry, M. (2018, August 1). How your vagina changes in your 30s, 40s and beyond. *Health.* https://www.health.com/condition/sexual-health/vagina-healthy-aging

Dailey, D. M. (1981). Sexual expression and aging. In F. J. Berghorn, D. E. Schafer, & Associates (Eds.), *The dynamics of aging* (pp. 311–330). Westview Press, Inc.

Danoff, D. (2015). *The ultimate guide to male sexual health: How to stay vital at any age.* Beyond Words.

Doll, G. M. (2013, July). Sexuality in nursing homes: Practice and policy. *Journal of Gerontological Nursing, 39*(7), 30–37 https://doi.org/10.3928/00989134-20130418-01

Doress-Worters, P. B., & Siegal, D. L. (1994). *The new ourselves, growing older: Women aging with knowledge and power.* Simon & Schuster.

Fabbre, V. D. (2014). Gender transitions in later life: The significance of time in queer aging. *Journal of Gerontological Social Work, 57,* 161–175. https://doi.org/10.1080/01634372.2013.855287

Fleming, K. C., Evans, J. M., & Chutka, D. S. (2003). A cultural and economic history of older age in America. *Mayo Clinic Proceedings, 78,* 914–921.

Forbes, M. K., Eaton, N. R., & Krueger, R. F. (2017). Sexual quality of life and aging: A prospective study of a nationally representative sample. *Journal Sex Research, 54*(2), 137–148. https://doi.org/10.1080/00224499.2016.1233315

Gore-Gorszewska, G. (2020). "Why not ask the doctor?" Barriers in help-seeking for sexual problems among older adults in Poland. *International Journal of Public Health, 65*(8), 1507–1515. https://doi.org/10.1007/s00038-020-01472-6

Gott, M., & Hinchliff, S. (2003). Barriers to seeking treatment for sexual problems in primary care: A qualitative study with older people. *Family Practice, 20*(6), 690–695. doi:10.1093/fampra/cmg612

Hofmeier, S. M., Runfola, C. D., Sala, M., Gagne, D. A., Brownley, K. A., & Bulik, C. M. (2017). Body image, aging, and identity in women over 50: The Gender and Body Image (GABI) study. *Journal of Women & Aging, 29*(1), 3–14. https://doi.org/10.1080/08952841.2015.1065140

Howe, N. (2014, August 13). The silent generation "The lucky few" (part 3 of 7). *Forbes.* https://www.forbes.com/sites/neilhowe/2014/08/13/the-silent-generation-the-lucky-few-part-3-of-7/?sh=2ad21b2c63bf

Huffpost. (2017, December 6). *7 cultures that celebrate aging and respect their elders.* https://www.huffpost.com/entry/what-other-cultures-can-teach_n_4834228

Hughes, C., & Fredenburg, B. (2020, July 24). How to help your adult children adjust to Dating. *Divorced Moms.com.* https://divorcedmoms.com/how-to-help-your-adult-children-adjust-to-you-dating/

Jankowski, G. S., Diedrichs, P. C., Williamson, H., Christopher, G., & Harcourt, D. (2014, April 28). Looking age-appropriate while growing old gracefully: A qualitative study of ageing and body image among older adults. *Journal of Health Psychology, 21*(4), 550–561. https://doi.org/10.1177/1359105314531468

Lakin, M., & Wood, H. (2018, June). Erectile dysfunction. *Cleveland Clinic: Center for Continuing Education.* http://www.clevelandclinicmeded.com/medicalpubs/disease management/endocrinology/erectile-dysfunction/

Langer-Most, O., & Langer, N., (2010). Aging and sexuality: How much do gynecologists know and care? *Journal of Women and Aging, 22,* 283–289.

Laumann, E., Nicolosi, A., Glasser, D., Paik, A., Gingell, C., Moreira, E., & Wang, T. (2005). Sexual problems among women and men aged 40–80 years: Prevalence and correlates identified in the global study of sexual attitudes and behaviors. *International Journal of Impotence Research, 1,* 39–57. https://doi.org/10.1038/sj.ijir.3901250

Levy, B. (2009). Stereotype embodiment. *Current Directions in Psychological Science, 18*(6), 332–336. https://doi.org/10.1111/j.1467-8721.2009.01662.x

Lindau, S. T., Schumm, L. P., Laumann, E. O., Levinson, W., O'Muircheartaigh, C. A., & Waite, L. J. (2007). A study of sexuality and health among older adults in the United States. *New England Journal of Medicine, 357*(8), 764–774.

Love & Harmony. (2010, January 20). Senior dating and dealing with adult children. *Eharmony.* https://www.eharmony.com/dating-advice/dating-tips/senior-dating-and-dealing-with-adult-children/

Mader, A. L. (2014). *Older adult experiences of their sexuality: A phenomenological inquiry* [unpublished doctoral dissertation]. Widener University, Chester, PA.

Mayo Clinic. (2020, June 9). *Hormone therapy: Is it right for you?* https://www.mayoclinic.org/diseases-conditions/menopause/in-depth/hormone-therapy/art-20046372

Memorial Sloan Kettering Cancer Center. (2018, December 18). *Pelvic floor muscle (Kegel) exercises for women to improve sexual health.* https://www.mskcc.org/cancer-care/patient-education/pelvic-floor-muscle-kegel-exercises-women-improve-sexual-health

Minois, G. (1989). *History of old age: From antiquity to the Renaissance.* University of Chicago Press.

Murphy, S. L., Xu, J., Kochanek, K. D., & Arias, E. (2018, November). Mortality in the United States, 2017. *CDC.* https://www.cdc.gov/nchs/products/databriefs/db328.htm

Nippoldt, T. B. (2020, April 14). Is the loss of sex drive normal as men get older? Mayo Clinic. https://www.mayoclinic.org/healthy-lifestyle/sexual-health/expert-answers/loss-of-sex-drive/faq-20058237

North American Menopause Society. (2020). *Decreased response and pleasure.* https://www.menopause.org/for-women/sexual-health-menopause-online/sexual-problems-at-midlife/decreased-response-and-pleasure

Parker-Pope, T. (2019, July 30). Why a woman's sex life declines after menopause (Hint: sometimes it's her partner). *The New York Times.* https://www.nytimes.com/2019/07/30/well/live/menopause-sex-decline-partner-husband-wife.html

Quinn-Nilas, C., Benson, L., Milhausen, R. R., Buchholz, A. C., & Goncalves, M. (2016). The relationship between body image and domains of sexual functioning among heterosexual, emerging adult women. *Sexual Medicine, 4*(3), e182–e189. https://doi.org/10.1016/j.esxm.2016.02.004

Rhode, J. (2018, May 1). *LGBTQ seniors face unique challenges.* Georgia Voice. https://thegavoice.com/community/features/lgbtq-seniors-face-unique-challenges/

Rienzo, B. A. (1985). The impact of aging on human sexuality. *Journal of School Health, 55*, 66–68. https://doi.org/10.1111/j.1746-1561.1985.tb04081.x

Rogers, P. (2019, October 23). Sex and aging. *Healthline.* https://www.healthline.com/health/healthy-sex-and-aging#takeaway

Snyder, R. J., & Zweig, R. A. (2010). Medical and psychology students' knowledge and attitudes regarding aging and sexuality. *Gerontology & Geriatrics Education, 31*, 235–255. https://doi.org/10.1080/02701960.2010.503132

United States Census Bureau. (2019, December 19). *2020 Census will help policymakers prepare for the incoming wave of aging boomers.* https://www.census.gov/library/stories/2019/12/by-2030-all-baby-boomers-will-be-age-65-orolder.html

Urology Care Foundation. (2018). *What is erectile dysfunction?* https://www.urologyhealth.org/urology-a-z/e/erectile-dysfunction-(ed)

Velez, A. (2020, May 18). Menopause is different for women of color. *Endocrine Web.* https://www.endocrineweb.com/menopause-different-women-color#:~:text=the%20research%20in%20SWAN%20shows,transition%20than%20white%20women%20do

Verrastro, V., Saladino,V., Petruccelli, F., & Eleuteri, S. (2020). Medical and health care professionals' sexuality education: State of the art and recommendations. *International Journal of Environmental Research and Public Health, 17*(7), 2186. https://doi.org/10.3390/ijerph17072186

Villines, Z. (2017, December 16). What you should know about retrograde ejaculation. *Medical News Today.* https://www.medicalnewstoday.com/articles/320332

Walz, T. (2002). Crones, dirty old men, sexy seniors: Representations of the sexuality of the older persons. *Journal of Aging and Identity, 7*(2), 99–112.

Weiss, G., Noorhasan, D., Schott, L. L., Powell, L., Randolph, Jr., J. F., & Johnston, J. M. (2009). Racial differences in women who have a hysterectomy for benign conditions. *Women's Health Issues, 19*(3), 202–210. https://www.ncbi.nlm.nih.gov/pmc/articles/PMC3786579/

Whiteman, H. (2015, January 11). Almost 1 in 5 hysterectomies are 'unnecessary', study finds. *Medical News Today.* https://www.medicalnewstoday.com/articles/287736

Witten, T. (2013). It's not all darkness: Robustness, resilience, and successful transgender aging. *LGBT Health, 1*(1), 24–33. https://doi.org/10.1089/lgbt.2013.0017

World Health Organization. (n.d.). *Female life expectancy.* https://www.who.int/gho/women_and_health/mortality/life_expectancy_text/en/#:~:text=Women%20generally%20live%20longer%20than,differences%20between%20men%20and%20women

10

Spirituality, Sexual Health, and EMDR Therapy

Jeanne C. Folks, DMin, LPC

LEARNING OBJECTIVES

- EMDR clinicians will recognize the importance of a client's personal spirituality and spiritual history in EMDR treatment.
- EMDR clinicians will master spiritual resource history taking.
- EMDR clinicians will understand the intersection of a client's spiritual and sexual wounds within the Adaptative Information Processing (AIP) model.
- EMDR clinicians will implement the use of unique client spiritual resources before, during, and after EMDR processing.

INTRODUCTION

Sex and spirituality can each create a sense of *belonging* or profound isolation. We can experience arriving, at long last, home, or feeling abandoned, adrift, lost, and unloved. Each has power to which the human mind, heart, and spirit are available and uniquely vulnerable. We can be elevated or wounded. A sexual experience can be deeply spiritual. A spiritual experience can be profoundly elemental, earthy, and sensory. Sexuality cannot be divorced from our spirituality either in potential glory or in potential destructive power. We carry wounds of direct assault to body and spirit. We also carry wounds created by the attempts of predation to force separation of our human and divine natures. We carry wounds of body and soul inextricably intertwined. This chapter explores the intersection of spiritualty and sexuality, woundedness within this intersection, and treatment of these wounds with eye movement desensitization and reprocessing (EMDR).

My Experience: Dichotomy of Spirituality and Humanity

In my early twenties, I migrated to the Episcopal church, from the rigid, judgmental Protestantism of my childhood. At that time, more than 40 years ago, women had only very recently been given the freedom to be ordained. During my years in seminary, like many students, I worked a number of jobs. I waitressed. I also worked as an artist's model, posing in art classes at a sister college. An older member of a women's prayer group I attended got wind of this and called the priest who was my sponsor for ordination. He gave me a choice. I could stop modeling immediately or he would stop sponsoring me.

I did not know it at the time, but that was the start of my withdrawal from the institutional church. I acceded to my sponsor's demand despite my confusion and disagreement. I could not understand why it was spiritually acceptable to work in a loud crowded bar and restaurant in a cheesy costume with men physically grabbing and verbally taunting me, but it was sinful for me to pose semi-nude in a room of serious art students where I was treated with exquisite respect. I further disconnected myself as a spiritual being from my earthly humanness. I lived in the ether, in chronic, low-grade dissociation as a way of being/not being.

There followed scores of reinforcing experiences, be it elderly ladies on retreat who told me I was "too pretty to become a priest" or a bishop breathing heavily and looming over me in private interviews. The message was reconfirmed and clear. Living in a physical body was highly problematic, especially for a young woman who loved the God she personally experienced. I was always, one way or another, being told to choose. I could be spiritual, or I could be sensual. I could not be both.

Seven years elapsed before the institutional church and I finally parted ways. I remained in a state of separation between body and soul for much longer. A lot of therapy, a 10-year battle with bulimia, more and better therapy and my own resolve to find True North helped me knit my being back together into a more cohesive, sensuous, and deeply spiritual being.

I know I am not alone. Although spiritual and sexual frames can be challenged in myriad ways, the resulting confusion, disorganization and injury are sadly, remarkably similar.

As the licensed professional counselor I am today, I am left with an urgent question that I will try to address in useful ways in this chapter: How do we as therapists help our clients knit their bodies and souls back together? How do we help them explore and heal, not just with delicacy and grace, but with earth and fire?

THE SENSUAL AND THE SACRED: THE INTERSECTION OF SEXUAL AND SPIRITUAL EXPERIENCE

We will explore five major spiritual themes, examining the journeys of five individuals.

1. **Longing for ecstasy:** Yet never satisfied. Seeking spiritual relatedness through sexual climax (Sophie).
2. **Guilt, fear and shame:** An over-externalized sense of God/Divine that creates a distracting, sexually repressive and often contentious noncorporeal relationship with self and others (Amanda).
3. **Free will, abdication, and embodiment:** An over-internalized sense of the Divine as a hiding place. Difficulty maintaining interest in sex when living a non-corporeal life. Addictive spiritual practice as a means of withdrawing from the world (Priya).
4. **Surrender and control:** Dominance and submission. The belief that God requires control of self and others. The only access to sexual release and spiritual connection is through pain (Sandy).
5. **Sacrifice, safety, and belonging:** Feeling wanted and cherished. A compromised internal sense of God and forced externalization—neither working. Impotence is one result (Hank).

The through-line for these themes is a sense of *relationality*. It is often more straightforward to see the relational components of sexuality. It is, in some ways, more difficult to see this in a person's spiritual life. The person who is avoiding God, hiding in God, angry at God, afraid of God, longing for God is in a profoundly relational experience (Clinton & Straub, 2014). We as therapists can miss the dysregulation of a client's spiritual relationship. If so, then we will almost certainly miss the dovetailing of that relationship with their sexual and interpersonal capacities (Pearlman & Saakvitne, 1995, pp. 55–73). As we will see, it is not always possible to heal one without reckoning the other.

These themes are far from exhaustive. Nevertheless, they feature frequent spiritual wounds and adaptive compromises that directly impact sexual practices and capacities. Knipe (2019) addresses the Adaptive Information Processes (AIP) model in relationship to psychological defenses (pp. 51–74). There are also overlapping themes in some of the case studies. Unrequited longings and the need for safety are through-lines, along with relationality, running throughout.

First, in addition to skills discussing sexual matters, we must have access to a client's spiritual vocabulary and to be able to elicit their spiritual story.

The Client's Language of Spirituality

For most of us, our training regarding history taking did not include inquiry of a client's spiritual beliefs, wounds, or resources. For years, my new client questionnaire included "religious affiliation." Sometimes that would be filled in with "Presbyterian," "Jewish," "Lapsed Something," "None," or it was left blank. I might inquire about the "lapsed," maybe ask if the client was active in their specified faith community. They would say yes or no. Often they would make some vague statement about, "I was raised Catholic, Universalist, etc., but I am not really into that anymore." That box would then be ticked in my mind and I would move on to social history, family of origin, inquire about medical history, medications, use of substances, and so on.

How much was lost/missed in those early initial consultations I will never know. I came to understand that asking about institutionalized belief systems is a fraction of the information available in most clients. Still, there is information even there. Noticing the energy with which a client answers the religious affiliation question can sometimes tip the therapist off to positive associations or dismissive defensiveness.

Spiritual typography is vast and complex. I learned to ask more and broader questions, questions that are far less confined and "pre-associated" with the past. To enter into dialogue around these issues with our clients, we must first have a shared lexicon (David et al., 2013).

How to Identify a Client's Broader and More Personal Spiritual Resources (or Their Absence)

Open-ended questions that can cast a wide net:

> Do you have any beliefs or a philosophy of life that serves you?
> How do you make major life-changing decisions?
> When the chips are down, what, if anything, do you turn to?
> Where do you go for sustenance when you feel the need to be renewed?
> What gives your life meaning? What gives you hope or a sense of purpose?

Some clients will be able to answer at least one of these questions with some ease and insight. Others may look at the therapist with skepticism, irritation, and/or confusion. This is all information. Questions such as these can identify depression, repression or potential dissociation when responses are consistently, "I don't know." "There's nothing to turn to. That's why I'm here." "Why are you asking me all these ridiculous questions? If I had the answers, I wouldn't need to be here."

If you are getting responses such as these, you are in a different kind of conversation, a conversation about injury, aloneness, isolation, and potential abandonment. Keep in mind that these too are deeply spiritual experiences although they may remain labeled in more "spiritually neutral" terms of pain, fear, anger, and resentment for some now, or permanently, in treatment.

Finding the ways in which a client formulates their personal belief system greatly helps the information gathering process. Some clients will shut this process of spiritual information gathering down a minute after it begins. This may be

Chapter 10 Spirituality, Sexual Health, and EMDR Therapy

because they do not conceptualize in spiritual terms or they just do not want to go there for a host of reasons that may show up later in treatment. Others will warm to open ended questions. Talk about talking about it. Ask, "How do you imagine it might feel if we talked in more detail about your spiritual beliefs, feelings, or practices?" "These can feel very private, very personal, and/or very complicated."

Keep in mind that, regardless of labels, these conceptualizations are indicators of *spiritual appropriation*. You will discover the way a client is able to take in comfort, support, access intuition, and inner knowing, and have a sense of connection to something larger than themselves.

What follows are potential questions and concepts that may help you in your spiritual resource interviewing with clients. It is really not that different from interviewing for sexual information. Ask open-ended questions first. Then, depending on the answers given, ask for more clarification. As therapists, we are good at following bread crumb trails.

Spiritual Language
"Do you have preferred words for your spiritual resource(s)?" With this question the therapist can begin to learn the client's spiritual language. It can help the therapist avoid the pitfalls of pronouns and unhelpful labels. Is the client comfortable with he/her/they, father/mother, grandfather/grandmother? Are there words or phrases that work better to avoid gender or role identification such as the Divine, the Sacred, the Wholly Other or Higher Power? All of Nature, Sacred Wind, the Heart of the Earth, or the Universe?

I am offering just a few examples here. Be curious. Keep asking yourself, out of nearly endless possibilities, why are a client's chosen words important to them? On rare occasion, a client will not want to speak their name for the Divine. This may be due to a religious prohibition, or it may be a client's personal fear of taint or intrusion by another. See if there is an alternate term that could be agreed upon, perhaps "spiritual resource." If the client has room, consider also asking about experiences of emotional robbery, where knowledge of what was treasured was used against them. That information can almost certainly lead to EMDR targets.

Spiritual Images
"Do you have a mental picture of your resource(s)?" This question can enlarge the conversation about language. Some clients have very concrete images, e.g., Jesus, Mary, Buddha, Wise One. These images can be welcoming, comforting, and forgiving. They can be a potential future resource for cognitive interweaves, which will be discussed further in this chapter.

Conversely, therapists need to be sensitive to the client's sacred image(s) potentially shifting out of the positive supportive role. Before or during EMDR processing, such images can express disapproval or judgment to a client, depending on the client's projections and transferences (Davies & Frawley, 1994). This does not necessarily negate the image as useful in the positive role of a resource. It does, however, potentially indicate an EMDR target. "When I have this particular thought, or engage in this particular behavior, I see Mary's face frowning." In this case, a negative cognition (NC) could be "I'm bad in Mary's sight."

Images can also be metaphorical and often come from the natural world: Wisdom Trees, Power Animals, the constancy of ocean waves or a representative image of the Universe, e.g., an infinite starry sky. Asking a client what they notice in their body when they call up the image will provide more information about the nature of the comfort and spiritual help they access.

Energy and the Senses
"How do you experience your resource?" "Does it radiate anything?" "Does it emit a vibration, a sound, a fragrance?" "Do you connect to your resource through sensation?" Some clients are less visual in their resources and more visceral. The noted meditation teacher Stephen Levine (2015) often talked about "Just the 'Ugh' in the core of our being." "That place in us that is uninjured and uninjurable." Sometimes it is a combination. "When you picture your resource are there sensations of warmth, lightness, or greater groundedness?" Is it more an experience of pure sensation? Being rocked, enveloped in safety or loving intention? Simply feeling connected to something more than oneself? Cataloging this information could be a big help in coming discussions of safe/calm place, fodder for interweaves and between session resources which will be discussed shortly.

Practices
"Are there practices or rituals that help you connect to your resource?" "Are there actions or activities that you engage in to access or deepen connection to your spiritual resources?" Just a few examples a client might share could be burning incense, playing certain music, movement or dance, creating an altar and/or dedicated space, the designation of specific times of day for prayer, reflection, or meditation. As the therapeutic relationship evolves, you may sufficiently understand the framework of your client's spirituality to gently offer suggestions, for example, "Would creating a dedicated space for meditation in your house be helpful?" At the beginning, however, remember you are gathering information from the client about their spiritual truth. You do not want to intrude, even with good intentions.

Spiritual Community (Then and Now)
"Is community or participation in a formal religion part of your spiritual life?" "Was it as a child?" "Did/does community help or complicate things, or both?" Relationships to spiritual communities can be robustly nurturing or very confusing. Sometimes, they are trauma inducing or trauma replicating. It is important to tread lightly here. When clients reply "It's complicated," it probably is. There may be anything from a general ambivalence to a trap door that, when sprung by the right trigger, will drop the client into enormous woundedness. The best guideline is the more the client prevaricates, the less the therapist pushes. Be patient. The EMDR targets will show up.

Spiritual/Sexual Wounds Are Potential EMDR Targets

Ask permission for exploration including of what is considered wrong or forbidden. Remember what was mentioned earlier about "talking about talking about it." For the sake of clarity, I have divided these spiritual wounds into five broad categories.

Institutional Wounds

Many of our clients grew up with some form of spiritual/religious instruction. Children have a large capacity for spiritual belief and trust (Richo, 2011, pp. 14–16). When spiritual beliefs are betrayed by abusive or inconsistent behavior by adults in relation to those beliefs, the trauma can be significant. For example, a child could be raised in a tradition that has a prohibition against divorce and then the child's parents do divorce. In Case Study 10.5 Hank gets deeply caught in just such a quagmire.

Spiritual institutions have the potential for serious abuses of power. There can be direct physical and/or sexual abuse by clergy or religious teachers (Walker et al., 2014, pp. 148–149, 179–181). This can be coupled with emotional abuse that takes advantage of the longing to belong to the community and a profound need to stay "in the good graces" of the Divine. The child may feel compelled to subsume their will to religious beliefs or religious leaders to protect themselves from physical dangers and/or cognitive dissonance. The enormity of confusion, disenfranchisement, and pain into adulthood can be incalculable.

Parental Wounds

The fusion of God and the punishing and/or rewarding parent can both seriously compromise the adult ability to appropriate a healthy, mature personal spirituality, and disrupt their interpersonal relationships, including sexuality—*doing the same thing with God that they experience with people*. Consider looking through this relational lens in formulating your EMDR plan. We will have an opportunity to do that in Case Study 10.1 of Sophie.

> *Our longing for love in relationships is for a secure attachment. In a secure attachment we neither cling nor run; we trust ourselves to welcome closeness without feeling engulfed, and to allow distancing without feeling abandoned. Then we maintain boundaries in our relationships, but they are not barriers to intimacy. (Richo, 2017, p. 53)*

Wounds of Abandonment

When the client views the Divine as all-knowing and all-powerful, painful questions can be carried obsessively. Common examples are "Where was God?" "Why didn't He/She/They save me?" In Case Study 10.3 of Priya, we will also have an opportunity to explore the converse of this, as she experiences the absence of the Divine in the world, only to be found in a secret place within.

Unlovability: Flaws, Made Wrong

The sense of being abandoned by the Divine can be turned against the self. "God has turned his back on me because I'm bad." "I couldn't fix things/make it stop. I was unworthy of help." "There's something fundamentally wrong with me. God would have saved a good person." With Amanda's Case Study (10.2), we will have the chance to investigate this type of combined spiritual and sexual struggle in detail.

Chosen to Suffer

One way people attempt to resolve the psychological and spiritual dilemmas of unlovability is to take on a rarified spiritual role in which sacrifice equals expression of love and devotion for the Divine. In this, there is no love without sacrifice. Difficulties with letting go of rarefied, spiritually elitist states/roles can feature prominently in EMDR treatment. Perceived spiritual messages from the Divine can be highly entrenched and can manifest as abdication of personal power. Conversely, perceived "otherness"—special knowing—being "chosen" can be fuel for narcissistic grandiosity (Knipe, 2019, p. 65). Sandy's Case Study (10.4) will prove an interesting expression of this theme, with a sexual kink as her road to spiritual reconnection.

EMDR APPLICATIONS

Safe Place—Protected Place—Comfortable Place—Peaceful Place—Calm Place

Building safe places has potential room for the addition of spiritual resources. Several cautions apply here. The correlation of spiritual resources and safety must come exclusively from the client. Do not give them *your* comfortable place. Comforting spiritual images are not generic and are not automatically transferable. Also, be aware that you may have learned, in your spiritual history taking, good reasons to leave spiritual resources out of calm place building. If your client has, for example ,unresolved anger or sense of injury in relation to their sense of the Divine, then that more likely qualifies as an EMDR target rather than a source of comfort.

Some examples of positive/useful calm place expressed by clients might include images of meeting a spiritual figure in a garden, being embraced by a spiritual figure, or a non-visual, comforting sensory response. This could include a sense of being warmed in Divine light or the intake of a Sacred Breath. Use the specific language you obtained in your spiritual resources interview to ask open ended questions, for example, "Is there a way (or someplace) you would like to meet (or spend time with) Jesus, your Spirit Animal, in Divine Light, and so on"

Install these images with bilateral stimulation (BLS), encouraging client observation of physical sensations and states of mind.

Integrating Spiritual Resources Between EMDR Sessions

Encouraging clients from the beginning of treatment to use their spiritual resources, if untainted, between sessions can be meaningful and helpful. Prayer, meditation, spiritual reflection, and/or reading of spiritual texts can increase a client's sense of meaning, purpose, and Divine participation in their healing journeys. As EMDR Therapy progresses, the recovery of lost or damaged spiritual practices can be both a support in the work and a benchmark of recovery. Exploring new, untried practices can be enlightening and strengthening (Boorstein et al., 2011, pp. 63–83).

Discussions between EMDR sessions with clients regarding referencing feelings and positive cognitions of spiritual/sensual connection experienced during EMDR processing can help build resources. Can the client put a "bookmark" in new feelings connected to "God does not hate me. I am his beloved child," "Sex is another way to feel the Divine close to me," or "The Living Air whispers her love to me as I walk in the woods"? Can they then call that feeling up daily, between sessions, and observe emotions, sensations, and self-beliefs?

Gratitude as a spiritual practice is a powerful, restorative tool (Neff & Germer, 2018, pp. 161–162, 164–165). The investigation of one's spiritual and sensual being brings with it, potentially, a sense of limitlessness—of oneness with creation and increasing well-being, stability, and safety. When clients have room to identify their blessings, encouraging them to do so mindfully can deepen the benefits of their gratitude. It can antidote despair. This is also true of feelings of loving partnership with the Divine and belonging (Kujawa-Holbrook, 2013, pp. 136–156).

Exploratory Questions

As with us all, clients can feel confusion about their own longings. The use of BLS without a protocol set up can be enormously useful in identifying and clarifying a client's deeper truth. For example, the client who says, "I wish I knew what I really want." Consider adding BLS while considering phrases such as, "I want more _____ in my life." "I'm open to knowing what more would feel like; what am I missing?" "What question am I trying to answer inside of me?"

With the addition of BLS there can be a cascade effect. When we begin to have an inkling about our longings it can open the door to knowing with more and more clarity. This can open a new channel of access for exploration. It is a foot in the door. "I long for _____." "I will feel more complete if I can experience_____."

The spiritual teacher, Oriah Mountain Dreamer (2007) references hearing the poet, David Whyte, suggest the following exercise. "It really does not matter if I ever get _____. What I really want is _____." With the addition of BLS, you will see this used to good effect with Sophie's Case Study.

Examples of Negative Cognitions

"I can never experience _____ because I _____." "If I enjoy sex too much, I'll lose my connection to God." "Sex is wrong." "God hates me." An instructive discussion of the links between trauma and damage to spiritualty can be found in Walker et al. (2014, pp. 148–150).

Cognitive Interweaves

Cognitive Interweaves are the friend of the spiritual investigation. Inquiry into the relationship between the client and their sense of their Higher Power during EMDR processing can keep the work moving forward. Interweaves introduce new information and vantage points that assist in shifting the trauma-laden neuropathways. An extensive categorized list of Interweaves and their usage has been compiled by other EMDR clinicians (Laliotis & Korn, 2020).

Spiritually focused Interweaves can help the client experience being understood and known, address issues of anger and justice, experience forgiveness and cleansing, and integrate past experiences into the present and future. Interweaves can support freedom to express despair, the sensory experience of reframed aloneness, and mine for additional supports and resources. They can help the client enlarge and expand their core beliefs.

The open-ended invitation to reflect can be so useful; for example, "How do you think God feels about this now?" "Where's the love connection?" "You see your Higher Power as omniscience and omnipresence—all seeing, all knowing. Does that make a difference?" "Things seem really stuck right now. What could happen if you asked Jesus to, 'Help me, help me, help me'?"

Use of Metaphors and Religious Imagery

Forms of the divine presence—Angels, Divine Light, Jesus, Mary, saints, the Buddha, prophets or sages—can help vivify spiritual dilemmas and generate resources (Leeds, 2009, p. 186). Metaphors such as abusers in remedial spiritual education or perpetrators taught to be good and own the pain they caused, can be helpful, especially if that perpetrator is now deceased. Seeing perpetrators as confused or injured children themselves can assist in understanding generational trauma that would benefit from spiritual Grace.

Examples of Positive Cognitions

As every experienced EMDR therapist knows, the identified positive cognition with which EMDR begins can change or significantly refine by the time desensitization and reprocessing are completed. Try not to let the client settle for "pretty good." Your client will feel (and you will most likely notice) when they drop into a deep peace that is core. The positive cognition will feel resonant and perfect. Here are some examples of where a client could end up, even if not stated by the client at the beginning of the protocol set up: "I can celebrate that I'm both a sexual and a spiritual being." "I open to a relationship filled with fire, not fear." "I can have an erection with confidence and joy." "God rejoices in all parts of me." "Celebrating all of my humanity honors God." As EMDR therapists also know, if the positive cognition (PC) is not forthcoming, there are often more targets to go.

Examples of EMDR Future Templates

The longer I work with EMDR the more I value EMDR Future Templates. This is the point at which adaptive reformulations solidify (Shapiro, 2018, pp. 204–207). Future templates allow the client to envision and practice their new conceptualizations in action. Please give Future Templates the time and attention your clients need. Much discussion is available in the EMDR literature about this crucial part of EMDR treatment (Leeds, 2009, pp. 197–202). Some possible examples for our purposes here:

> Enjoying sex with abandon.
> Engaging in sexual activity without fear or apology.
> Having sexual feelings during spiritual practices and feeling integrated.
> Enjoying feelings of spiritual transcendence during sex.
> Feeling acceptance and approval from a Higher Power for being fully human.
> Being in a more integrated relationship between God and humanity.

THERAPIST SELF-AWARENESS AND BUILDING TRUST

Eckhart Tolle asks the question, "Can I be the space for this?" (Tolle, 2008). In the case of either spirituality or sexuality, you, the therapist, might have work of your own to do in order to feel comfortable raising these issues. Having a mutually agreed lexicon for spirituality with your client can make it easier to also address sexuality and find that lexicon as well. (Further guidance can be found in Chapter 3 regarding discussions of sexual issues with your clients.) Obtain whatever clinical support or consultation you need to raise and explore issues of sexuality without eroticizing the therapy relationship. Pearlman and Saakvitne (1995) offer a useful discussion of erotic or sexual responses in the therapeutic relationship (pp. 208–211). Just as the therapist handles their own sexual arousal while allowing the client to graphically explore, the therapist holds the sacred space while the client explores their spiritual dilemmas. It is important to stay mindful and to recognize what is yours and what is the client's. In either case, try to avoid self-condemnation for your own humanity and seek consultation when necessary (Davies & Frawley, 1994).

If you have your own dearly held spiritual beliefs, keeping track of the counter-transferential need to "protect" the Divine is crucial. If I, as both a therapist and a spiritually aware being, have a sense of the Divine as something much larger than myself, then does God really need me to protect His/Her/Their reputation or image? This may not work for you, but what I tell myself when I feel the urge to say to a client, "Oh no! God loves everybody" is that "God is tough. He can take it." Clients can rage, assault, and/or blame God for past injuries and heartbreak. They can conversely adore, idealize, and/or abdicate their power to a Higher Authority. Just as we do not want to either referee or take sides in a client's family squabbles, let us not participate in these spiritual conflicts either.

Clients can use sacred text as indictment or support. If you have knowledge of a client's preferred spiritual texts, try to avoid getting "showy," "knowy," or "teachy." You will be playing "dueling scriptures" before you know it. When a client quotes religious text and then says something like, "This means I'm going to hell," it can be so tempting to say, "I really don't think it means that." Better, "I'd never thought of that interpretation. Tell me more." Consider asking, "How do you think God feels about this?"

On the other hand, a nonbeliever (or different believer) therapist may experience a counter-transferential wish to debunk a client's belief. This can be particularly true if the client's belief strikes the therapist as naïve, superstitious, or fantastical. Resist. You and your client are going to need that information and how it is held by the client for the EMDR therapy to come. I have seen a client's theology mature or evolve during the course of treatment. I have also seen it enlarge in their awareness as it has always been held by them. In either case, just as with their sexuality, it is theirs and theirs alone. Consider reflecting on the question, "Can I do this work with clients without developing a spiritual attunement?"

It is worth repeating that the therapist must contain both humor and enthusiasm as the client explores and takes risks. Be careful with humor that can touch the client's fear of mockery or humiliation. Be careful of enthusiasm that can be experienced as pressure. Again, talk about talking about it.

Chapter 10　Spirituality, Sexual Health, and EMDR Therapy　279

CASE STUDIES

Case Study 10.1: Sophie: Longing for Ecstasy, Even at the Price of Adult Intimacy

Ecstasy is a transcendent experience of limitless joy, wonder, and exquisite sensation eagerly sought, yet elusive in human experience. Much has been written about unbridled, expansive spiritual experiences and ultimate sexual encounters. One of the leaders in the field of mind-body-spirit medicine, Deepak Chopra (2006), writes, "Ecstasy is a primordial energy state. To experience ecstasy, we must satisfy our physical, sensual, mythical, and spiritual needs. In the return of ecstasy, we can say with Solomon, 'I have become like Paradise'" (p. 159). With Sophie, we will see her depth of longing for a spiritual experience on a collision course with her sex life. In her quest for ecstasy she objectified her partners. She was never satisfied. Ultimately, she was lost on every front.

Sophie, a 33-year-old ciswoman artist, came into therapy seeking help with her sexual relationships, reporting them as "good, but never fully satisfying." She reported, "I just don't know what's wrong. I have mind-blowing sex, but then I feel disappointed soon after. My partners leave because they don't feel like they make me happy."

On the intake questionnaire, to the open question, "As far as I'm concerned, God is _____," she stated, "limitless." She described her parents as "nonjudgmental and supportive," but also "remarkably lacking in curiosity and rather dull." Her childhood was physically safe but greatly lacking in joy, adventure, or intellectual stimulation. Sophie became a dreamer and, if there were stimulating teachers with exciting lessons at school, she was no longer present enough to notice. The one exception was art. Painting helped her feel expansive and expressive, although not more personally interactive.

When Sophie became sexually active in her late teens she discovered that during orgasm she experienced a transcendent freedom that felt liberating. "It felt like what I'd been looking for my whole life." "It feels like, for a moment, I am one with the Universe. I guess I might call it God." As the work unfolded, it also became clear that Sophie found people to be boring and sexual ecstasy short lived.

Not unlike a runner's high, Sophie experienced and loved the biochemical release experienced during sexual climax. For additional reading, Safron (2016) offers a well-researched discussion of both the neurophenomenology of sexual trance and the neurophenomenology of orgasm (p. 5). Elevating dopamine and flooding the system with endorphins to induce ecstatic trance states is practiced in many religious traditions (Chopra, 2006, pp. 125–126, 156–159). This can be accomplished through dance, ascetical practices, and the use of hallucinogens, as well as sexual practices combined with meditation as in the Tantric tradition. For Sophie, however, her experience of ecstasy/spiritual transcendence lasted only as long as her multiple orgasms and did not translate to a more pervasive spiritual awareness or a deepening of interpersonal intimacy. Nevertheless, her longing for transcendence was abiding. It was about this that she realized she was curious.

The Canadian meditation teacher, Oriah Mountain Dreamer, eloquently addresses the topic of longing: "That in longing, there is intent, a seeking." Much of what Sophie had been experiencing is what Dreamer would identify as craving "which holds dissatisfaction with what we have right now and the inability to be at peace with it." "Craving is always tinged with fear," the fear of not enough, of never feeling full or fulfilled. Longing is often buried beneath craving. It is a wanting for things to be different. It asks the question, 'How do I want to live?" rather than, "What do I want to have?," even if that is ecstatic experiences (Dreamer, 2007).

Sophie was willing to work with an exercise, referenced by Dreamer (2007), developed by the Irish American poet, David Whyte with the addition of bilateral stimulation (BLS). Whyte invites people to examine the statements, "It does not interest me if I ever have _____. What I really long for is _____." This exploration, deepened with BLS, was challenging at first, but Sophie was intrigued with entertaining the thought, "It doesn't interest me if I ever have another orgasm." It took time, however, until she was able to formulate her response, "What I really long for is a feeling of limitless connection."

Of course, Sophie wants and deserves sexual climax. Nevertheless, orgasms were not getting her where she wanted to go in a comprehensive, integrated way. She was dismissive of people and disinterested in complex, interpersonal intimacy. She did not feel a cohesive connection to the Divine. Longings remained under the surface of her sexual experiences. She was able to see this and was willing to continue her exploration through EMDR therapy.

With the negative cognition, "People are not worth my time. I'm better off on my own," Sophie felt the sensation of her heart aching and feeling restricted. This led to a memory of her birthday party at age 10. "There was a cake and presents, mostly clothes. Three girls from my class were invited. I don't know how they were chosen. There were no games planned. It was so dull, my heart hurt then. I can feel it hurting now, a squeezing in my chest."

Through desensitization, Sophie discharged much of her heartache. She could see the fatigue in her high school–educated father who worked two, often three jobs. She could see low-grade chronic depression in her mother. Sadness loosened the ache in her heart and she could weep for her parents and their "dull" struggle.

During Reprocessing, Sophie was able to look more closely at their faces as they viewed her work that hung at a recent art show. She could see, through their tired eyes, pride in her creativity, and she reached the positive cognitions of, "I know they loved me. They did the best they could. They gave me all they had."

Using exploratory questions coupled with BLS, it became more and more clear that what she was experiencing was primarily a spiritual crisis. She had concluded that orgasm was her exclusive tool for a feeling of ecstatic expansiveness. She would energetically "leave" her sexual partners to "fly free." Yet, in so doing, she missed the deeper intimacy of a shared experience with another person. Her sexual partners were a means to an end for her. Her partners would leave when they saw this, and it became clear that she had little interest in the ordinary matters of shared daily life.

Sophie became open to the possibility that *more* connection with her sexual partner would result in *less* boredom. With BLS guiding the exploratory question, "How will I know I'm more in touch with myself?" Sophie had the responses: "As I continue my journey of discovery I welcome partnership" and "I'll look in people's eyes as they look at my paintings and like what I see."

With the BLS-guided question, "How will I know I'm more in touch with another person?" Sophie responded with, "I will have orgasms and let it be a shared experience with my partner." "I will feel my ecstasy increase rather than feeling limited." Work with Future Templates significantly strengthened this.

Sophie's shifted understanding of her parents' love and devotion to her are helping her feel safe to be fully human. She is coming to believe being human and interconnected is good and that the Divine wants that for her. She increasingly feels that transcendent sexual experiences do not have to separate us; rather, they can facilitate connection both to the Divine and to each other. Pema Chödrön, an American Tibetan Buddhist nun, puts it well, "To the degree that we look clearly and compassionately at ourselves, we feel confident and fearless about looking into someone else's eyes" (Chödrön, 2016, p. 76).

Case Study 10.2: Amanda: Guilt, Fear, Shame—the Unforgivable—Sexual Repression

Contemporary theologian and teacher of Centering Prayer, Cynthia Bourgeault (2016) reflects on the "sorrow of being" through examination of the anonymous fourteenth century mystic, author of *The Cloud of Unknowing*, who states, ". . . what we are really dealing with is a fourteenth-century forerunner of what today would be called the phenomenology of consciousness—and specifically consciousness at the key transition point where it shifts from brain-centered to heart-centered cognition" (p. 198).

Detached from her body and with a sense of God totally externalized, Amanda demonstrates not agnosticism, but rather, a relationship with God in conflict. A fateful decision in her youth left her shut down and cut off from her sensuous self and any inner sense of the Divine as resource.

Amanda, a 34-year-old ciswoman, grew up with parents who loved her but also held her, and themselves, to intense and specific standards of moral rectitude. Being good equaled following rules that earned God's favor. God was perceived as easily disappointed and brought to grief and alienated by human frailty and failure (Walker et al., 2014, pp. 237–238).

During her late teen and college years, Amanda rebelled against the pressures of these rigid standards through abuse of alcohol and promiscuity. In her junior year of college, Amanda's roommate, Belinda, died of alcohol poisoning after attending a frat party Amanda had persuaded her to attend.

Amanda broke off communication with her family, dropped out of school, and lived a nomadic, alcohol-fueled lifestyle for the next few years. In her early thirties, Amanda wound up working for an aging couple on their small farm. The couple ran a nondenominational, conservative Christian home church and saw Amanda as a spiritual project they felt called to undertake.

With the influence of her deeply religious employers, who had given her work when no one else would, Amanda achieved sobriety and started attending the couple's home church meetings. The familiarity of love and rigid theology drew Amanda in. She struggled more and more with a combination of guilt over her choices in college and emerging sexual urges that alcohol had suppressed. She committed to a celibate lifestyle and engaged in rigorous spiritual practices of fasting multiple days per month, praying on her knees for 2 hours daily and allowing herself only 5 hours of sleep per night under one thin blanket regardless of the temperature. All this was in service of her repentance and "road back to God."

Amanda came into treatment after her elderly employers sold their farm, the husband went into a nursing facility, and the home church disbanded.

Her presenting concern was that she would "go to hell for sure if she began drinking or became sexually active again." Sexual activity was the strongest of the two concerns. "I'm a sexual deviant. I need help getting my sexual feelings under control." "I have to put them in their place." She saw nothing wrong with her ascetical practices. Her concern was that "they're not working." She was overwhelmed with guilt, fear, and longing.

Perceiving the Divine as completely separate from inner experience presents unique challenges to treatment (Clinton & Straub, 2014). In EMDR therapy the task is to reference the adult self as resource (Knipe, 2019, pp. 27–43). In Amanda's case, her adult was preoccupied with God's "otherness" as well as God being, in her experience, in the parental role of "hater of all that's sensuous and free." Amanda experienced God as the deeply aggrieved and chronically alienated parent. She correlated proof of devotion with sensations of potential connection through self-inflicted physical pain and ordeals in a bid for Divine approval and acceptance.

Corporal discipline in religious traditions can take many forms. Sleep deprivation and vigils, fasting, flogging, hair shirts, heat/cold exposure, and stress positions such as prolonged kneeling are just a few examples. These practices can be expressions of devotion and/or avenues to altered states of consciousness (Walker et al., 2014, pp. 89–90). They can also, paradoxically, be used to repress, deny, detract from, or circumvent body sensations and emotional awareness. Both or either are paths of passionate expression and human experience.

For Amanda, it was the latter. Her acts of spiritual rigor were aids to shutting down access to her painful inner experiences of guilt and shame (Neff & Germer, 2018, pp. 121–128) rather than engaging in acts of sacrifice intended as expressions of love and devotion for the Divine. She was caught in the belief not just that she had "done bad" but that she was bad. She lived under the shame-driven threat of rejection, exile, and unending isolation if she gave in to "unholy" desires.

Fear of exile leads many to deny their truth and obliterate "unauthorized" longings in order to maintain often tenuous and/or abusive connection with God and with people. Healthy connection does not extract a price, most certainly not in terms of power and control over another. Sexual and spiritual rebellion are often attempts to break away from toxic control while greatly risking the need to belong.

Amanda's negative cognitions included, "I'm a sexual deviant." "I am bad." "I deserve to be punished." "God is disgusted with me." "There is no connection without sacrifice." and "It's my fault Belinda is dead."

Given these potential negative cognitions, there was a temptation to go immediately with a goal of rehabilitating Amanda's relationship with God. In truth, however, this was a case of intense traumatic bereavement

(Pearlman et al., 2014, pp. 69–90). It was crucial for Amanda to cultivate an observing ego capable of mercy, a potent spiritual value.

Working with the negative cognition of "It's my fault Belinda is dead" allowed Amanda to grieve the depth of her regret over her roommate's death. Amanda was able to view the young woman she had once been, longing to love God with freedom rather than through a gauntlet of rules, and to forgive herself for wanting freedom from rigidity. She came to a positive cognition of "Belinda and I were both young. We both made choices. I can honor her life and my own." Amanda took comfort in an early version of Niebuhr's Serenity Prayer, "O God, give us the serenity to accept what cannot be changed, the courage to change what can be changed, and the wisdom to know the one from the other" (Burrow, 2007) and envisioned it as a supportive tool during EMDR Future Template processing.

More room developed for Amanda to work through her remaining negative cognitions with more spaciousness and compassion. As her heart enlarged toward herself, the heart of God seemed to spontaneously enlarge toward her as well. As the poet Mark Nepo (2016) puts it, "Like a worried glassblower trying to refigure his clear and shattered heart, I have cut myself on all that I was, surprised at the wisdom hiding in the edges" (p. 41).

Case Study 10.3: Priya: Free Will, Abdication and Embodiment— Hiding and Craving Safety

Unlike Amanda, Priya had an over-internalized sense of the Divine. Her childhood experiences of power abuse led her to passive cooperation with others. She found what felt to her like peace through meditation. Vietnamese Buddhist monk, Thich Nhat Hanh, stresses the value of meditation as providing direction toward enlightenment. He states, "If you don't have a direction to go, you are lost. You cannot be happy. To know where to go is very important. If you don't know where to go, you will suffer a lot. And this is the nature of faith as understood in the Buddha's teaching" (Hanh, 1999, p. 119). We will see that even a beautiful spiritual practice can be misappropriated, as Priya creates a hiding place from the world and her corporal/sexual self through addiction to meditation.

Priya is a 26-year-old ciswoman who suffered ongoing childhood sexual abuse by a babysitter and his friends. To cope, she dissociated into a space of deeply internalized spiritual awareness. Priya stopped fighting back and would go limp. Her perpetrators would then lose interest and leave her alone.

"Your will is my will" became Priya's motto. Her injury was inflicted through the abuse of power and the negation of the will versus free choices (Shapiro, 2018, p. 295). Priya adaptively learned to avoid conflict and to abdicate her will to the wants and needs of others. She sought an inner, otherworldly experience of the Divine as her safety. "The Universal Divine is my hiding place. So much better than the world." Priya would go on long, silent meditation retreats at a local Buddhist meditation center which she found comforting, yet her life was robotic and unfulfilling.

Priya's experience of the Universal Divine was deeply internalized yet she was disconnected from her executive, adult functioning. She was passive and had trouble making even simple life decisions. She looked for "signs" from the Universe regarding her choices, signs that only she would internally recognize. She would get confused and frightened that she might miss or misinterpret the signs the Universe was sending her. Priya accepted each next thing that came into her life as the Universal Divine will for her.

When she came into therapy, Priya had had a brief sexual encounter with a young woman she met at the Buddhist center. In her confusion and agitation, she stated, "I don't even know how it happened. It just did." "Shanti said she wanted to kiss me, and I just said okay. One thing led to another." "Now I can't meditate. I'm spinning and I can't focus on anything."

Priya did not/could not understand why her abdication to Divine Guidance (Richo, 2011, pp. 99–102) was not working for her. She kept waiting for rescue in the form of more definitive instruction and felt hurt and scared that it did not seem to be showing up. She had no capacity to understand free will or the role of free will in adult functioning or adult spirituality (Richo, 2011, pp. 22–25). Her passivity masqueraded as devotion, when, in actuality, it was an adaptive reflex of self-protection that kept her appropriation of adult free will from actualizing.

As most therapists know, addictions are not exclusively the province of substances. Priya had an addictive attachment to meditation. David Richo (2017) speaks to human longing as expanding our focus and addiction as contracting. "Addiction is attached to the object of desire. Behind the desire might be a longing we gave up on" (Richo, 2017, p. 33). For Priya, her addition was to oblivion. Her longing was for safety and freedom from fear.

Priya struggled with a tension of opposites. Until she could find freedom to be self-determining, she would not have a robust connection to herself or the Divine. Priya expressed a desire to make her own decisions in life. She, at times, could see that meditation was not all she wanted from life. With explanation and practice, Priya was able to understand and maintain dual attention and was able to watch herself retreat into meditation to find the Divine only there. She wanted to find the Divine in the world as well and knew her early abuse experiences were in the way.

EMDR therapy with Priya began with a series of negative cognitions: "I'm not safe in this world." "I must always say yes and cooperate with everyone, or I'll die." "I can only know God in secret." "I can only be alive within." "There is no place for me on earth." "If others make all the decisions, I'll be safe." Priya frequently had dissociative body sensations of "folding inward" and "going foggy." Up until this point she had associated the latter with a highly desirable meditative state.

As Priya progressed through her memories of sexual abuse, she came to embrace her personal power. She was able to sympathize with and be angry on behalf of the unprotected child she had been. She welcomed the positive cognitions of "I'm entitled to give permission" and "I can say no," refined from "I'm allowed to say no" (Laliotis, 2021). Other positive cognitions developed and installed for Priya included:

"I can have a sexual relationship and be safe."
"I have good instincts. I can explore relationships with trustworthy people who don't want to control me."
"I can feel the support of the Divine Universe as I make my own choices in life,"
"It's good to live in my body."
"I'm welcome on the planet."

Priya cultivated a new understanding of yielding as the opposite of holding, clenching, or abdicating. She came to see opening and letting go as a profound act of free will to be chosen after she had personally assessed risk. She used two Sanskrit mantras to reflect upon and embrace the Divine within her and, equally, in others and the world— Om Namo Bhagavate Vasudevaya, meaning, "I bow down to the Lord who resides in the hearts of all beings" (Narayanan, 2018) and Lokah Samastah Sukhino Bhavantu, meaning "may all beings everywhere be happy and free" (Murphy, 2018).

Case Study 10.4: Sandy: Surrender and Control—Dominance and Submission

With an avoidant attachment style, fearing engulfment, and idealized defenses, we will see in Sandy, a high powered, corporate perfectionist whose sole connection to God was duty. Sandy used control to manage both her sexual and spiritual life. The Jewish philosopher Martin Buber (1958) juxtaposes the I-Thou and the I-It relationships. In the former, human beings

Chapter 10   Spirituality, Sexual Health, and EMDR Therapy

relate to one another with authenticity and without objectification. In the I-It relationship (in which Sandy was stuck) people relate to each other as objects, devoid of connection. Sandy would find, as Buber (1958) suggests, that "all real living is meeting" (p. 11).

Sandy grew up in a family of high achievers. Financial success correlated to personal value and emotions were treated as impediments to material gain. With a surgeon father and attorney mother, Sandy had minimal physical access to her parents and even less emotional access. She received attention and approval for straight As and athletic awards, and cold condemnation for the slightest hint of failure.

A CPA and CFO of a large company, Sandy came into therapy reporting "a recurring, disturbing dream" that was distracting her from her work. She found this "unacceptable" and wanted swift assistance to make the dream stop.

Upon inquiry regarding her spiritual resources, Sandy reported an internalized sense of God, even a partnership, devoid of humanity and shared human experience. She reported a sense of spiritual obligation of service to others through maintaining a level of excellence in her own achievements that she believed others could not maintain. She reported a belief that "most people are weak and give up excellence too easily." Her perceived "otherness," special knowing of true excellence and being "chosen" felt at the same time grandiose and highly burdensome (Knipe, 2019, p. 65).

When asked how she coped with that stressful burden, she calmly reported, without embarrassment, that she hired a professional disciplinarian to spank her to tears. Manually achieving release, Sandy let go of control in order to attain orgasm. It was not her direct action. It was "done for her." Ironically, by being the "employer" of the disciplinarian, Sandy got to exercise control while getting help giving it up. She had the control of requesting, in very specific ways, what she wanted and did not want from a spanking experience. She reported trust that the use of a safe word would be respected because she was dealing with a professional and paying significant amounts of money for a service. The business nature of the arrangement left her free of the emotional entanglements of relationship while obtaining the stress relief she craved.

Sandy came into treatment to explore her troubling dream, however, and did not want to digress from her goal. She reported in her dream reliving a memory of a beloved puppy she had briefly at age seven. With no explanation, one day the puppy was gone when she returned home from school. When she pressed her father, he stated she was "getting attached to it" and that emotional distraction would keep her from being successful in life. He made clear that "God expects our highest achievements."

Through some preliminary exploratory questions with bilateral stimulation (BLS) such as, "Did I learn anything about power and self-control from my father?" "Do these spanking experiences build me up or tear me down?" (Richo, 2017), and "What am I really seeking?" (Dreamer, 2007), it became clear that Sandy's puppy dream had far-reaching implications. It was a perfect example of pervasive messages she received about her rarified spiritual obligations and the inadmissibility of her emotional needs.

Sandy's first negative cognition in relation to her dream was, "If I'm not in control, I will fail God." Her initial body sensations were of systemic muscle tension and rigidity. In processing her dream, Sandy saw more connections with messages from childhood. She worked with additional negative cognitions including, "People will only do what I make them do," "My feelings are irrelevant," and "If I care, I'll be derailed."

Sandy's positive cognitions progressed incrementally:

"I can loosen control by inches."
"When I feel safe, I can open."
"I can discern trustworthiness in others."
"Loving my puppy was a good thing."
"I can grieve and remember connection."
"I need and deserve care and support."
"God would like me to have human connection."
"It's safe to breathe. It's safe to feel."

Through EMDR, Sandy also came to the realization that she was engaging in experiments of trust, exploring limits, and even intimacy, through her spanking fetish. She was able to observe the sensation of being held and protected by her partner, even while that partner was also administering pain. She could see in her experience a *breaking open—not breaking down*. Eventually, she could see that negotiation is an act of intimacy. She came to understand that exercises in dominance and submission were not the end of her sexual and spiritual journeys, but rather, the beginning. She realized that allowing trust and responsibility to be shared engendered a positive sensation of connection measured in a release of muscle tension separate from her orgasms. She had a glimpse of yielding as an act of spiritual opening and orgasm as only one small road to getting there.

While still hard-hitting in the corporate world, Sandy reported a softening of the ruthlessness toward herself and others, and that it was never her true nature. Sandy continued sessions with her professional partner but with considerably more awareness that included, not just instructions given, but mindful negotiation, mutual trust and respect. As Buber (n.d.) put it so well, "A person cannot approach the divine by reaching beyond the human. To become human is, what this individual person, has been created for."

Chapter 10 Spirituality, Sexual Health, and EMDR Therapy

Case Study 10.5: Hank: Sacrifice, Safety, and Belonging

Hank's spiritual life was derailed by childhood circumstance, leading to lifelong spiritual disconnection. In addition to painful spiritual alienation, this also had significant relational and sexual consequences in terms of anxious attachment and sexual repression. Best known for his work in the field of comparative mythology, Joseph Campbell (2003), speaks eloquently of the hero's journey. At the start of treatment, Hank's is a hero's spiritual journey interrupted. He will come, in some ways, full circle, back to his beginning with far greater wisdom and perspective. He eventually finds true Francis of Assisi's belief, also a traveler on the hero's quest, "The journey is essential to the dream" (Assisi, n.d.).

A 45-year-old soft-spoken cisman CPA, Hank's doctor referred him to therapy to "reduce his stress." On further investigation, Hank confided that he had sought medical assistance for erectile dysfunction. When his measured hormone levels were in normal range, his doctor looked to other causes. Hank was overweight, had high blood pressure, and frequent headaches, in addition to his sexual impotency.

In a 10-year marriage with no children, Hank described his wife as "a good woman who finds me disappointing, but she tries not to complain."

An only child, Hank grew up with criticism from his father who had stereotypical masculine expectations for his son. Hank experienced his dad as impossible to please and chronically disappointed in him. Hank liked to swim and play tennis. He hated team sports and the ethos surrounding them. He was deeply interested in his religion classes in Catholic school. He worried a lot about sin and the exhortation to "honor thy parents." Although he never mentioned it to his parents, Hank secretly fantasied about becoming a priest. His father, however, was already chronically annoyed by Hank, "with his wimpy head in the clouds." Hank's dream had no legs to stand on.

When Hank was 14, his father left Hank, his two younger siblings, and his mother. As the therapy progressed with Hank, it became clear that he blamed himself for his father leaving his mother. He felt that it was his fault for not being "the son his father could be proud of." Hank's mother fueled this belief by telling Hank that he now "had to step up and be the man of the house."

Major complex issues became clear in the work with Hank. He had a fused sense of God and the disappointed parent. Hank had an arrested "young" conceptualization of the Divine. He believed he had both made a sacrifice for his family, which God required, and, at the same time, defied his calling from God to the priesthood. In a way, he spiritually "shorted out." Consequently, Hank struggled with feelings of being adrift, belonging nowhere to no one, even his wife. He felt unlovable and had a skewed self-perception as a failure and unworthy of connections both Divine and human.

These experiences were the foundation for a sequential list of EMDR targets addressing Hanks's injured understanding of masculinity and his compromised spiritual life.

Hank resonated with the negative cognitions, "I'm bad and worthless," "I'm not a spiritual or a sexual being," "I have failed God's charge," and "I try so hard and fail so completely." As Hank processed memories of confrontations with his father and damaging internalized messages, he began to untangle the past and present. He could see with compassion the impossible corner into which he'd been painted as a teenager. "In the context of trauma psychotherapy, therapists may sometimes use God concepts grounded in sacred writings to counter negative God images that clients have developed as a result of past abuse" (Walker et al., 2014, p. 9). Hank began having strong recollections of specific scriptures that he appropriated for comfort, healing and spiritual/emotional reorganization. "Lord, only say the word and my soul shall be healed," *Matthew 8* (New International Version Bible, 2021) and, ultimately, "Sing to the LORD a new song; sing to the LORD, all the earth. Sing to the LORD, praise his name; proclaim his salvation day after day...For great is the LORD and most worthy of praise," *Psalm 96* (New International Version Bible, 2021).

Over a period of many months, Hank marshaled these buried scriptures of his youth and vivified his personal value as a sexual being. He slowly began to change his diet and to walk at a local nature preserve. He lost weight and his overall health improved. He still struggled at times with impotence, however, incremental improvements were enormously encouraging for him and well tolerated. He and his wife entered couples' counseling and the reorganization of their relationship was hopeful.

As EMDR progressed, Hank's positive cognitions were triumphant:

"I am worthy."
"It's a privilege and gift to be in charge of my own life."
"I can still serve God and others."
"The pilgrimage I've been on has taught me so much. I can serve in new and better ways."
"I can fully embrace my humanity. I can live my life today as a married man and be whole."
"I can thrive in my marriage and enjoy making love to my wife."
"I am pleasing in the sight of God."

Near the end of his treatment, Hank consulted the priest of his local parish to explore his rebirth of faith (Hanh, 1999, pp. 66–93). His story was met with compassion and understanding. Hank was invited to be a lector, reading scripture passages during services which he was attending with joy and increasingly less emotional conflict.

At his final session, Hank reflected on the well-known quote from St. Augustine as the Early Church Father reflected on his own journey to God, "You have made us for yourself, O Lord, and our heart is restless until it rests in you" (St. Augustine of Hyppo: Confessions, n.d.).

CONCLUSION

This chapter examined the intersection of sexual and spiritual wounds, frequently, inextricably intertwined. Although far from comprehensively covering all possible permutations, through the case studies, we have seen clients out of balance both sexually and spiritually due to trauma. Presentations differed significantly. Some experienced the Divine solely externally, some solely internally. We saw clients use spirituality to hide from the world and/or from themselves as sexual beings. Others we saw using their sexuality as a means of backing away from or moving more deeply into their spiritual self. In every case, we saw how a client's spiritual being and sexuality could be inextricable intertwined. All experienced relational wounds, pain, and disenfranchised isolation of one kind or another. Links between client woundedness and their access to the Divine as a resource were explored.

This chapter described skills to elicit spiritual information from clients through spiritually sensitive dialogue and inquiry. The use of spiritual resources in treatment planning, EMDR processing, as well as post EMDR integration, was also explained. Looking through the lens of EMDR therapy, we saw how working with the unique spiritual sensibilities of individual clients, and, ultimately, the connectedness that affords, can facilitate healing on multiple levels of mind, body, and spirit.

Healing sexual trauma is healing a sacred wound because that process brings us into being more human. Into being able to access these deep primordial, creative and regenerative energies because ultimately, the sexual energy is the energy of creative aliveness. And this is the most sacred experience that I believe a human being can have. (Levine, 2014)

REFERENCES

Assisi, F. (n.d.). *The journey is essential to the dream.* https://www.quotetab.com/quote/by-francis-of-assisi/the-journey-is-essential-to-the-dream

Boorstein, S., Fisher, N, & Rinpoche, T. (2011). *Solid ground: Buddhist wisdom for difficult times.* Parallax Press.

Bourgeault, C. (2016). *The heart of centering prayer: Nondual Christianity in theory and practice*. Shambhala.
Buber, M. (n.d.). *A person cannot approach the divine by reaching beyond the human*. https://www.inspiringquotes.us/quotes/ZecW_B8rkPmFd
Buber, M. (1958). *I and thou* (2nd ed.). Charles Schribner's Sons.
Burrow, R., Jr. (2007). The serenity prayer: Faith and politics in times of peace and war. *Encounter, 68*(4), 70.
Campbell, J. (2003). *The hero's journey: Joseph Campbell on his life and work* (Vol. 7). New World Library.
Chödrön, P. (2016). *When things fall apart: Heart advice for difficult times*. Shambhala Publications.
Chopra, D. (2006). *Kama Sutra: Including the seven spiritual laws of love*. Virgin Books.
Clinton, T., & Straub, J. (2014). *God Attachment: Why you believe, at, and feel the way you do about God*. Howard Books.
David, E. B., Moriarty, G. I., & Mauch, J. C. (2013). God images and god concepts: Definitions, developments, and dynamics. *Psychology of Religion and Spirituality*. https://doi.org/10.1037/a0029289
Davies, J. M., & Frawley, M. G. (1994). *Treating the adult survivor of childhood sexual abuse: A psychoanalytic perspective*. Basic Books.
Dreamer, O. M. (2007). *Your Heart's Prayer: Following the thread of desire into a deeper life*. (O. M. Dreamer, Narr.) [Audiobook]. Sounds True. https://amzn.to/3sY045x
Hanh, T. N. (1999). *Going home: Jesus and Buddha as brothers*. Riverhead Books.
Knipe, J. (2019). *EMDR toolbox: Theory and treatment of complex PTSD and dissociation* (2nd ed.). Springer Publishing.
Kujawa-Holbrook, S. A. (2013). *The sacred art: Journey to the center of the heart (The art of spiritual living)*. Skylight Paths.
Laliotis, D. (2021). *The dance of attachment: An advanced EDR clinical course*. License# CT 000152.
Laliotis, D., & Korn, D. (2020). *An EMDR therapy primer: From practicum to practice* (3rd ed.). Springer Publishing.
Leeds, A. M. (2009). *A guide to the standard EMDR protocols for clinicians, supervisors, and consultants*. Springer Publishing.
Levine, P. A. (2014). *Sexual healing: Transforming the sacred* (P. A. Levine Narr.) [Audiobook]. Sounds True. https://amzn.to/3uxnSh7
Levine, S. (2015). *Exploring sacred emptiness* (S. Levine, Narr.) [Audiobook]. Sounds True. https://amzn.to/3fzHooQ
Murphy, A. (2018, April 18). *What is the meaning of Lokah Samastah Sukhino Bhavantu*. Gaia. https://www.gaia.com/article/what-is-the-meaning-of-lokah-samastah-sukhino-bhavantu
Narayanan, A. S. (2018, January 16). Vishnu mantra meaning and benefits. *The Times of India*. https://timesofindia.indiatimes.com/religion/mantras-chants/vishnu-mantra-meaning-and-benefits/articleshow/68205198.cms
Neff, K., & Germer, C. (2018). *The mindful self-compassion workbook: A proven way to accept yourself, build inner strength, and thrive*. Guilford Press.
Nepo, M. (2016). *The way under the way: The place of true meeting*. Sounds True.
New International Version Bible. (2021). *The NIV Bible*. https://www.thenivbible.com (Original work published 1985)

Pearlman, L. A., & Saakvitne, K. W. (1995). *Trauma and the therapist: Countertransference and vicarious traumatization in psychotherapy with incest survivors*. W. W. Norton & Company.

Pearlman, L. A., Wortman, C. B., Feuer, C. A., & Farber, C. H. (2014). *Treating traumatic bereavement: A practitioner's guide*. The Guilford Press.

Richo, D. (2011). *How to be an adult in faith and spirituality*. Paulist Press.

Richo, D. (2017). *The five longings*. Shambala.

Safron, A. (2016). What is orgasm? A model of sexual trance and climax via rhythmic entrainment. *Socioaffective Neuroscience & Psychology, 6*, 31763. https://doi.org/10.3402/snp.v6.31763

Shapiro, F. (2018). *Eye movement desensitization and reprocessing (EMDR) therapy: Basic principles, protocols, and procedures* (3rd ed.). The Guilford Press.

St. Augustine of Hyppo: Confessions. (n.d.). Lib 1, 1–2, 2.5, 5: CSEL 33, 1–5.

Tolle, E. (2008, February 6). *Can I be the space for this?* [Video]. YouTube. https://www.youtube.com/watch?v=Lx526pO9UV0&ab_channel=EckhartTolle

Walker, D. F., Courtois, C. A., Aten, J. D., & William, H. (Eds.). (2015). *Spiritually oriented psychotherapy for trauma*. American Psychological Association.

ADDITIONAL READING

Chödrön, P. (2002). *The places that scare you: A guide to fearlessness in difficult times.* Shambhala Publications.

Ciocca, G., Limoncin, E., Di Tommaso, S., Mollaioli, D., Gravina, G. L., Marcozzi, A., & Jannini, E. A. (2015). Attachment styles and sexual dysfunctions: A case–control study of female and male sexuality. *International Journal of Impotence Research, 27*(3), 81–85. https://doi.org/10.1038/ijir.2014.33

Dreamer, O. M. (2005). *What we ache for: Creativity and the unfolding of your soul.* HarperOne.

Frankl, V. E. (1986). *The doctor and the soul: From psychotherapy to logotherapy.* Intage.

Frankl, V. E. (2006). *Man's search for meaning* (I. Lasch Trans.). Beacon Press.

Hensley, B. (2015). *An EMDR therapy primer second edition: From practicum to practice.* Springer Publishing.

Levine, P. A. (2010). *In an unspoken voice: How the body releases trauma and restores goodness.* North Atlantic Books.

Merton, T. (1966, June 3). *Is the world a problem? Ambiguities in the secular.* Commonweal. https://www.commonwealmagazine.org/world-problem

Rumi, J. A. D. (2004). *The essential Rumi, new expanded edition* (C. Barks, J. Moyne, Trans.). HarperOne. (Original work written in 13th century).

Siegel, I. R. (2017). *The sacred path of the therapist: Modern healing, ancient wisdom and client transformation.* W. W. Norton & Company.

van der Kolk, B. A. (1996). *The body keeps the score: Approaches to the psychobiology of posttraumatic stress disorder.* The Guilford Press.

Wesselmann, D., & Potter, A. E. (2009). Change in adult attachment status following treatment with EMDR: Three case studies. *Journal of EMDR Practice and Research, 3*(3), 178–191. http://doi.org/10.1891/1933-3196.3.3.178

Whyte, D. (1996). *The heart aroused: Poetry and the preservation of the soul in corporate America.* Currency Press.

11

Sexual Health Resources for EMDR Therapists and Their Clients

Stephanie Baird, LMHC

LEARNING OBJECTIVES

- This chapter provides EMDR clinicians with current sexual health related websites, podcasts, television shows, videos, books for professionals and clients
- This chapter also provides EMDR clinicians with educational and training programs available for further professional learning.

INTRODUCTION

This final resource chapter is not meant to be an exhaustive sexual health resource or take the place of dedicated sexual health education. My hope is that this book validates and encourages you, the EMDR therapist most likely contacted for treating sexual trauma, to embrace positive sexual health as an important and essential part of life both for yourself, as a trusted professional, and for your clients seeking care. May this book encourage ongoing exploration, acquisition, and sharing of knowledge, helping to demystify sexuality, counteract erotophobia, and encourage sexual well-being and empowerment for all.

Sexual Health Websites, Television, Podcasts, and Video Resources

Useful videos and podcasts have been popping up on YouTube, Vimeo, and other media and educational forums. Our younger clients also prefer information viewed through social media platforms such as Instagram or Tick Tock. It can be very helpful to share a link with a client struggling over a particular issue. Clients may have validating and/or normalizing "aha" moments from this psychoeducation.

Anatomical and Physiological Genital Information

These videos illustrate the anatomy and pathways of some sexual organs:

- BioDigital Human: http://www.biodigital.com/
- Betty Dodson: The Internal Clitoris. http://videosift.com/video/Anatomy-of-the-Clitoris
- Sperm pathway: https://www.youtube.com/watch?v=v22CjFYizi0
- Foreskin anatomy (uncircumcised erection): https://www.youtube.com/watch?v=NWaBToX5s90
- Unwanted arousal: This TED Talk beautifully explains "The Truth About Unwanted Arousal" (Emily Nagoski). https://www.youtube.com/watch?v=L-q-tSHo9Ho

Many survivors of sexual assault report signs of physiological arousal during the assault (vaginal lubrication, erections, orgasms, etc.). These are automatic physiological reactions to sexual stimulation and have no correlation with whether the survivor wanted that sexual interaction.

Sexual Consent

Consent is a basic sexual health right and has gained much more attention since the #metoo movement.

Consent: It's as Simple as Tea: This video uses the metaphor of making someone tea to help explain consent: https://www.youtube.com/watch?v=QDhKM8qWWBM

FRIES: This video describes enthusiastic consent and its five elements, helping to promote empowered and pleasurable sex: (Freely Given, Reversible, Informed, Enthusiastic, Specific). https://www.youtube.com/watch?v=pgydDscVnVQ

Chapter 11 Sexual Health Resources for EMDR Therapists

Sex Educational Websites for Kids and Teens

Amaze.org: This site has many age-appropriate videos and short lessons for kids. Their mission: "AMAZE envisions a world that recognizes child and adolescent sexual development as natural and healthy, a world in which young people everywhere are supported and affirmed and the adults in their lives communicate openly and honestly with them about puberty, reproduction, relationships, sex and sexuality."

Scarleteen.com ("sex ed for the real world"): This is a treasure trove of age-appropriate content for teen "inclusive, comprehensive, and supportive sexuality and relationship info." A quick glance at their homepage netted these topics "gender, sexual identity, disability, abuse, sexual politics," and quarantine-relevant articles on "How to Actually Date Yourself!" and "Self-Care and Social Distance."

Planned Parenthood: https://www.plannedparenthood.org/learn/teens (age-appropriate information related to teen sexuality and relationships)

Go Ask Alice website: https://goaskalice.columbia.edu/: Health website for kids, with expert information, including sexual health.

Real Talk mobile app (health and sex ed for teens)

Sex Educational Websites for Adults

The Omgyes.com website. Disclosure: This is a pay site with a one-time fee ($49 at last check) for Season 1, which includes "practical techniques to enhance clitoral pleasure…(with) over 60 short videos, 12 touchable simulations, and dozens of infographics." No matter at what "sexpert" level your client might be, if they are interested in female-bodied pleasure, they will learn something new. Their practical pleasure techniques include "layering, hinting, signaling, surprise, orbiting, multiples, edging," and so on. Their information is research and science derived, and they state that the one-time fee contributes to ongoing research.

Sexsmartfilms.com: "Promoting sexual literacy." Educational films about sex and sex therapy.

A Woman's Touch: www.sexualityresources.com (Educational web resource by Ellen Barnard with excellent holistic sexual health information for all genders, including natural vaginal renewal for menopausal individuals)

Aging and Sexual Health

American Psychological Association: *Aging and Sexual Health Resource Guide* bit.ly/2PkoDW2

American Society on Aging: *Sexuality, Intimacy, and Aging: It's Time to Talk* bit.ly/2LBdhLj

National Institute on Aging: *Sexuality in Later Life* bit.ly/2P8gcgF

Our Better Half podcast (www.ourbetterhalf.net): This podcast has been produced since around 2010 and focuses on sex over the age of 50, most episodes interviewing someone prominent in the field of sexuality.

Safer Sex for Seniors: safersex4seniors.org

SAGE: sageusa.org: Country's oldest and largest organization dedicated to improving lives of LGBTQ older adults offering services, support, and resources for LGBT older adults and their caregivers.

Pelvic, Vulvar, and Urology Resources

American Physical Therapist Association (Apta.org): Clients can search this website of physical therapists to locate a pelvic floor specialist in their area.

National Vulvodynia Association (nva.org): Information on vulvar health.

Urology Care Foundation (urologyhealth.org): Includes information on erectile dysfunction and other urological conditions.

Sexual Health Experts and Activists Websites

Thankfully the field of sex-positive educators, commentators, and creators continues to expand since the Kinsey's initial foray back in the 1950s. This is a very short list of my favorite activists/educators not mentioned elsewhere.

Susie Bright: Susie has been promoting sex-positive living since the early 1980s, and was one of the first prominent bisexual activist/educators to be referred to as a "sex-positive feminist." She has written many books, delivered lectures across the country, appeared in films, and maintains a weekly podcast, and referred to by many as a "national treasure." You can locate her books on Amazon or other book sites.

Betty Dodson (DodsonandRoss.com): Website and videos on Bodysex, orgasm instruction, and so on. Although Betty Dodson is now deceased, her work carries on.

Joe Kort, PhD, LMSW (Joekort.com): Joe Kort is a leading sex therapist/educator/consultant with the podcast smartsexsmartlove.com. He has written books for therapists on working with LGBTQ clients as well self-help books for gay men.

Carol Queen: "Author, editor, sociologist and sexologist active in the sex-positive feminism movement" (Wikipedia.com) with many published books on sex, activism, and porn.

Dan Savage (Savagelovecast.com): This is a long-running sex advice podcast by the well-known Dan Savage.

Tristan Taormino (tristantaormino.com): Tristan, sex educator, write, media maker, consultant, believes "everyone deserves sex education that is consent-focused, inclusive, pleasure-oriented, accessible, and trauma-informed."

Sex-Positive Retail and Educational Websites

Goodvibes.com (sex toys AND feminist-oriented information): Good Vibrations began in 1977 when feminist sex activist Joani Blank opened her first sex toy store in San Francisco to provide high quality products, originally geared toward women's bodies. I remember receiving their catalogues in the mail in the 90s, examining with delight all the types of toys and props solely made for pleasure! They have online ordering plus 10 physical locations (mostly in California plus two in the Boston-area). Their San Francisco Polk Street location features the Vibrator Museum, which was closed due to "seismic retrofitting" around 2019. Good Vibrations was a worker-owned co-op for about 14 years, later becoming a corporation in 2006. In 1995 they declared May International Masturbation Month, as a "sex-positive response to the firing of then-Surgeon General Dr. Joycelyn Elders." If you search through their website, you can check out all the categories of toys for sale (i.e., gender play, vibrators, bondage, etc.), plus look under their "sex info" tab for lots of free information, sex tips, and tricks. Good Vibrations also carries many erotic fiction and non-fiction books for your inspiration (e.g., best women's erotica, best lesbian erotica, books on orgasm, feminist porn, polyamory).

Babes in Toyland https://www.babeland.com/: This sex toy store opened in 1993 in response to the lack of female-centered sex toy stores in the Seattle area. They have since gone on to open three more stores in the New York City area. All of their inventory is available via its website, which also contains sexual health information.

Smitten Kitten https://www.smittenkittenonline.com/: This newer, progressive sex toy store and website opened in 2003 to promote and facilitate non-toxic sex toy use for everyone. While based in Minneapolis (hosting local events), everything can be ordered online. They also started the website Badvibes.org in 2004 to help combat toxic materials used in sex toys and promote transparency in the sex toy industry.

LGBQ Educational and Information Websites

Bisexuality, Bi.org
Bisexual Resource Center, Biresource.net
Diverse Elders Coalition, diverseelders.org
Highlander Research and Education Center, highlandercenter.org
Human Rights Campaign, HRC.org
Lesbian Hermstory Archives, lesbianherstoryarchives.org
LGBTQ Student Resources, GLSEN.org
Making Gay History, makinggayhistory.com
National Black Justice Coalition, nbjc.org
National Center for Transgender Equality, transequality.org

National LGBTQ Task Force, thetaskforce.org
National Resource Center on LGBT Aging, lgbtagingcenter.org
Old Lesbian Oral Herstory Project, olohp.org
Older Lesbians Organizing for Change, oloc.org
PFLAG (formerly known as Parents, Families, and Friends of Lesbians and Gays), Pflag.org
Sage: Advocacy and Services for LGBT Elders, sageusa.org
Stonewall Veterans Association, stonewallvets.org
The Trevor Project, thetrevorproject.org—"saving young LGBT lives"

Gender, Transgender, Intersex Educational and Information Websites

Cisgender Privilege: https://projecthumanities.asu.edu/content/cisgender-privilege-checklist
Complexity of Sex Determination: https://blogs.scientificamerican.com/sa-visual/visualizing-sex-as-a-spectrum/
Gender Neutral Terms: https://nonbinary.wiki/w/index.php?title=Gender_neutral_language_in_English&mobileaction=t oggle_view_desktop
Intersex: https://isna.org/faq/what_is_intersex/
Judith Butler: Your behavior creates your gender: https://www.youtube.com/watch?v=Bo7o2LYATDc&t=28s
List of Gender Words: https://anagnori.tumblr.com/post/72143410400/glossary-of-transgender-non-binary-and
National Children's THRIVE Program: www.nationwidehildrens.org/thrive
National Resource for Transgender Equality: www.transequality.org
Transgender Gender-Variant & Intersex Justice Project: tgijp.org
TransProud: www.transproud.com
Trans Student Educational Resources: www.transstudent.org
Why Pronouns Matter: https://www.youtube.com/watch?v=N_yBGQqg7kM&feature=youtu.be
World Professional Association for Transgender Health. (2011). *Standards of care for the health of transsexual, transgender, and gender nonconforming people* (7th ed.). World Professional Association for Transgender Health. https://www.wpath.org/publications/soc ("The overall goal of the standards of care is to provide clinical guidance for the health professionals to assist transsexual, transgender, and gender nonconforming people with safe and effective pathways to achieving lasting personal comfort with their gendered selves…")

LBGTQ and Spirituality Websites

Baptist: Association of Welcoming and Affirming Baptists, awab.org
Faithfully LGBT: faithfullylgbt.com, Testimonies of LGBTQ Christians.
Judaism: Reformjudaism.org, Has LGBTQ resources such as LBTQ Equality and Gender Expression.
Muslims for Progressive Values, mpvusa.org
Roman Catholic, dignitiyusa.org

Fidelity and Affairs

Many of us will work with clients recovering from being on either end of an affair.

- "Rethinking Infidelity…A TED Talk for Anyone Who Has Ever Loved" by Esther Perel (https://www.youtube.com/watch?v=P2AUat93a8Q) This TED Talk covers questions folks may have about how this could have happened to them.
- "The secret to desire in a long-term relationship": TED Talk by Esther Perel. https://www.ted.com/talks/esther_perel_the_secret_to_desire_in_a_long _term_relationship?language=en
- "Where Shall We Begin" podcast by Esther Perel (estherperel.com/podcast). This podcast focuses on couples and sexuality, featuring a diversity of couples presenting their sexual concerns (each couple receiving one session of help) for Ester Perel's piercing explorations.

CNM and/or Polyamory Websites

Polyamory Glossary: https://www.morethantwo.com/polyglossary.html
Loving More: https://www.lovingmorenonprofit.org/

BDSM and Kink Websites

FetLife.com: This is a social media website for kink-interested individuals. Not all individual profiles are "vetted." There are many instructional and educational events listed as well.
kinkacademy.com: Website with 2000+ videos plus experts on kink topics ranging from bondage to wrestling.
https://slutphd.com/archives-2/: The writer of this blog is an active kinkster AND studies kink (etc.) for a living.
https://www.stefanosandshay.com/: Shay and her partner, Stefanos, are well-known kink/BDSM educators.
fetishflea.com: New England leather alliance.
fanfair.info: Annual Transgender week in Cape Cod, oriented to kink/BDSM.

Sex-Positive Television Series

Akwafina is Nora from Queens (HBO, 2020-): Hilarious comedy with vagina- and vibrator-friendly scenes, diverse racial casting (including LGBTQ).

The Bisexual (Hulu, 2018): Comedy/drama that explores one woman coming to terms with her bisexuality.

Bridgerton (Netflix, 2020-): Romance series with diverse racial casting and fairly realistic erotic scenes.

Broad City (Comedy Central, Hulu, 2014–2019): Hilarious comedy, very vagina and queer friendly.

Grace and Frankie (Netflix, 2015-): Hilarious comedy depicting two older ciswomen who make lube, vibrators, and other inventions for the aging population. Great role modeling of elders and positive sexuality. Positive LGBT depictions. A+ casting: Jane Fonda, Lily Tomlin, Sam Waterson, Martin Sheen.

Insecure (HBO, 2015-)

L Word: Generation Q (Showtime, 2019-): Modern drama, realistic depiction of lesbians.

Master of None, Season 3 (Netflix, 2021): Dramedy. This season nearly exclusively focuses on the sexual and emotional relationship between two Black lesbians.

Motherland: Fort Salem (Freeform, 2020-): Diverse, mostly female casting depicting empowered ciswomen. LGBT friendly.

Mrs. Fletcher (HBO, 2019-): Positive exploration of middle-aged mother finally exploring her sexuality.

Sens8 (Netflix, 2015–2018): Sci-fi thriller by the Wachowski siblings. Positive depictions of LGBTQ sexuality, diverse cast.

Sex Education (Netflix, 2019-): Comedy series where the son of a sex therapist ends up providing his high school peers with proxy sex therapy.

Tales of the City (Netflix 2019 reboot): Serial drama with diverse LGBTQ casting.

We Are Who We Are (HBO, 2020): Incredible drama set in Italy on an American military base depicting the teen children of military exploring gender and sexuality.

Shrill (Hulu, 2019-present): Body positive dramedy with BIPOC and LGBTQ casting.

Pornography Resources

Some clients will present with complaints of feeing like they watch too much porn, or that their partner watches too much porn. Research is showing both some very specific benefits (couples who openly discuss porn likes and dislikes correlate with better overall sexual communication and satisfaction) as well as detriments for many (losing self-esteem due to comparing oneself to unrealistic standards, activities, adaptation to "super stimulus," etc.). Here are a number of resources that can help provide clarity and perspective on the influence of porn on our clients' sexual health.

- *Real Sex vs. Porn Sex Video:* https://www.youtube.com/watch?v=q64hTNEj6KQ
- Pew Internet Project. *Health Fact Sheet.* Pew Research Center: http://www.pewinternet.org/fact-sheets/health-fact-sheet/
- Corinna, H. (2018). *Making sense of sexual media.* http://www.scarleteen.com/article/politics_sexuality_etc/making_sense_of_sexual_media
- Gottman, J., & Gottman, J. (2016). *An open letter on porn.* https://www.gottman.com/blog/an-open-letter-on-porn/: In this letter pre-eminent relationship researchers discuss their concerns and the research related to porn viewing, read all the way through to their update.
- Yourbrainonporn.com. This website advertises itself as a clearinghouse of scientific research and information regarding the impact of porn on the brain, originally developed by Gary Wilson. While AASECT denounces the pathologizing of porn use and states there is no scientific evidence for "porn addiction," clients with "out of control" usage have reported feeling helped by this website.
- *Make Love Not Porn:* http://Makelovenotporn.com. This website features real world folks sharing their sexual selves and interactions, often in very different ways from the porn industry. This site is a membership site and viewers pay the participants with membership and fees.
- *Feminist-approved porn list:* https://www.reddit.com/r/chickflixxx/. This reddit page is for women-identified folks to post links to their favorite feminist erotica and porn. This running list helps to normalize female-bodied pleasure and desire among "regular" (non-porn industry) folk, showing female pleasure as hot, crucial, and beautiful. One caveat, sex educators often emphasize the importance of paying for porn in order to honor and pay the sex worker for the time and effort they put into putting themselves out there.
- erikalust.com. This website promotes feminist ethical porn. Erika Lust made her first indie erotic short film in 2004 (*The Good Girl,* ironically) and hasn't looked back. She promotes ethics, cinematic quality, and empowerment of women in her erotic films. Her website contains her own film catalogue, plus other directors' films she has selected for their ethical and artistic sensibilities. This is porn your clients can feel very good about paying for and watching.

Sexual Health Phone Apps

Bwom: Assists with pelvic health, oriented toward those with uteruses.

Clue Period and Health Tracker: Awesome menstruation and health tracker app that has many categories folks can respond to each day, including unprotected sex, high sex interest, mood-related, bowel movement, and so on. Many options are free.

Eve: "Savvy period and sex tracker."

Gottman Card Decks: "Helpful questions, statements, and ideas for improving your relationship."

My Sex Doctor: "Targeted at young adults, this app wants to 'start a welcome and long-due revolution, one where you no longer have to risk embarrassment.'"

Sexual Health Books
Professional Resources

Betchen, S., & Davidson, H. (2018). *Master conflict therapy: A new model for practicing couples and sex therapy.* Routledge.

Bruess, C. E., & Schroeder, E. (2018). *Sexuality education: Theory and practice* (7th ed.). ETR.

Buehler, S. (2021). *What every mental health professional needs to know about sex, third edition.* Springer Publishing Company.

Chang, S. C., Singh, A. A., & Dickey, L M. (2018). *A clinician's guide to gender-affirming care.* Context Press. (First in-depth book for therapists who work with transgender clients.)

Constantinides, D. M., Sennott, S. L., & Chandler, D. (2019). *Sex therapy with erotically marginalized clients: Nine principles of clinical support.* Routledge.

Davis, M. (2019). *Our whole lives: Sexuality education for older adults.* UUA.

DeFur, K., & Johnson, A. (2017). *Our whole lives, second edition: Sexuality education for grades 4–6.* UUA.

Gambescia, A., Weeks, G., & Hertlein, K. (2021). *A clinician's guide to systemic sex therapy, 3rd edition.* Routledge. (AASECT award-winning book.)

Hall, K., & Binik, Y. (2020). *Principles and practice of sex therapy* (6th ed.). Guilford.

Kleinplatz, P. (2012). *New directions in sex therapy: Innovations and alternatives.* Routledge. (AASECT award-winning book.)

Lev, A. (2013). *Transgender emergence: Therapeutic guidelines for working with gender-variant people and their families.* Taylor & Francis.

Levine, S. B. (Ed.). (2015). *Handbook of clinical sexuality for mental health professionals.* Brunner-Routledge.

Nelson, T. (2019). *Integrative sex & couples therapy: A therapist's guide to new and innovative approaches.* Pesi Publishing and Media.

Ogden, G. (2018). *Expanding the practice of sex therapy: The neuro update edition.* Routledge. (Ogden's book expands upon her 4-D Wheel of Sex Therapy, with this edition bringing relevant neuropsychological developments including the mention of EMDR.)

Shahbaz, C. (2017). *Becoming a kink aware therapist, 1st edition.* Routledge.

Weiner, L., & Avery-Clark, C. (2017). *Sensate focus in sex therapy: The illustrated manual.* Routledge.

Wilson, P. (2014). *Our whole lives: Sexual education for grades 7–9* (2nd ed.). UUAC.

General Sex-Positive Information

Bader, M. (2003). *Arousal: The secret logic of sexual fantasies.* St. Martin's Griffin.

Blank, J. (1997). *First person sexual: Women and men write about self-pleasuring.* Down There Press.

Brown, A. M. (2019). *Pleasure activism: The politics of feeling good.* AK Press. (This is an extraordinary recent release that looks at the intersection of pleasure, sexuality, race [a construct], and activism.)

Chapter 11 Sexual Health Resources for EMDR Therapists

Dischiavo, R. (2016). *The deep yes: The lost art of true receiving*. Spanda Press. (This is a great book to refer clients to, particularly our clients that have trouble "receiving" and enjoying pleasure.)

Dodson, B. (1996). *Sex for one: The joy of self-loving*. Random House. (Betty Dodson, the "mother of masturbation," wrote the first edition of this sentinel book "Sex for One" in 1987 and it has been a game-changer for the orgasm-challenged, helping many folks [mostly with clitorises and vulvas] learn to have orgasms.)

Janssen, E., & Bancroft, J. (2007). The dual control model: The role of sexual inhibition and excitation in sexual arousal and behavior. In E. Janssen (Ed.), *The psychophysiology of sex* (p. 197). Indiana University Press.

Joannides, P. (2017). *Guide to getting it on,* unzipped V.9.0. Goofy Foot Press. (Revised and updated illustrated editions are published nearly every year. Consider it a modern bible on everything sexuality-related. Comprehensive reference book for clients and our offices.)

Klein, M., & Robbins, R. (1999). *Let me count the ways*. Jeremy P. Tarcher. (Explains how to make sex more enjoyable focusing on sensuality and *outercourse* [not intercourse].)

Kleinplatz, P. J. & Menard, A. D. (2020). *Magnificent sex: Lessons from extraordinary lovers*. Routledge.

Komisaruk, B., Whipple., B., Nasserzadeh, S., & Beyer-Flores, C. (2010). *The orgasm answer guide*. Johns Hopkins University Press.

Kort, J. (2019). *Erotic orientation: Helping couples and individuals understand their sexual lives*. Smart Sex, Smart Love Books.

Lehmiller, J. (2018). *Tell me what you want: The science of sexual desire and how it can help improve your sex life*. Da Capo Lifelong Books.

Moen, E., & Nolan, M. (2018). *Drawn to sex, volume 1: The basics*. Erika Moen Comics and Illustration, LLC.

Moen, E., & Nolan, M. (2020). *Drawn to sex, volume 2: Our bodies and health*. Erika Moen Comics and Illustration, LLC. (These illustrated guides can be helpful sex educational resources for our more intellectually challenged clients.)

Morin, J. (1996). *The erotic mind: Unlocking the inner sources of passion and fulfillment*. Harper Perennial. (A seminal and revolutionary book changing the way people think about sex.)

Morin, J. (1998). *Anal pleasure and health: A Guide for men and women*. Down There Press.

Ogden, G. (2008). *The return of desire: A guide to rediscovering your sexual passion*. Trumpeter

Perry, F. (2019). *How to have feminist sex: A fairly graphic guide*. Penguin Random House. (This is my favorite go-to illustrated book for feminist-oriented sexual pleasure.)

Queen, C., & Rednour, S. (2015). *The sex & pleasure book: Good vibrations guide to great sex for everyone*. Barnaby LTD.

Taormino, T. (2010). *The big book of sex toys*. Quiver Books.

Yeshe, L. T. (2010). *Introduction to tantra: The transformation of desire*. Readhowyouwant.com.

General Sexuality History and/or Science

D'Emilio, J., & Freedman, E. B. (2012). *Intimate matters: A history of sexuality in America, 3rd edition*. University of Chicago Press.

Foucault, M. (1980). *The history of sexuality, volume I*. Vintage.

Roach, M. (2009). *Bonk: The curious coupling of sex and science*. Canongate Books.

Healing From Sexual Trauma

Bass, E. (2008). *The courage to heal: A guide for women survivors of child sexual abuse, 20th anniversary edition*. Harper Collins.

Cohn, R. (2011). *Coming home to passion: Restoring loving sexuality in couples with histories of childhood trauma and neglect, 1st edition*. Praeger.

Levine, P. (2010). *In an unspoken voice: How the body releases trauma and restores goodness*. North Atlantic books.

Lew, M. (2004). *Victims no longer: The classic guide for men recovering from sexual child abuse*. Harper Perennial.

Porges, S. (2011). *The polyvagal theory: Neurophysiological foundations of emotions, attachments, communication, and self-regulation*. W. W. Norton.

Maltz, W. (2012). *The Sexual healing journey: A guide for survivors of sexual abuse, 3rd Edition revised and updated*. William Morrow Paperbacks.

Saakvitne, K., Gamble, S. J., Pearlman, L., & Lev, B. T. (2000). *Risking connection: A curriculum for working with survivors of childhood abuse*. Sidran Press.

Shapiro, F. (2013). *Getting past your past: Take control of your life with self-help techniques from EMDR therapy*. Rodale Books.

Van der kolk, B. (2015). *The body keeps the score: Brain, mind, and body in the healing of trauma*. Penguin Books.

Clitoris, Vagina, and/or Female-Identified Related Sexual Health

Brotto, L. (2018). *Better sex through mindfulness: How women can cultivate desire*. Greystone Books.

Cass, V. (2007). *The elusive orgasm: A woman's guide to why she can't and how she can orgasm*. DeCapo Press.

Diamond, L. (2009). *Sexual fluidity: Understanding women's love and desires*. Harvard University Press.

Enright, L. (2019). *The vagina: A reeducation*. Allen and Unwin.

Ensler, E. (2001). *The vagina monologues*. Villiard.

Goldstein, A., Pukall, C. F., Goldstein, I. (2011). *When sex hurts: A woman's guide to banishing sexual pain*. De Capo Press.

Hite, S. (1976). *The Hite report: A nationwide study of female sexuality*. Macmillan.

Kinsey, A. C., Pomeroy, W., Baxter, M., Clyde, E., & Gebhard, P. H. (1953). *Sexual behavior in the human female*. W.B. Saunders.

Mintz, L. (2018). *Becoming cliterate: Why orgasm equality matters and how to get it*. HarperOne.

Nagoski, E. (2019). *Come as you are workbook: A practical guide to the science of sex*. Simon & Schuster. (This is the companion workbook to *Come as You Are*, with handy worksheets, questionnaires, and suggested assignments.)

Nagoski, E. (2021). *Come as you are: Revised and updated*. Simon & Schuster. (This book has some of the best current information on how to help people with clitorises, vulvas, and vaginas experience orgasm and pleasure [and to help those that care about clitorises and vaginas, etc.].)

Newman, F. (2012). *The whole lesbian sex book: A passionate guide for all of us*. Cleis Press. (Covers bisexual and transwomen; has detailed drawings.)

Resh, E. (2013). *Women, sex, power, and pleasure.* Hay House.
Stendhal, R. (2011). *True secrets of lesbian desire: Keeping sex alive in long-term relationships.* North Atlantic Books.
Sugrue, D., Foley, S., & Kope, S. (2012). *Sex matters for women: A complete guide to taking care of your sexual self.* Guilford Press.
Taormino, T. (2011). *The secrets of great g-spot orgasms and female ejaculation.* Quiver Books.
Thomashauer, R. (2018). *Pussy: A reclamation.* Hay House.
Wolf, N. (2012). *Vagina: A new biography, revised and updated.* Harper Collins.

Penis and/or Male-Identified Sexual Health

Chia, M., Abrams, A., & Douglas, A. (2001). *The multi-orgasmic man: Sexual secrets every man should know.* Harper Collins.
Danoff, D. (2015). *The ultimate guide to male sexual health: How to stay vital at any age.* Beyond Words. (This book is especially helpful for our aging clients who may be struggling with physical changes.)
Glickman, C., & Emirzian, A. (2013). *The ultimate guide to prostrate pleasure: Erotic exploration for men and their partners.* Cleis Press.
Haberman, H. (2001). *The family jewels: A guide to male genital play and torment.* Greenery Press.
Kinsey, A., Charles, P., Wardell, B., & Martin, C. E. (1948). *Sexual behavior in the human male.* W.B. Saunders.
McCarthy, B., & Metz, M. (2004) *Coping with erectile dysfunction.* New Harbinger Publications. (This classic book is often recommended to clients struggling with erections.)
Metz, M., & McCarthy, B. (2004). *Coping with premature ejaculation: How to overcome PE, please your partner and have great sex.* New Harbinger Publications.
Spitz, A. (2018). *The penis book: A doctor's complete guide to the penis--from size to function and everything in between.* Rodale.

Lesbian and Gay Specific Resources, Memoirs, History and Activism

Acquaviva, K. (2017). *LGBTQ-inclusive hospice and palliative care: A practical guide to transforming professional practice.* Harrington Park Press.
Andrews, M. (1996). *The preacher's son.* Window Books.
Baker, M.-J., & Scheele, J. (2016). *Queer: A graphic history.* Icon Books.
Bechdel, A. (2006). *Fun home: A family tragicomic.* Mariner Books.
Bronski, M. (2011). *A queer history of the United States.* Beacon Press.
Carter, D. (2010). *Stonewall: The riots that sparked the gay revolution.* Griffin.
Faderman, L. (1991). *Odd girls and twilight lovers: A history of lesbian life in twentieth-century America.* Columbia University Press.
Fleishman, J. (2020). *The stonewall generation: LGBTQ elders on sex, activism, and aging.* UUAC. (This recently published book interviews LGBTQ elders "who came of age around the time of the Stonewall Riots" and is a treasure-trove of LGBTQ liberation history.)
Frank, N. (2009). *Unfriendly fire: How the gay ban undermines the military and weakens America.* Thomas Dunne Books.

Johnson, E. P. (Ed.). (2016). *No tea, no shade: New writings in black queer studies*. Duke University Press.
Kort, J. (2018). *Cracking the erotic code: Helping gay men understand their sexual fantasies*. Smart Sex, Smart Love Books.
Kort, J. (2018). *LGBTQ clients in therapy: Clinical issues and treatment strategies*. W. W. Norton and Co.
Marcus, E. (2002). *Making gay history: The half-century fight for lesbian and gay equal rights*. Harper Perennial.
Mogul, J. L., Ritchie, A. J., & Whitlock, K. (2012). *Queer (in)justice: The criminalization of LGBT people in the United States*. Beacon Press.
New York Library. (2019). *The Stonewall reader*. Penguin Classics.
Roughgarden, J. (2004). *Evolution's rainbow: Diversity, gender, and sexuality in nature and people*. University of California Press.
Shilts, R. (2007). *And the band played on: Politics, people and the AIDS epidemic, twentieth anniversary edition*. St. Martin's Press.
Vaid, U. (2013). *Irresistible revolution: Confronting race class and the assumptions of LGBT politics*. Magnus Books.
Williams, W. (1992). *The spirit and the flesh: Sexual diversity in American Indian culture*. Beacon Press.

Bisexuality Specific Resources, Memoirs, History, and Activism

Andrew, E. (2000). *Swinging on the garden gate*. Skinner House Books.
Beauchemin, F. (Ed.). (2016). *How queer!: Personal narratives from bisexual, pansexual, polysexual, sexually-fluid, and other non-monosexual perspectives*. Our Own Authority.
Bisexual Anthology Collective. (1998). *Plural desires: Writing bisexual women's realities*. Sister Vision Press.
Burleson, W. (2005). *Bi America: Myths, truths, and struggles of an invisible community*. Routledge.
Eisner, S. (2013). *Bi: Notes for a bisexual revolution*. Seal Press.
Harrad, K. (Ed.). (2018). *Claiming the b in LGBT*. Thorntree Press.
Hutchins, L., & Ka'ahumanu, L. (Eds.). (1994) *Bi any other name: Bisexual people speak out*. Alyson Books.
Kolodny, D. (Ed.). (2000). *Blessed bi spirit: Bisexual people of faith*. Bloomsbury Academic.
Ochs, R. (2001). *Bisexual resource guide*. Bisexual Resource Center.
Ochs, R., & Rowley, S. L. (2005). *Getting bi*. Bisexual Resource Center.
Ochs, R., & Williams, S. (2014). *RECOGNIZE: The voices of bisexual men*. Bisexual Resource Center.
Orndorff, K. (Ed.). (1999). *Bi lives: Bisexual women tell their stories*. See Sharp Press.

Transgender Specific Resources, Memoirs, History, Activism, and Education

Bornstein, K. (2013). *My new gender workbook: A step-by-step guide to achieving world peace through gender anarchy and sex positivity 2nd edition*. Routledge.
Bornstein, K., & Bergman, S. B. (2010). *Gender outlaws: The next generation*. Seal Press.
Chang, S. C., Singh, A. A., & Dickey, L M. (2018). *A clinician's guide to gender-affirming care*. Context Press. (First in-depth book for therapists who work with transgender clients.)

Duron, L. (2013). *Raising my rainbow: Adventures in raising a fabulous, gender creative son.* Broadway Books.

Erickson-Schroth, L. (Ed.). (2022). *Trans bodies, trans selves: A resource by and for transgender communities.* Oxford University Press.

Feinberg, L. (1996). *Transgender warriors: Making history from Joan of Arc to Rupaul.* Beacon Press.

Feinberg, L. (1999). *Trans liberation: Beyond pink or blue.* Beacon Press.

Feinberg, L. (2004). *Stone butch blues* (3rd printing). Alyson Publications. (Categorized as "fiction," reads like a memoir).

Green, E., & Maurer, L. (2015). *The teaching transgender toolkit.* Planned Parenthood of the Southern Finger Lakes.

Iantaffi, A. (2017). *How to understand your gender: A practical guide for exploring who you are.* Jessica Kingsley Publishers.

Lev, A. I., & Gottlieb, A. R. (2019). *Families in transition: Parent perspectives on raising gender diverse children, adolescents, and young adults.* Harrington Park Press

Rajunov, M., & Duane, A. S. (2019). *Nonbinary: Memoirs of gender and identity.* Columbia University Press.

Sennott, S. L. (2011). Gender disorder as gender oppression: A transfeminist approach to rethinking the pathologization of gender non-conformity. *Women & Therapy, 34,* 93–113.

Shlasko, D. (2017). *Trans allyship workbook: Building skills to support trans people in our lives.* Think Again Training.

Singh, A. A., & Dickey, L. M. (2017). Affirmative counseling with transgender and gender nonconforming clients. In K. A. DeBord, A. R. Fischer, K. J. Bieschke, & R. M. Perez (Eds.), *Handbook of sexual orientation and gender diversity in counseling and psychotherapy* (pp. 157–182). American Psychological Association. https://doi.org/10.1037/15959-007

Snorton, C. R. (2017). *Black on both sides: A racial history of trans identity.* University of Minnesota Press.

Stryker, S. (2017). *Transgender history: The roots of today's revolution.* Seal Press.

Wilchins, R. (2017). *TRANS/gressive: How transgender activists took on gay rights, feminism, the media, congress...and won!* Riverdale Avenue Books.

Body Image

Bacon, L. (2010). *Health at every size: The surprising truth about your weight, revised and updated.* Benbella Books. (My "go to" book for clients struggling with weight-related self-esteem issues.)

Queen, C. (2013). *Exhibitionism for the shy* (2nd ed.). Down There Press. (First edition published 1995)

Age-Appropriate Sex and Sexuality Development Books for Children

Harris, R., & Emberley, M. (1999, 2014). *It's so amazing!: A book about eggs, sperm, birth, babies, and families.* Candlewick Press.

Saltz, G., & Cravath, L. A. (2008). *Amazing you: Getting smart about your private parts.* Puffin Books.

Sanders, J. (2016). *My body! What I say goes!: A book to empower and teach children about personal body safety, feelings, safe and unsafe touch, private parts, secrets and surprises, consent, and respectful relationships.* Educate2Empower Publishing.

Silverberg, C., & Smyth, F. (2018). *What makes a baby.* Triangle Square.

Spelman, C. M., & Weidner, T. (1997). *Your body belongs to you.* Albert Whitman and Co.

Age-Appropriate Sex and Sexuality Development Books for Teens

Corinna, H. (2016). *S.E.X.: The all-you-need-to-know sexuality guide to get you through your teens and twenties,* second edition. De Capo Lifelong Books.

Hasler, N. (2010). *SEX: A book for teens.* Zest Books.

Lang, J. (2018). *Consent: The new rules of sex education: Every teen's guide to healthy sexual relationships.* Althea Press.

Planned Parenthood. (2019). *In case you're curious: Questions about sex from young people with answers from the experts.* Viva Editions.

Sex Education Resource Books for Parents and Caregivers

Brand, A. (2021). *Stop sweating and start talking: How to make sex chats with your kids easier than you think.* Wise Ink Creative Publishing.

Sex and Aging

Brick, P., Lunquist, J., Sandak, A., & Taverner, B. (2009). *Older, wiser, sexually smarter: 30 sex ed lessons for adults only.* Planned Parenthood of Greater Northern New Jersey.

Doll, G. A. (2012). *Sexuality and long-term care: Understanding and supporting the needs of older adults.* Health Professions Press.

Price, J. (2006). *Better than I ever expected: Straight talk about sex after sixty.* Seal Press.

Price, J. (2011). *Naked at our age: Talking out loud about senior sex.* Seal Press.

Price, J. (2014). *The ultimate guide to sex after 50.* Cleis Press.

Sex and Cultural and Racial Diversity

Boykin, K. (2005). *Beyond the down-low: Sex, lies, and denial in black America.* Carroll and Graff.

Carol, J. (2009). *Sexuality now: Embracing diversity.* Cengage Learning.

King, J. L. (2004). *On the down low: A journey into the lives of straight Black men who sleep with men.* Broadway Books.

Moultrie, M. (2017). *Passionate and pious: Religious media and black women's sexuality.* Duke University Press.

Myers, N. J. (2003). *Black hearts: The development of black sexuality in America.* Trafford Publishing.

Staples, R. (2006). *Exploring black sexuality.* Rowman and Littlefield Publishers.

Sex and Disabilities

Buehler, S. (2011). *Sex, love, and mental illness: A couple's guide to staying connected.* Praeger.

Katz, A. (2009). *Sex when you're sick: Reclaiming sexual health after illness or injury.* Praeger.

Kaufman, M., Silverberg, C., & Odette, F. (2007). *The ultimate guide to sex and disability.* Cleis Press.

Kroll, K., & Klein, E. L. (2001). *Enabling romance: A guide to love, sex, and relationships for people with disabilities (and the people who care about them).* United Spinal Association.

McRuer, R., & Mollow, A. (Eds.). 2012. *Sex and disability.* Duke University Press.

Schovr, L., & Jensen, S. (1988). *Sexuality and chronic illness: A comprehensive approach.* Guilford Press.

Sex and Spirituality

Bolz-Weber, N. (2019). *Shameless: A sexual reformation.* Convergent Books.

Brownson, J. V. (2015). *Reframing the church's debate of same sex relationships.* Erdmanns.

Klein, L. K. (2018). *Pure: Inside the evangelical movement that shamed generations of young women and how I broke free.* Atria Books and Simon and Shuster.

Seller, T. (2017). *Sex, god, and the conservative church: Erasing shame from sexual intimacy.* Routledge.

Stayton, W. (2020). *Sinless sex: A challenge to religions.* Luminare Press.

Committed (Mostly Monogamous) Relationships, Affairs, and Sexual Health

Perel, E. (2009). *Mating in captivity: Unlocking erotic intelligence.* Harper Collins.

Perel, E. (2017). *The state of affairs: Rethinking infidelity.* Harper Collins.

Schnarch, D. (2011). *Intimacy and desire: Awaken the passion in your relationship.* Beaufort Books.

Schnarch, D. (2011). *Passionate marriage: Keeping love and intimacy alive in committed relationships.* Beaufort Books.

Polyamory, Open Relationships, and Consensual Non-Monogamy

Easton, D. (2009). *The ethical slut: A practical guide to polyamory, open relationships, and other adventures.* Celestial Arts.

Fern, J. (2020). *Polysecure: Attachment, trauma and consensual nonmonogamy.* Thorntree Press.

Labriola, K. (2013). *The jealousy workbook: Exercises and insights for managing open relationships.* Greenery Press.

Sheff, E. (2013). *The polyamorists next door.* Rowman & Littlefield.

Sheff, E., & Wolf, T. (2015). *Stories from the polycule.* Thorntree Press.

Taormino, T. (2008). *Opening up: A guide to creating and sustaining open relationships.* Cleis Press.

Veaux, F., & Rickert, E. (2014). *More than two: A practical guide to ethical polyamory.* Thorntree Press.

Wolf, T. (2016). *Ask me about polyamory: The best of kimchi cuddles.* Thorntree Press.

BDSM/Kink-Related Lay and Professional Books

Bader, M. J. (2002). *Arousal: The secret logic of sexual fantasies*. Thomas Dunne Books.

Baldwin, G. (2003). *Ties that bind: SM/leather/fetish/erotic style: Issues, commentary, and advice* (2nd ed.). Daedalus Publishing Company.

Beckmann, A. (2009). *The social construction of sexuality and perversion: Deconstructing sadomasochism*. Palgrave Macmillan.

Brame, G. G., Brame, W. D., & Jacobs, J. (1993). *Different loving: The world of sexual dominance and submission*. Villard Books.

Easton, D., & Liszt, C. A. (2000). *When someone you love is kinky*. Greenery Press.

Harrington, L. (2009). *Sacred kink*. Mystic Productions, LLC.

Kaldrea, R., & Tenpenny, J. (2009). *Dear Raven and Joshua: Questions and answers about master/slave relationships*. Alfred Press.

Kleinplatz, P., & Moser, C. (Eds.). (2006). *Sadomasochism: Powerful pleasures*. Harrington Park Press.

Langdridge, D., & Marker, M. (Eds.). (2007). *Safe, sane, and consensual: Contemporary perspectives on sadomasochism*. Palgrave Macmillan.

Midori. (2005). *Wild side sex: The book of kink: Educational, sensual, and entertaining essays*. Daedalus Publishing.

Newmahr, S. (2011). *Playing on the edge: Sadomasochism, risk, and intimacy*. Indiana University Press.

Sadie, S. (Ed.). (2007) *Spiritual transformation through BDSM: Stories and submissions from fellow travellers*. Ephemera Bound Publishing.

Stein, D., & Schachter, D. (2009). *Ask the man who owns him: The real lives of gay masters and slaves*. Perfectbound Press.

Thompson, M. (Ed.). (2004). *Leatherfolk: Radical sex, people, politics, and practice* (3rd ed.). Daedalus.

BDSM/KINK Beginner's Manuals

Bannon, R. (1993). *Learning the ropes: A basic guide to safe and fun S/M lovemaking*. Daedalus Publishing Company.

Califia, P. (2001). *Sensuous magic: A guide to S/M for adventurous couples* (2nd ed.). Cleis Press.

Easton, D., & Hardy, J. W. (2001). *The new bottoming book*. Greenery Press.

Easton, D., & Hardy, J. W. (2003). *The new topping book*. Greenery Press.

Green, L. (1998). *The sexually dominant woman: A workbook for nervous beginners* (2nd ed.). Greenery Press.

Henkin, W. A., & Holiday, S. (2003). *Consensual sadomasochism: How to talk about it & how to do it safely* (2nd ed.). Daedalus Publishing Company.

Jacques, T., Dale, D., Hamilton, M., & Sniffer. (1993). *On the safe edge: A manual for SM play*. Whole SM Publishing Corporation.

Ortman, D. M., & Sprott, R. A. (2013). *Sexual outsiders: Understanding BDSM sexualities and communities*. Rowman & Littlefield Publishers.

Rinella, J. (2004). *The complete slave: Creating and living an erotic dominant/submissive lifestyle* (2nd ed.). Daedalus Publishing Company.

Taormino, T. (2012). *The ultimate guide to kink*. Cleis Press.
Taormino, T. (2013). *50 shades of kink: An introduction to BDSM*. Cleis Press.
Varrin, C. (2004). *Female dominance: Rituals and practice*. Citadel Publishing.
Warren, J. (2000). *The loving dominant* (2nd ed.). Greenery Press.

Out of Control Sexual Behavior

Braun-Harvey, D., & Vigorito, M. (2016) *Treating out of control sexual behavior: Rethinking sex addiction*. Springer Publishing Company.

Pornography and Sex-Work History and Activism

Delacoste, F. (1998). *Sex work: Writings by women in the sex industry* (2nd ed.). Cleis Press.
Ley, D. (2016). *Ethical porn for dicks: A man s guide to responsible viewing pleasure*. ThreeL Media.
Rogers, V. (2016). *We need to talk about pornography: A resource to educate young people about the potential impact of pornography and sexualized images on relationships body image and self-esteem*. Jessica Kingsley Publishers.
Smith, M., & Mac, J. (2018). *Revolting prostitutes: The fight for sex workers' rights*. Verso.
Taormino, T. (2002). *True lust: Adventures in sex, porn, and perversion*. Cleis Press.
Taormino, T., Perrenas-Shimzu, C. Penley, C., & Miller-Young, M. (Eds.). (2013). *The feminist porn book: The politics of producing pleasure*. The Feminist Press.

Sex-Positive Erotic Fiction Books

Brent, B., & Queen, C. (2000). *Best bisexual erotica*. Black Books.
Bright, S. (1997–2003). *Best American erotica* (Annual Series). Touchstone.
Califa, P. (1988). *Macho sluts*. Alyson Publications.
Foster, E. (2016). *How not to fall* (Belhaven series). Kensington. (These are written by a sex educator ["Emily Foster" is the author's nom de plume for this series] and portray sex-positive hot depictions of feminist cis-gender heterosexual erotic interactions, from accurate naming of body parts, to realistic descriptions of the nuances of sexual desire and interest. Anyone with a geeky bent will also enjoy the neurophysiological terms scattered throughout. This series deliberately counteracts the misinformation and harmful stereotype perpetuations in the *50 Shades of Grey* series.)
Herotica series (feminist erotica series from 1993 to 2003), often edited by Susie Bright or Marcy Sheiner. Down There Press.
Kwon, R. O., & Greenwell, G. (2021). *Kink stories*. Simon and Shuster.
Queen, C., & Schimel, L. (1996). *Switch hitters: Lesbians write gay erotica and gay men write lesbian erotica*. Cleis Press.
Rosen, R. (2018). *Best gay erotica of the year, Volume 4*. Down There Press.
Sexsmith, S. (2021). *Best lesbian erotica of the year, volume 6*. Cleis Press.
Taormino, T. (2011). *Sometimes she lets me: Best butch/femme erotica*. Cleis Press.
Taormino, T. (2011). *Take me there: Trans and genderqueer erotica*. Cleis Press.

Sexual Health Training Programs

Organizations Offering Sexual Health and Sexuality-Related Workshops, CEUs, and Professional Training

- *American Association of Sexuality Educators, Counselors, and Therapists* (AASECT) www.aasect.org: Annual conference, trainings.
- *The Center for Sexual Pleasure and Health* www.thecsph.org: Providence, Rhode Island: Offers sexual health trainings, workshops and information. CSPH offers the mandatory Sexual Attitude Reassessment (SAR) class for proceeding with any kind of sex educator or counselor certification.
- *Integrative Psychiatry and Sexuality Counseling Associates* www.thriveintegrativepsych.com: Evelyn Resh, CSC, CNM, MPH, MSN, and associates provide medical and psychiatric consultation, treatment, and trainings.
- *Institute for Sexuality Education and Enlightenment* (ISEE at instituteforsexuality.com): Offers dozens of webinars related to a multitude of sexuality and sexual health topics. In-person trainings are generally offered a couple times of year in Massachusetts and Oregon. ISEE offers the mandatory Sexual Attitude Reassessment (SAR) class for proceeding with any kind of sex educator or counselor certification.
- *NSTA* www.northamptonsextherapy.com: Jassy Casella Timberlake, LMFT provides sex therapy and supervision and has a wealth of experience informed by decades of work.
- *Safer Society* safersocietypress.org: Mission is to provide services and resources for preventative and restorative responses to sexual and social violence.
- *Society for Sex Therapy and Research* www.sstarnet.org: International organization lists sex therapists, sex researchers, and has an annual conference.
- *South Shore Sexual Health Center* www.sssexualhealthcenter.com (Massachusetts): Offers sexual health and sex therapy supervision, consultation, classes, trainings, workshops, and events, etc. Offers the mandatory Sexual Attitude Reassessment (SAR) class.
- *Stop it now! Stopitnow.org*: Offers child sexual abuse prevention trainings.
- www.Ourshine.org (Ashley Mader, PhD): Provides consultation, trainings, and workshops related to aging and sexuality. Sex therapist specializing in older adults and aging. Provides consultation and general sex therapy and education trainings and consultation. Former co-host of podcast on sex and aging "Our Better Half."

Sexuality-Related Educational Certificates and Programs

Institute for Sexuality Education and Enlightenment (ISEE): Certification Programs in Sex Educator, Sex Counselor, AASECT-Approved Sex Therapist, and an ACES certificate (Advancing Clinical Excellence in Sexuality), instituteforsexuality.com

Institute of Somatic Sexology https://instituteofsomaticsexology.com/courses/certificate-in-sexological-bodywork

The Masters & Johnson Institute, St. Louis, Missouri: Does not have an academic program, but provides training programs involving workshops and, through special arrangements, practicum in residence that focus on recovery from sexual trauma.

Robert Wood Johnson Medical School, Piscataway, New Jersey: Post-graduate training in relationship and sex therapy. Offers a week-long sexuality course (40 hours) that's not offered by any other program (counts as graduate credit if individual writes a paper).

Rutgers University—Post-Graduate Training Program in Sex Therapy—Department of Psychiatry/Medical School, Piscataway, New Jersey: Hosts a 10-month course, which meets for 2 hours on a weekly basis. Covers both assessment and treatment of all sexual dysfunctions. The second semester of the course offers supervision of participants' cases.

Southern Connecticut State University, New Haven, Connecticut: Graduate course in Human Sexuality, including a 15-hour SAR.

Sex Educator Training Programs

Institute for Sexuality Education and Enlightenment (ISEE): Certification Program in Sex Educator (instituteforsexuality.com).

Our Whole Lives (OWL) Sexuality Education Curricula (uua.org/re/owl): "Honest, accurate information about sexuality changes lives. It dismantles stereotypes and assumptions, builds self-acceptance and self-esteem, fosters healthy relationships, improves decision-making, and has the potential to save lives. For these reasons and more, we are proud to offer Our Whole Lives (OWL), a comprehensive, lifespan sexuality education curricula for use in both secular settings and faith communities." (uua.org/re/owl) Curricula covers grades K-1, 4–6, 7–9, 10–12, Young Adult, Adult, and Older Adult. Most recent publications include: Davis, Melanie (2019). *Our whole lives: Sexuality education for older adults.* UUA and deFur, K., & Johnson, A. (2017). *Our whole lives, second edition: Sexuality education for grades 4–6.* UUA.

Planned Parenthood: https://www.plannedparenthood.org/learn/for-educators: Planned Parenthood is the largest provider of sex education in the United States. Each state-affiliated Planned Parenthood offers various trainings for professionals and sex educators. For example, here is information on trainings in Massachusetts: https://www.plannedparenthood.org/planned-parenthood-massachusetts/local-training-education/professionals.

Graduate Level Sexuality Programs

American Academy of Clinical Sexologists[2] Maimonides University, North Miami, Florida. PhD inpastoral clinical sexology. Prepares students for sex therapy certification in Florida (a requirement in Florida if wanting to practice in this statestate). Emphasizes the importance of religion in providing therapy.

Columbia University – Mailman School of Public Health[1] New York, New York; MPH in sexuality and health. Equips students with skills needed to address health issues, for example, reproductive health, and child and adolescent health, related to sexuality through interdepartmental studies. (Note: Students applying for the program are expected to have worked for 2 years in the field of public health, which can include undergraduate volunteer/practicum experiences.)

Hofstra University – Interdisciplinary Studies/Marriage & Family Counseling[2] New York, New york. MA in interdisciplinary studies/marriage and family counseling (plus family counseling certification. Provides skills needed for marriage/family counseling and introduces students to sexuality education, counseling and research.

Indiana University – Kinsey Institute[1] Bloomington, Indiana.PhD minor in human sexuality; majors include counseling, education, health behavior, psychology, and sociology. Offers research programs investigating a variety of sex topics and a summer institute for students who are not involved with the university. Houses one of the largest library holdings on human sexuality, as well as a sexuality art museum. Hosts seminars on sexuality and holds special events.

Institute for Advanced Study of Human Sexuality[3] San Francisco, California. MA, MPH, EdD, PhD, DHS (Doctor of Human Sexuality), plus certification options – human sexuality. Seeks to train sexologists. Offers long-distance learning. Certificate programs are unique to the Institute, for example, erotology. Also, the master's program allows students to travel to Paris or China for a cultural perspective on public health.

San Francisco State University Program in Human Sexuality[1] San Francisco, California. MA in human sexuality. Provides a foundation for sex counseling, teaching, and research. Specializes in gay, lesbian, and bisexual studies. Houses the Institute on Sexuality, Social Inequality, and Health, the National Sexuality Resource Center, and the Center for Research on Gender and Sexuality, plus has a summer institute.

University of Connecticut – Center for HIV Intervention & Prevention – Psychology Department[1] Storrs, Connecticut. MA, PhD in social psychology with a specialization in HIV prevention. Conducts HIV risk dynamics and prevention research.

Chapter 11 Sexual Health Resources for EMDR Therapists

University of Guelph – Department of Family Relations & Applied Nutrition[1,2] Guelph, Ontario, Canada. MSc in couple and family therapy; PhD in family relations and human development. Emphasizes child/adolescent development, social/personality development, parent-child relations, social gerontology, human sexuality, and marriage/family therapy.

University of Hawaii – Human Sexuality Program – Department of Social Work; Pacific Center for Sex and Society - Department of Anatomy and Reproductive Biology[1,2] Honolulu, Hawaii. MA, PhD specializes in human sexuality counseling. Houses the Pacific Center for Sex and Society, which provides research opportunities.

University of Minnesota – Department of Family Social Science[1,2] St. Paul, Minnesota. MA, PhD in family social science; MFT certification for clinical track. Specializes in marriage/family and sex therapy.

University of New Brunswick – Department of Psychology[1,2] Fredericton, New Brunswick, Canada. PhD in psychology. Prepares students for clinical or experimental psychology involving human sexuality.

University of Quebec – Department of Sexology[2] Montreal, Quebec, Canada. BA, MA in sexology. Focuses on sex education. Master's level encompasses sex therapy and research, plus more advanced sex education.

University of Utah – Department of Psychology[1,2] Salt Lake City, Utah. PhD in clinical psychology. Emphasizes human sexuality in research and clinical work.

University of Wisconsin – Departments of Psychology & Sociology[1] Madison, Wisconsin. PhD in psychology or sociology. Focuses on human sexuality, especially sex research. Part of a consortium where a student may study at University of Chicago, University of Minnesota or Wisconsin.

Widener University – Human Sexuality Program[2] Wayne, Pennsylvania. MEd, EdD in human sexuality education/clinical sexuality. Prepares professionals for sex education, consulting, research, and counseling. Also offers joint degree programs with Social work or Clinical Psychology. Program is both distance and work friendly in that human sexuality courses are offered on weekends. One semester course is generally two weekends. Also provides opportunity to study abroad.

[1] Program reflecting training primarily as a researcher
[2] Program reflecting a practitioner model/clinical skills.
[3] Program reflecting general sexology.

Internship and Post-Doctoral Programs

University of California – Center for AIDS Prevention Studies San Francisco, California. Grants traineeships in AIDS Prevention Studies.

University of Minnesota – Department of Family Practice & Community Health Minneapolis, Minnesota. Fellowships in human sexuality, dysfunction and disease prevention for post-doctorates in clinical psychology. Conducts sexuality research, provides sex education, offers clinical services for sexual and relationship problems, and promotes community sexual health via community health initiatives. Houses the Center for Sexual Health and the Center for HIV/STI Intervention & Prevention Studies.

SUMMARY

Thank you for showing curiosity, courage, intention, and personal and professional growth in the face of our continuing erotophobic culture by obtaining and reading this book. If this is your first official/professional foray into increasing sexual health knowledge and competence, then I thank you deeply for choosing this book as your jumping off point. If this is not your first rodeo in this arena, then I certainly welcome any and all feedback to improve this book as a whole (including this chapter).

I sincerely hope that all the material encountered in this book, while hopefully satisfying immediate questions and clinical dilemmas (particularly regarding the integration of EMDR therapy and sexual health), also leave you with an overwhelming thirst and hunger for the continued pursuit, digestion, and application of positive sexual health, sexual pleasure principles, and inalienable sexual rights. If this book has indeed properly done its job to whet your whistle, then may this last Resource Chapter encourage a fun, dynamic, and pleasurable lifelong sexual health knowledge acquisition. Engaging and positive resources for everyone (and just about every kind of learner) under the sun is listed in this chapter. May these recommended podcasts, TED Talks, websites, books, and educational programs bring hope and clarity to you and your clients.

Lastly, as mentioned in the chapter introduction, sexual health information can change quickly. Always strive to find the most updated website, book, TED Talk, and so on, to share with clients.

Now, boldly go forth armed and ready to share more sexual health knowledge than 99% of the U.S. population!

Index

AASECT. *See* American Association of Sexuality Educators, Counselors and Therapists
ableism, 219
abortion, 41
ACEs. *See* adverse childhood experiences
Adaptive Information Processing (AIP) Model, 15–16, 269
Adolescent-Dissociative Experiences Scale, 103
adverse childhood experiences (ACEs), 232, 234
AFAB. *See* assigned-female-at-birth
Affect Bridge, 103–104
ageism, 256–257, 259
aging, 244
  books, 310
  EMDR and, 260–261
    case study, 261–262
  and health care providers, 259–260
  history of, 244
  LGBTQ, 253–255
  loss of a partner, 257–259
  men, sexual health of
    benign prostate hypertrophy, 252
    body image, 252–253
    ejaculation, 251–252
    erections, 249–251
    sexual desire, 251
  older adult sexuality experiences, 244–245
  relationship of older adults
    family influence, 257–258
    in nursing homes, 258, 259
  resources, 297–298
  Sexually Transmitted Infections, 245
  social influence on, 256–257
  stereotypes, 256–257
  transgender, 254–255
  women, sexual health of
    body image, 249
    hysterectomies and oophorectomies, 247–249
    menopause, 246–247
AIP. *See* Adaptive Information Processing Model
Akwafina is Nora from Queens (TV series), 302
aloe vera, 46
AMAB. *See* assigned-male-at-birth
Amaze.org, 297
ambiguous genitalia. *See* intersex
American Academy of Clinical Sexologists, 316
American Association of Sexuality Educators, Counselors and Therapists (AASECT), 8, 118–119, 144–145, 314
American Physical Therapist Association, 298
American Psychological Association (APA), 193, 213, 297

American Society for Reproductive Medicine, 206
American Society on Aging, 297
anal sex, 40, 46
anger, 174, 178
anticipatory anxiety, current sexual difficulties due to, 112–113
anti-depressants, impact on ejaculation, 251, 252
Antisocial Personality Disorder (APD), 233
APA. *See* American Psychological Association
APD. *See* Antisocial Personality Disorder
arousal, 41, 55, 63. *See also* desire
   clitoris during, 71
   disorders, 79–81
   dual control model, 42–43, 50, 55–57
   during EMDR sessions, 102–103, 105
   four-stage model of, 62
   and lubrication, 69
   sexual arousal template, 48
   in survivors of childhood abuse, 72
   willingness model, 42
arousal concordance, 44
arousal nonconcordance, 44, 50
asexuals, 196
assessment (EMDR phase 3), 109–110
assigned-female-at-birth (AFAB), 169
assigned-male-at-birth (AMAB), 169
assigned-sex-at-birth, 169
Association of Welcoming and Affirming Baptists, 301
Astroglide, 45
audio bilateral stimulation, 32, 147
audio porn, 144, 164
avocado oil, 46
Avodart, 252

Babes in Toyland, 299
Baby Boomers, 244–245, 253
Backdoor balm, 46
bacterial vaginosis, 86
Badvibes.org website, 45
Bancroft, John, 42, 50, 55
barium rings, 40
Basson, Rosemary, 41, 56, 63–64, 79

BDSM, 224, 237
   beginner's manuals, 241, 312–313
   books, 312
   case study, 227–228
   consent in, 226–227
   risk-aware consensual kink, 226
   safe, sane, and consensual, 226
   websites, 301
benign prostate hypertrophy (BPH), 252
Better Health Channel, 222
bilateral stimulation (BLS), 15, 18, 32, 105, 108, 109, 110, 111, 118, 129, 147, 275, 280, 281, 288
BioDigital Human, 296
bi.org, 299
birth control sponges, 41
Bisexual, The (TV series), 302
Bisexual Resource Center, 299
bisexuality, 194–195, 308
BLS. *See* bilateral stimulation
body dysmorphic disorder, 139
body image, 139–141, 205, 209
   of aging men, 252–253
   of aging women, 249
   books, 309
body scan (EMDR phase 6), 111, 185
bondage, BDSM, 225
Boston Public Health Commission, 143, 163
botulinum toxin type A injections, for dyspareunia, 86
BPH. *See* benign prostate hypertrophy
breasts, 32, 35
Bridgerton (TV series), 302
Bright, Susie, 5, 298
Broad City (TV series), 302
bubble/shield boundary resource, 106–107, 127
Burke, Tarana, 5
butterfly hug tapping, 32, 147
Bwom app, 303

calm place, 105, 274–275
CBT. *See* cognitive-behavioral therapy
Center for Sexual Pleasure and Health, The (CSPH), 314

central nervous system, 42–43, 55
cerebral palsy, 220–221
cervical cancer, 85
cervical caps, 41
cervix, 32
CETs. *See* core erotic themes
childbirth, 86, 203–204
children
    adverse childhood experiences, 232, 234
    books for, 309–310
    child sexual abusers, 233, 234
    childhood sexual abuse, 72, 124, 136, 140, 178, 232–233, 237
    exposure to pornography, 145–147
circles of sexuality, 11, 12, 16–17, 115–116
cisgender, 169
client history (EMDR phase 1), 103–104
clitoris, 30
    clitoral orgasm, 32, 82, 153
    clitoral stimulation, 82
    nonerect, 70
    during sexual arousal, 71
closure (EMDR phase 7), 111–112
Clue Period and Health Tracker app, 303
CNM. *See* consensual non-monogamy
cognitive distortions, 234
cognitive interweaves, 173, 174, 178, 276
cognitive restructuring, 80
cognitive-behavioral therapy (CBT), 73–74
    for desire disorders, 78
    for dyspareunia, 86
Columbia University, 316
Come as You Are Workbook, The: A Practical Guide to the Science of Sex (Nagoski), 43, 81, 153
comfortable place, 274
common humanity, 108, 128
communication
    deficits, 75, 76
    of sexual concerns, between health care providers and older adults, 260
    training, 80
compersion, 200
condoms, 40, 41
Conference Room/Meeting Place, 124

consensual non-monogamy (CNM), 200–201, 202–203, 301, 311
consent, sexual, 6–7, 21–22, 25, 175, 258
    in kink/BDSM, 226–290
    resources, 296
container exercise, 105–106
    self-compassion container, 107–109, 128–129
conversion therapy, 193
Coping With Erectile Dysfunction (Metz & McCarthy), 80, 154
Coping With Premature Ejaculation (Metz & McCarthy), 83
core erotic themes (CETs), 48, 49, 225, 229
corpus cavernosum, 37
corpus spongiosum, 37
corrective sexual education, 67–71
couples-based sex therapy, 63, 75–77, 87
CravEx Protocol, 119
CSPH. *See* Center for Sexual Pleasure and Health, The
cultural competence, 9, 218
cultural humility, 218
culture, 17
    construct of sexuality, 62
    and desire disorders, 78
    expectations
        of men, 176, 177
        of women, 172, 174
    and gender, 168
    and menopause, 247
    and sexual health, 5–6
    sexual myths, 68
    victim blaming, 172

dating, 116–117
Declaration of Sexual Pleasure, 4, 24–25
Declaration of Sexual Rights, 3, 24
deep breathing, 85
dehydroepiandrosterone (DHEA) cream, 40
delayed ejaculation, 83–84, 251
dementia, and sexual consent, 258
demisexuals, 196–197, 198
dental dams, 40
Department of Defense, 177

depression, 117–118
desensitization (EMDR phase 4), 110
desire, 41, 55, 63. *See also* arousal
   and aging
      men, 251
      women, 246, 249
   disorders, 78–79
   dual control model, 42–43, 50, 55–57
   impact of relational factors on, 78–79
   responsive, 41–42, 50, 56, 79
   spontaneous, 41, 42, 50, 56, 79
   willingness model, 42
DeTUR (Desensitization of Triggers and Urge Reprocessing) Protocol, 119
Developmental Needs Meeting System (DNMS), 124, 236
DHEA. *See* dehydroepiandrosterone cream
Diagnostic and Statistical Manual (DSM-5), 78, 84, 229, 233
diaphragms, 41
DignityUSA, 301
directed masturbation, 81, 82
disabilities, people with. *See* marginalized populations
discipline, BDSM, 225
disgust, 174–175
dissociation, 103
   Conference Room/Meeting Place, 124
   Developmental Needs Meeting System, 124
   and gender dysphoria, 183–184
   management of, 123–124
Dissociative Experiences Scale, 103
Dissociative Experiences Scale II, 183
Diverse Elders Coalition, 299
DNMS. *See* Developmental Needs Meeting System
Dodson, Betty, 31, 32, 298
domination, BDSM, 225
Drawn to Sex (Moen & Nolan), 221
DSM-5. *See* Diagnostic and Statistical Manual
dual control model of sexual response, 42–43, 50, 55–57
dyspareunia, 84, 86

EAP. *See* Employee Assistance Programs
early ejaculation. *See* premature ejaculation
eating disorders, 139
ecstasy, 279–281
ED. *See* erectile dysfunction
edgeplay, 226
egg whites, 46
ejaculation, 152
   changes, and aging, 251–252
   delayed, 83–84, 251
   premature, 83, 112
   retrograde, 251
embryonic development, 28
EMDR. *See* Eye Movement Desensitization and Reprocessing
EMDR International Association (EMDRIA), 193, 213
EMDR Sexual Dysfunction Protocol, 102, 137
EMDRIA. *See* EMDR International Association
emotions, 13, 124, 224
   emotional intimacy, 41, 43, 56, 261–262
   and men, 177–178
   and TGNC people, 182–183
   and women, 173–176
Employee Assistance Programs (EAP), 177
endometriosis, 86
enlarged prostate. *See* benign prostate hypertrophy (BPH)
erectile dysfunction (ED), 80–81, 143, 164, 249–251
erikalust.com, 303
erotic fiction books, sex-positive, 313
erotic templates, 48–49, 50
erotically marginalized populations, 224, 237
   fetishes and paraphilias, 228–229
   kink/BDSM, 224, 225
      consent in, 226–227
   trauma reenactment *vs.* trauma play, 224–225
erotophobia, 5, 6, 136
estrogen, 39–40, 246–247
estrogen creams, 247, 248

Index

ethical pornography, 142, 144, 163, 164, 303
ETR (Education, Training and Research), 11
Eve app, 303
excitement (sexual arousal), 41, 62
extended orgasm, 153
external urethral orifice, 29
Eye Movement Desensitization and Reprocessing (EMDR), 2, 14–15, 17–18, 30, 31, 32, 125
  assessment, 109–110
  body scan, 111
  client history and treatment planning, 103–104
  closure, 111–112
  and cultural/individual factors interfering sexual health, 5–6
  current sexual difficulties due to anticipatory anxiety, 112–113
  desensitization, 110
  erotic templates, 48–49, 50
  future templates, 48, 112, 116, 117, 118, 132–138, 141, 154, 178
    sexual health, 133–138
  guidelines for working with sexual dysfunction clients, 102–103
  increasing sexuality-related self-esteem with, 140–141
  installation, 111
  with men, 176–179
  negative sexual socialization/lack of sexuality education, targets related to, 16
  and pornography, 144–145
    case studies, 145–147
  preparation and resourcing, 105–107
  protocol, 102–113
  re-evaluation, 112
  related to dual control model, 43
  sexual health case studies, 115–118
  sexual health targets
    past targets, 114
    present targets, 114
  sexual trauma survivors, 74
  and SOCE, 193–194, 213
  Strengthening a Confident and Joyful Sexual Self resource, 140, 147–151, 154, 157–159
  with TGNC people, 179–186
  with women, 171–176

Faithfully LGBT, 301
family planning clinics, 40
fanfair.info, 301
Feeling State Addiction Protocol (FSAP), 119–123, 144
female genital mutilation (FGM), 30
female orgasmic disorder, 81–82
Female Sexual Arousal Disorder (FSAD), 79–80
female sexuality, myths about, 68
female-identified sex offenders, 232
feminism, 5
feminist sex therapy, 63–65
fertility, 203–207, 209–210, 214
fetishes, 228–229, 237
fetishflea.com, 301
FetLife.com, 301
FGM. See female genital mutilation
float-back technique, 103–104
fluid-bonded relationship, 200
FOSTA law, 229
4-Dimensional Wheel of sexual health (Ogden), 13–15, 17–18, 116
frenulum, 36
Freud, Sigmund, 171, 176
FRIES (Freely, Reversible, Informed, Enthusiastic, Specific), 7, 21–22, 25
FSAD. See Female Sexual Arousal Disorder
FSAP. See Feeling State Addiction Protocol
future templates, EMDR, 48, 112, 116, 117, 118, 132, 141, 154, 178
  infertility, 206
  script, 133
  sexual health, 133–134
    case studies, 134–138
  spirituality, 277

GAB. *See* Global Advisory Board for Sexual Health and Wellbeing
Gage, Suzann, 70
gender, 165–167, 186
   bias, 173
   educational and information websites, 300
   -inclusive intake questions, 181
   inequality, and orgasm gap, 66
   language related to, 168–169
   men, EMDR with, 176–179
   and pregnancy loss, 208
   self-reflection, 170–171
   vs. sex, 167–168
   as a social construct, 167, 168
   TGNC people, EMDR with, 179–186
   women, EMDR with, 171–176
gender binary, 169
gender dysphoria, 183–184, 185, 186
gender identity, 165, 167, 169
gender nonconforming, 169
gender presentation/expression, 169
gender pronouns, 169, 181
Gender Unicorn, 195
genital numbness, 31
Genito-Pelvic Pain/Penetration disorder (GPPPD), 84
ghee butter, 46
Global Advisory Board for Sexual Health and Wellbeing (GAB), 4
GLSEN.org, 299
Go Ask Alice, 297
Good Clean Love, 45
good sex, conditions for, 71–72
Goodvibes.com, 299
Gottman Card Decks app, 303
Gottman Institute, 143, 163–164
GPPPD. *See* Genito-Pelvic Pain/Penetration disorder
Grace and Frankie (TV series), 302
graduate level sexuality programs, 316–317
gratitude, 275
greysexuals, 196
grief, 282–284
   and infertility, 207
   and pregnancy loss, 209, 210
G-spot area, 34

Handbook for EMDR Clients (Luber), 103
Healing Circle, 124, 236
healing from trauma, phases of, 4
health care providers, and aging sexual health, 259–260
health insurance, 172, 180
Hebrew Home Nursing Home, 258
heteronormativity, 200
Highlander Research and Education Center, 299
hippocampus, 74
HIV, 40
Hofstra University, 316
hormone replacement therapy (HRT), 186, 246–247
hot flash, 246
HRT. *See* hormone replacement therapy
HSDD. *See* hypoactive sexual desire disorder
Human Rights Campaign, 299
humectants, 45
hymen, 33
hypoactive sexual desire disorder (HSDD), 78, 79
hysterectomy, 247–249
hysteria, 171

ID. *See* intellectual disabilities, people with
inclusivity, 11
Indiana University, 316
infertility, 204. *See also* pregnancy loss
   and body image, 205
   grief, 207
   negative cognitions, 205–206
   partner relationship system concerning, 205
   preparation and resources, 206
   questionnaire, 207
   reassessment and EMDR future templates, 206
Infertility Protocol with EMDR, 204–207, 214
infidelity, 202–203, 301
informed consent, 103
inhibited ejaculation. *See* delayed ejaculation

Insecure (TV series), 302
installation (EMDR phase 5), 111
Institute for Advanced Study of Human Sexuality, 316
Institute for Sexuality Education and Enlightenment (ISEE), 314, 315
Institute of Somatic Sexology, 315
Integrative Psychiatry and Sexuality Counseling Associates, 314
intellectual disabilities (ID), people with, 222
   EMDR for, 222–224
   sexual health rights for, 222
InterAct, 39
internalized ageism, 256, 259
internet pornography, 5, 48–49
internship and post-doctoral programs, 317–318
interpersonal violence
   against men, 178–179
   against women, 172, 173
intersex, 28–29, 38–39, 167, 300
Intersex Society of North America, 38
intimate justice, 22
ISEE. *See* Institute for Sexuality Education and Enlightenment

Janssen, Erick, 42, 50, 55
Johnson, Virginia E., 41, 55, 62, 75, 82, 83
Judd, Ashley, 5
justice, 11, 22

Kaplan, Helen Singer, 41, 55, 63
Kegel exercises, 35, 152
kink, 224, 237
   beginner's manuals, 241, 312–313
   books, 312
   consent in, 226–227
   websites, 301
kinkacademy.com, 301
Kinsey, Alfred, 41, 55, 194
Kinsey Scale, 194–195
Klein Sexual Orientation Grid, 195
Kort, Joe, 298

L Word: Generation Q (TV series), 302
labia, 31
labial fusion, 35
labiaplasty, 31
language, 192
   gender, 168–169, 208
   spiritual, 271
   and TGNC clients, 181–182, 185–186
laughter curtain, 256
Lesbian Hermstory Archives, 299
LGBTQ people, 194. *See also* marginalized populations; transgender and gender non-conforming (TGNC) people
   aging of, 253–255
   books, 307–308
   educational and information websites, 301
lightstream resource, 109
Loulan, Joanne, 42
lubrication, 50, 79
   oil-based, 46
   vaginal, 33–34, 44–46, 68–69
   water-based, 34, 40, 45, 246

MacLelland, Sarah, 22
Make Love Not Porn, 303
Making Gay History, 299
male sexuality, myths about, 68
male-identified sex offenders, 232, 234
Maltz, Wendy, 74–75
man-slut, 7, 21
manual sex, 41
marginalized populations, 217–218, 237. *See also* transgender and gender non-conforming (TGNC) people
   books, 310–311
   erotically, 224–229, 237
   intellectual disabilities, people with, 222–224
   neurodiverse populations, 221
   physically, 218–221
   principles to consider when working with, 218
   sex offenders, 232–236, 237
   sex work, 229–232, 237, 313

masochism, BDSM, 225
Master of None (TV series), 302
Masters, William H., 41, 55, 62, 75, 82, 83
Masters & Johnson Institute, The, 315
masturbation
   directed, 81, 82
   mutual, 41
   therapeutic, 153
medical trauma, 37
men
   aging, sexual health of
      benign prostate hypertrophy, 252
      body image, 252–253
      ejaculation, 251–252
      erections, 249
      sexual desire, 251
   EMDR with, 176
      access issues, 176–177
      emotional and behavioral considerations, 177–178
      interpersonal violence, 178–179
men who have sex with men (MSM), 194
menarche, 35
menopause, 35–36, 246–247
menstruation, 35
mental health professionals, 260
metaphors, 276
#metoo movement, 5, 6, 21
microaggressions, 192
microbicides, lubricants with, 45
mindfulness, 108, 128, 152–153
monogamy, 200
Motherland: Fort Salem (TV series), 302
Mrs. Fletcher (TV series), 302
MSM. *See* men who have sex with men
Multi-Orgasmic Man, The (Chia & Abrams), 154
Muslims for Progressive Values, 301
mutual masturbation, 41
My Sex Doctor app, 304

nagaimo, 46
Nagoski, Emily, 42–43, 55–56, 147, 153
NAMS. *See* North American Menopause Society

National Black Justice Coalition, 299
National Center for Transgender Equality, 299, 300
National Children's, 300
National Institute on Aging, 297
National LGBTQ Task Force, 300
National Resource Center on LGBT Aging, 300
National Vulvodynia Association, 298
NC. *See* negative cognition
negative cognition (NC), 110, 113, 205–206, 276
neurodiverse populations, 221
new relationship energy (NRE), 202
New View of a Woman's Body, A (Gage), 70
New View of Women's Sexual Problems, 64–65, 69, 86–87
nipples, 32
"no means no" concept, 7, 21
nonbinary identity, 169
North American Menopause Society (NAMS), 246
Northampton Sex Therapy Associates (NSTA), 58, 64, 87, 314
NRE. *See* new relationship energy
NSTA. *See* Northampton Sex Therapy Associates
nursing homes, older adults in
   relationships, 258, 259
   transgender people, 254

offense drivers model, 234
Office of Population Affairs, 2, 18
Office of the Surgeon General, 2, 18
Ogden, Gina, 13–15
oil-based lubricants, 46
Old Lesbian Oral Herstory Project, 300
older adults. *See* aging
Older Lesbians Organizing for Change, 300
olive oil, 46
Omgyes.com, 297
omnisexuals, 195
oophorectomy, 247–249
oral sex, 41, 116

Orenstein, Peggy, 22, 23, 30
orgasm, 32, 41, 55, 62, 63, 279–281
   and aging women, 246
   clitoral, 32, 82, 153
   disorders, 81–84
   extended, 153
   faking, 66
   quality, 46
orgasm gap, 66–67, 87
osmolality of lubricants, 45
Our Better Half podcast, 298
Our Whole Lives (OWL), 10–11, 143, 163, 219, 315
   assumptions, 11
   circles of sexuality, 11, 12, 16–17, 115–116
   program values, 10–11
out of control sexual behaviors, 118–119
   books, 313
   case study, 121–122
   Feeling State Addiction Protocol (FSAP), 119–123
outercourse, 41
ovaries, 32
OWL. *See* Our Whole Lives

pansexuals, 195
paraphiliac disorder, 229, 237
paraphilias, 228–229, 237
Partner Engagers, 47, 48, 58–59
PC. *See* positive cognition
PDE5. *See* phosphodiesterase-5 inhibitors
peaceful place, 274–275
pedophilia, 233
pelvic floor, 34–35, 246
pelvic floor physical therapy, 34–35
penis, 32, 36–37
   chambers, 37
   erections, 153–154
   medical trauma related to, 37
peri-menopause, 35
perineum, 29, 37
PFLAG, 300
PGE-1. *See* prostaglandin-E1
PH level of lubricants, 45

phosphodiesterase-5 (PDE5) inhibitors, 80, 250–251
physical therapy (PT)
   for dyspareunia, 86
   pelvic floor, 34–35
physically marginalized populations, 218–221
Pillai-Friedman, Sabitha, 102, 137
Planned Parenthood, 40, 297, 315–316
   FRIES (Freely, Reversible, Informed, Enthusiastic, Specific), 7, 21–22, 25
   model of sexual health, 11–13
plateau (sexual arousal), 41, 62
pleasure. *See* sexual pleasure
PLISSIT (Permission, Limited Information, Specific Suggestions, Intensive Therapy) model, 9–10, 17, 30, 124
polyamory, 200–201, 301, 311
polysemicity, 9, 224
polysexuals, 195
porn literacy, 142–143, 145, 163, 164
porn-induced erectile dysfunction, 143, 164
pornography, 31, 44, 121–122, 162–164
   audio porn, 144, 164
   books, 313
   definition of, 141, 162
   and EMDR, 144–145
      case studies, 145–147
   ethical, 142, 144, 163, 164, 303
   exposure of children to, 145–147
   impact on sexual health, 141–144, 164
   internet pornography, 5, 48–49
   resources, 302–303
positive cognition (PC), 110, 111, 113–114, 277
post-traumatic stress disorder (PTSD), 74, 115–116, 135, 172, 197–198, 222, 224, 228
preemptive radical inclusion (PRI), 197
Pre-Exposure Prophylaxis (PrEP), 40
pregnancy, 35, 214
   loss, 207–208, 213
      clinical observations and insights, 209
      EMDR targets, 210
      impact on sexual health, 210–212

pregnancy (*cont.*)
　　intake information gathering, 208–209
　　language, 208
　　and partners, 213
　　sexual intimacy and fertility concerns, 209–210
　　prevention, 40–41, 49
premature ejaculation, 83, 112
PrEP. *See* Pre-Exposure Prophylaxis
preparation (EMDR phase 2), 105–107, 207
PRI. *See* preemptive radical inclusion
primary female orgasmic disorder, 81
progesterone, 39
Proscar, 252
prostaglandin-E1 (PGE-1), 251
prostate, 38
protected place, 274–275
psychoeducation, 12, 37, 67, 80, 82, 83, 107, 117, 118, 124, 174, 177
psychological cliterodectomy, 22, 30
PT. *See* physical therapy
PTSD. *See* post-traumatic stress disorder
puberty, 35

Queen, Carol, 5, 298
queer, 197

RACK. *See* risk-aware consensual kink
rape culture, 172
RDI. *See* Resource and Development Installation
Real Talk app, 297
re-evaluation (EMDR phase 8), 112
reformjudaism.org, 301
relationship satisfaction, 41, 56
relationship status, 214
　　case study, 202–203
　　compersion, 200
　　consensual non-monogamy/polyamory, 200–201
　　heteronormativity and romonormativity, 200
　　infidelity, 202–203
　　monogamy, 200
　　new relationship energy, 202
　　singlehood, 199
relaxation training, for vaginismus, 85
religious imagery, 276
resolution (sexual arousal), 41, 62
Resolve, 206
Resource and Development Installation (RDI), 106, 141
　　books, 304–313
　　phone apps, 303–304
　　training programs, 314–318
　　websites, television, podcasts, and videos, 296–303
resourcing (EMDR phase 2), 105–107, 184–185
Responsible Sex Ed Institute, 142, 163
responsive desire, 41–42, 50, 56, 79
retrograde ejaculation, 251
risk-aware consensual kink (RACK), 226
Robert Wood Johnson Medical School, 315
Role Enactors, 47, 48, 58–59
role models, 178
romonormativity, 200
Rutgers University, 315

sadism, BDSM, 225
safe, sane, and consensual (SSC), 226
safe place, 274–275
Safer Sex for Seniors, 298
Safer Society, 314
SAGE, 298, 300
same gender loving, 194
San Francisco State University, 316
SAR. *See* Sexual Attitude Reassessment
Savage, Dan, 298
Scarleteen.com, 297
scrotum, 36, 37
secondary female orgasmic disorder, 82
seduction theory, 171
self-compassion container exercise, 107–109, 128–129
self-esteem
　　impact of social media on, 139, 141

of neurodiverse individuals, 221
sexuality-related, 140–141
self-kindness, 108, 128
self-objectification, 22
self-reflection, 8, 170–171
self-worth, 10
seminal vesicles, 38
Sens8 (TV series), 302
sensate focus technique, 75–76, 80, 87
 environment/setting, 76
 goals of, 76
 instructions, 76–77
 timing/scheduling, 76
SES. *See* Sexual Excitation System
SESTA law, 142, 163, 229
sex
 conditions for good sex, 71–72
 definition of, 3
 responsible sexual choices, 11
sex assumed at birth, 169
sex cam work, 231–232
sex chromosomes, 28
Sex Education (TV series), 302
sex educator training programs, 315–316
Sex for One: The Joy of Self-Loving (Dodson), 31, 32
sex hormones, 39–40
sex offenders, 232–236, 237
 case study, 235–236
 clients with background of sexual offending, 234–235
 EMDR with, 234
 female-identified, 232
 male-identified, 232, 234
 offense drivers model, 234
sex therapy, 6, 86–87
 common sexual problems reported in, 65–67
 couples-based, 63, 75–77, 87
 feminist, 63–65
 frameworks, 62–65
 New View of Women's Sexual Problems, 64–65, 69, 86–87
 with sexual trauma survivors, 72–73
  trauma processing, 73–74
  treatment of sexual problems, 74–75

sex trafficking, 229, 230, 237
sex work, 229–232, 237, 313
sexological worldview, 8–9
sex-positive books, 304–305, 313
sex-positive television series, 302
Sexsmartfilms.com, 297
sexual abuse, 145, 233
 adolescent, 31
 childhood, 72, 124, 136, 140, 178, 232, 237
 in nursing homes, 254
sexual activity, definition of, 3
sexual and affectional orientation, 191–192, 213–214
 asexuals and greysexuals, 196
 bisexuality/pansexuals/polysexuals/omnisexuals, 194–196
 case study, 197–199
 demisexuals, 196–197, 198
 denouncing SOCE, 193–194, 213
 MSM/same gender loving categories, 194
 preemptive radical inclusion, 197
 queer, 197
sexual and reproductive anatomy, 28, 49, 70–71
 clitoris, 30
 external
  estrogen-dominant body, 29–32
  testosterone-dominant body, 36–37
 G-spot area, 34
 in utero, 28
 internal
  estrogen-dominant body, 32–35
  testosterone-dominant body, 37–38
 intersex, 38–39
 labia, 31
 menopause, 35–36
 menstruation, 35
 nipples, 32
 pelvic floor, 34–35
 penis, 36–37
  chambers, 37
 perineum, 37
 resources, 296
 scrotum, 36, 37

sexual and reproductive anatomy (*cont.*)
    seminal vesicles and prostate, 38
    sex hormones, 39–40
    testes, 38
    vagina, 29, 33–34
sexual arousal template, 48
sexual assault, 2, 16, 172
Sexual Attitude Reassessment (SAR), 8
sexual avoidance, 64, 136–138
sexual desire. *See* desire
sexual dysfunction(s), 63
    arousal disorders, 79–81
    desire disorders, 78–79
    diagnosis and treatment approaches for, 77–86
    EMDR Sexual Dysfunction Protocol, 102, 137
    orgasm disorders, 81–84
    sexual pain disorders, 84–86
    treatment, 75–77
Sexual Excitation System (SES), 42, 43, 55, 56
sexual fantasy training, 80
Sexual Healing Journey, The (Maltz), 75
sexual health, 2, 10, 18–19
    books, 304–313
    case studies, 16–18, 115–118
    comfort of EMDR therapists with addressing, 8
    consent, 6–7, 21–22
    considerations, TGNC clients, 185–186
    cultural and individual factors interfering, 5–6
    Declaration on Sexual Pleasure, 4, 24–25
    Declaration of Sexual Rights, 3, 24
    definition of, 2
    EMDR future templates, 133–138
    EMDR part targets related to, 114
    EMDR present targets related to, 114–115
    experts/activists websites, 298
    4-Dimensional Wheel (Ogden), 13–15, 17–18, 116
    genital numbness, 31
    impact of pornography on, 141–144, 164
    impact of pregnancy loss on, 210–212
    and infertility, 204–207
    integration into AIP, 15–16
    of older adults, and health care providers, 259–260
    Our Whole Lives (OWL), 10–11, 143, 163, 219, 315
    phone apps, 303
    Planned Parenthood model, 11–13
    PLISSIT model, 9–10, 17, 30, 124
    positive and negative cognitions, 113–114
    positive models of, 10–13
    rights, for people with intellectual disabilities, 222–224
    sexological worldview of EMDR therapists, 8–9
    training programs, 314–318
sexual history, 260
Sexual History Questionnaire, The (NSTA), 64, 87, 90–100, 103
Sexual Inhibition System (SIS), 42, 43, 55–56
sexual intimacy, 146, 209–210, 211, 261–262
sexual motivation linked to emotional/physical satisfaction, 41, 56
sexual myths, 68
sexual orientation change efforts (SOCE), 193–194, 213
sexual pain disorders, 84–86
sexual personality styles, 46–48, 50, 58–59
sexual pleasure, 4, 22–23, 24–25, 41, 82
    and clitoris, 30
    Declaration of Sexual Pleasure, 4, 24–25
    and pregnancy, 209–210
    resources for improving, 152–154
sexual problems. *See also* sexual dysfunction(s)
    New View of Women's Sexual Problems, 64–65, 69, 86–87
    orgasm gap, 66–67, 87
    reported in sex therapy, 65–67
sexual research, 41–42
sexual response, 63–64
    dual control model, 42–43, 50, 55–57
    willingness model, 42

Index **331**

sexual revolution, 5
sexual rights, 3, 24, 258
sexual stimuli, 41, 44, 56
Sexual Styles Survey, 47, 52–54
Sexual Trancers, 46, 47, 48, 58–59
sexual trauma, 2, 31, 104
   books, 306
   case study, 16, 115–116
   and lack of sexual desire, 43
   resources for healing from, 306
   self-help resources for survivors of, 74–75
   survivors, sex therapy with, 72–73
      trauma processing, 73–74
      treatment of sexual problems, 74–75
sexuality education, 221, 222
   corrective, 67–71
   lack of, 16
   Our Whole Lives (OWL), 10–11, 143, 163, 219, 315
   Planned Parenthood model, 11–13
   SIECUS, 11–12, 13, 17
   UNESCO, 11, 12
   websites
      for adults, 297
      for kids and teens, 297
Sexuality Information and Education Council of the United States (SIECUS), 11–12, 13, 17
sexuality-related educational certificates and programs, 315
Sexually Transmitted Infections (STIs), 40, 49, 245
Shapiro, Francine, 15
SIECUS. *See* Sexuality Information and Education Council of the United States
sildenafil (Viagra), 80, 250
Silent Generation, 244
singlehood, 199
SIS. *See* Sexual Inhibition System
Slippery Stuff Liquid, 45
Sliquid Organics, 45
slut-shaming, 7, 21
Smitten Kitten, 299
smittenkittenonline.com, 46

SOCE. *See* sexual orientation change efforts
social media, 132, 139, 141
social model of disability, 219
Society for Sex Therapy and Research, 314
South Shore Sexual Health Center, 314
Southern Connecticut State University, 315
spermicide, 41
spiral resource, 109
spiritual appropriation, 271
spiritual wounds
   chosen to suffer, 273
   institutional wounds, 272
   parental wounds, 272
   unlovability, 274
   wounds of abandonment, 272
spirituality, 267–268
   books, 311
   case studies
      free will, abdication and embodiment, 284–286
      guilt/fear/shame, 282–284
      longing for ecstasy, 279–281
      sacrifice, safety, and belonging, 289–291
      surrender and control, 286–288
   EMDR applications
      cognitive interweaves, 276
      exploratory questions, 275–276, 281, 288
      future templates, 277
      integration of spiritual resources between sessions, 275
      metaphors and religious imagery, 276
      negative cognitions, 276
      positive cognitions, 277
      safe place, 274–275
   energy and senses, 272
   identification of spiritual resources of clients, 270–272
   practices, 272, 284
   sacred/religious texts, 278
   spiritual community, 272
   spiritual images, 271–272
   spiritual language, 271

spirituality (*cont.*)
  therapist self-awareness and trust building, 277–278
  websites, 301
spontaneous desire, 41, 42, 50, 56, 79
SSC. *See* safe, sane, and consensual
Start Strong curriculum, 143, 163
Stendra, 250
stillbirth, 210–212
stimulation, sexual, 31, 33, 34, 44, 46, 82
STIs. *See* Sexually Transmitted Infections
Stonewall Veterans Association, 300
Stop it now!, 314
Storms Sexuality Axis, 195
Strengthening a Confident and Joyful Sexual Self resource, 140, 147–148, 154, 157–159
  case study, 150–151
  client worksheet, 160–161
  script for EMDR clinicians, 148–150, 157–159
Subjective Units of Distress Scale (SUDS), 17, 18, 110, 211, 212
submission, BDSM, 225
SUDS. *See* Subjective Units of Distress Scale
supernormal stimuli, 142, 143, 162, 164
sweet almond oil, 46

tadalafil (Cialis), 80, 250
Tales of the City (TV series), 302
Taormino, Tristan, 5, 298
testes, 38
testosterone, 35, 39
TF-CBT. *See* Trauma-Focused Cognitive Behavioral Therapy
TGNC. *See* transgender and gender non-conforming people
therapeutic masturbation, 153
therapists, EMDR
  comfort with addressing sexual health, 8–9
  education of, 8
  self-awareness, 277–278
  self-reflection, 8
    gender self-reflection, 170–171

sexological worldview of, 8–9
therapeutic gender match, 177
therapeutic relationship, 73, 102, 277–278
theratappers, 147
THRIVE Program, National Children's, 300
Timberlake, Jassy Casella, 314
toxic masculinity, 177, 178
Trans Student Educational Resources, 300
transgender and gender non-conforming (TGNC) people, 169. *See also* marginalized populations
  EMDR with, 179
    access issues, 180–181
    body attention scan, 185
    emotional and behavioral considerations, 182–183
    gender dysphoria and implications for dissociation, 183–184
    practicing language, 181–182
    resourcing and imagery considerations, 184–185
    sexual health considerations, 185–186
Transgender Gender-Variant & Intersex Justice Project, 300
transgender people, 116–117, 134, 168
  aging of, 254–255
  body image of, 139
  books, 308–309
  definition of, 169
  educational and information websites, 300
TransProud, 300
trauma play, 224–225
trauma reenactment, 224–225
Trauma-Focused Cognitive Behavioral Therapy (TF-CBT), 73–74
treatment planning (EMDR phase 1), 103–104
Trevor Project, The, 300
trust in therapeutic relationship, 73, 277–278

UNESCO. *See* United Nations Educational, Scientific and Cultural Organizations

United Nations Educational, Scientific and Cultural Organizations (UNESCO), 11, 12
University of California, 317
University of Connecticut, 316
University of Guelph, 317
University of Hawaii, 317
University of Minnesota, 317
University of New Brunswick, 317
University of Quebec, 317
University of Utah, 317
University of Wisconsin, 317
urethra, 29, 32, 36
Urology Care Foundation, 298

VA. *See* Veterans Affairs
vagina, 29, 33–34
    lubrication, 33–34, 44–46, 68–69
    progressive dilation program, 85
vaginal atrophy, 246
vaginal dryness, 246, 257
vaginal orgasms, 32
vaginal rejuvenation, 34
vaginismus, 84–85
vaginoplasty, 31
Validity of Cognition (VOC), 110, 111, 211
vanilla, 224
vardenafil (Levitra, Staxyn), 80, 250
Veterans Affairs (VA), 177
vibrators, 82
victim blaming, 172, 175
virgin coconut oil, 46
Vitamin E cream, 40
VOC. *See* Validity of Cognition
vulva, 29, 33

WAS. *See* World Association for Sexual Health

water-based lubrication, 34, 40, 45, 246
We Are Who We Are (TV series), 302
Weinstein, Harvey, 5
Westheimer, Ruth, 5
WHO. *See* World Health Organization
Widener University, 317
willingness model, 42
Woman' Touch, A, 297
women
    aging, sexual health of, 260
    body image, 249
    hysterectomies and oophorectomies, 247–249
    menopause, 246–247
    EMDR with, 171–172
    access issues, 172
    emotional and behavioral considerations, 173–176
    interaction with legal systems, 173
    saying no to others, 175–176
women who have sex with women (WSW), 194
World Association for Sexual Health (WAS), 3, 18, 24
    Declaration of Sexual Pleasure, 4, 24–25
    Declaration of Sexual Rights, 3, 24
World Health Organization (WHO), 2, 18, 30, 257
World Professional Association for Transgender Health, 300
worldview, sexological, 8–9
WSW. *See* women who have sex with women
www.ourshine.org, 314

yeast infection, 86
Your Brain on Porn program, 143, 303

www.ingramcontent.com/pod-product-compliance
Ingram Content Group UK Ltd.
Pitfield, Milton Keynes, MK11 3LW, UK
UKHW021837210426
RIPUK00021B/345